# CAMBRIDGE MONOGRAPHS ON APPLIED AND COMPUTATIONAL MATHEMATICS



33 **Mathematical Modelling of the Human Cardiovascular System**

The *Cambridge Monographs on Applied and Computational Mathematics* series reflects the crucial role of mathematical and computational techniques in contemporary science. The series publishes expositions on all aspects of applicable and numerical mathematics, with an emphasis on new developments in this fast-moving area of research.

State-of-the-art methods and algorithms as well as modern mathematical descriptions of physical and mechanical ideas are presented in a manner suited to graduate research students and professionals alike. Sound pedagogical presentation is a prerequisite. It is intended that books in the series will serve to inform a new generation of researchers.

A complete list of books in the series can be found at
www.cambridge.org/mathematics.
Recent titles include the following:

19. Matrix preconditioning techniques and applications, *Ke Chen*
20. Greedy approximation, *Vladimir Temlyakov*
21. Spectral methods for time-dependent problems, *Jan Hesthaven, Sigal Gottlieb & David Gottlieb*
22. The mathematical foundations of mixing, *Rob Sturman, Julio M. Ottino & Stephen Wiggins*
23. Curve and surface reconstruction, *Tamal K. Dey*
24. Learning theory, *Felipe Cucker & Ding Xuan Zhou*
25. Algebraic geometry and statistical learning theory, *Sumio Watanabe*
26. A practical guide to the invariant calculus, *Elizabeth Louise Mansfield*
27. Difference equations by differential equation methods, *Peter E. Hydon*
28. Multiscale methods for Fredholm integral equations, *Zhongying Chen, Charles A. Micchelli & Yuesheng Xu*
29. Partial differential equation methods for image inpainting, *Carola-Bibiane Schönlieb*
30. Volterra integral equations, *Hermann Brunner*
31. Symmetry, phase modulation and nonlinear waves, *Thomas J. Bridges*
32. Multivariate approximation, *V. Temlyakov*
33. Mathematical modelling of the human cardiovascular system, *Alfio Quarteroni, Luca Dede', Andrea Manzoni & Christian Vergara*
34. Numerical bifurcation analysis of maps, *Yuri A. Kuznetsov & Hil G.E. Meijer*

# Mathematical Modelling of the Human Cardiovascular System

## Data, Numerical Approximation, Clinical Applications

ALFIO QUARTERONI
*Politecnico di Milano and École Polytechnique Fédérale de Lausanne (EPFL)*

LUCA DEDE'
*Politecnico di Milano*

ANDREA MANZONI
*Politecnico di Milano*

CHRISTIAN VERGARA
*Politecnico di Milano*

CAMBRIDGE
UNIVERSITY PRESS

**CAMBRIDGE**
**UNIVERSITY PRESS**

University Printing House, Cambridge CB2 8BS, United Kingdom

One Liberty Plaza, 20th Floor, New York, NY 10006, USA

477 Williamstown Road, Port Melbourne, VIC 3207, Australia

314–321, 3rd Floor, Plot 3, Splendor Forum, Jasola District Centre, New Delhi – 110025, India

79 Anson Road, #06–04/06, Singapore 079906

Cambridge University Press is part of the University of Cambridge.

It furthers the University's mission by disseminating knowledge in the pursuit of education, learning, and research at the highest international levels of excellence.

www.cambridge.org
Information on this title: www.cambridge.org/9781108480390
DOI: 10.1017/9781108616096



First published 2019

Printed and bound in Great Britain by Clays Ltd, Elcograf S.p.A.

*A catalogue record for this publication is available from the British Library.*

*Library of Congress Cataloging-in-Publication Data*
Names: Quarteroni, Alfio, author.
Title: Mathematical modelling of the human cardiovascular system : data, numerical approximation, clinical applications / Alfio Quarteroni, Politecnico di Milano, Luca Dede', Politecnico di Milano, Andrea Manzoni, Politecnico di Milano, Christiana, Vergara Politecnico di Milano.
Description: New York, NY : Cambridge University Press, [2019] | Series: Cambridge monographs on applied and computational mathematics series | Includes bibliographical references and index.
Identifiers: LCCN 2018050818 | ISBN 9781108480390 (alk. paper)
Subjects: LCSH: Cardiovascular system – Mathematical models.
Classification: LCC QP105 .Q83 2019 | DDC 612.1–dc23
LC record available at https://lccn.loc.gov/2018050818

ISBN 978-1-108-48039-0 Hardback

# Contents

# Introduction

This book is devoted to the mathematical and numerical modelling of the cardiovascular system, a research topic that has attracted remarkable interest from both the mathematical and bioengineering communities over the past 25 years. The driving motivation for this interest is the increasing impact of cardiovascular diseases in our lives. According to Mozaffarian *et al.* (2015), cardiovascular diseases are the major cause of death worldwide, leading to more than 17.3 million deaths per year, a number that is expected to grow to more than 23.6 million by 2030. In Europe this now corresponds to nearly half of all deaths (47%).

We focus on the two principal components of the cardiovascular system: *arterial circulation* and *heart function*, with its electrical and mechanical activities, blood flow in its chambers, and valve dynamics. Geometric complexity, the lack of data to feed the mathematical models, and the multiphysics and multiscale nature of the processes at hand present major challenges when trying to reproduce both function and dysfunction.

Owing to its composite nature, the cardiovascular system is first modelled by means of stand-alone *core components*, each describing a single functionality, for example arterial fluid dynamics, the electrical activity of the heart, and the fluid dynamics in the left ventricle. Each core model needs careful mathematical analysis and efficient numerical approximation, often via specifically devised methods. The next step is integration of the core models into global, coupled integrated models suitable for describing a meaningful and coherent part of the cardiovascular system – or even the entire system. This step requires the introduction of suitable coupling conditions, as well as novel numerical strategies for a stable, robust and computationally effective solution of the global problem.

Clinical data play a decisive role in models of the cardiovascular system, and at the same time dealing with data represents a formidable challenge.

Clinical radiological images (such as *computer tomography* and *magnetic resonance imaging*) are necessary to construct the computational domains wherein the mathematical models (very often based upon a system of differential equations) are defined. The procedure of geometric reconstruction is difficult and, especially for the heart, requires advanced mathematical and numerical tools. Standard radiological images can sometimes be useless: some cardiovascular components may be smaller than the spatial resolution of the imaging device (this is the case for the Purkinje network, for example); in other cases the elevated brightness gap between fluid and vessel wall makes the detection of the latter very hard. Boundary data that feed the mathematical models are also difficult to obtain. When the computational domain results from an artificial truncation, specific physical quantities (*e.g.* fluid velocity or pressure) should be provided at those locations of the arterial tree corresponding to the artificial boundaries. However, this would require invasive measurements that cannot be easily carried out. In some specific circumstances, this calls for suitable parameter identification and data assimilation techniques. Finally, the huge inter- and intra-patient data variability and uncertainty are further sources of concern regarding model calibration and validation.

In spite of all these difficulties, a wealth of models has already been successfully used to address both physiological and pathological instances. The aim is, on one hand, a better understanding of the physical and quantitative processes governing the cardiovascular system, and on the other hand the opening of new frontiers in therapeutic planning and the design of implantable devices (*e.g.* medical stents, cardiac defibrillators, ventricular assisted devices and prosthetic valves).

The literature on the mathematical and numerical modelling of the cardiovascular system is huge, as readers will see by browsing our references, a tiny subset of the total. In the following chapters we will provide a perspective on the main contributions to this field. Here, among the several books, monographs and review papers published so far, we mention Formaggia, Quarteroni and Veneziani (2009*a*), Taylor and Figueroa (2009) and Quarteroni, Veneziani and Vergara (2016*c*) for the circulatory system, and Peskin (2002), Smith, Nickerson, Crampin and Hunter (2004), Colli Franzone, Pavarino and Scacchi (2014), Quarteroni (2015) and Quarteroni, Lassila, Rossi and Ruiz-Baier (2017) for the heart.

The book consists of three main parts: in Part 1 we model the *arterial circulation* (Chapters 1, 2 and 4), in Part 2 we model the *heart function* (Chapters 5, 6 and 7), and in Part 3 we treat *inverse problems* and include *uncertainty* (Chapters 8, 9, 10 and 11). Both Parts 1 and 2 consist of an introductory section on physiology (Chapters 1 and 5), a section describing the available data and their use (Chapters 2 and 6), and a final section on mathematical and numerical modelling (Chapters 4 and 7). In Part 3 we begin by emphasizing the need to move beyond a single (forward) simulation in some applications (Chapter 8). This represents the common denominator of three topics recently applied to cardiovascular mathematics: *control and optimization* (Chapter 9), *parameter estimation* (Chapter 10) and *uncertainty quantification* (Chapter 11).

When appropriate (in particular in Chapters 4, 7, 9, 10 and 11), we report some numerical results to highlight the effectiveness of the numerical strategies presented here. Unless otherwise specified, all the numerical results presented in this book have been obtained using the finite element library LifeV; see www.lifev.org for more details.

*Disclaimers.* This book is based upon the review paper A. Quarteroni, A. Manzoni and C. Vergara (2017), 'The cardiovascular system: mathematical modelling, numerical algorithms and clinical applications', *Acta Numerica*, 365–390. Several slight (and sometimes more substantial) additions have been made throughout.

Despite the fact that it is 280 pages long,[1] several topics related to the cardiovascular system have not been addressed. Among others, we mention the *venous system* (essential if one wants to consider a closed-loop model of the cardiovascular system, and playing a crucial role in some specific pathologies: see *e.g.* Toro 2016), the *metabolic system* (D'Angelo 2007), the *respiratory system* (Maury 2013, Wall, Wiechert, Comerford and Rausch 2010, Trenhago *et al.* 2016), the *cerebro-spinal fluid circulation* (Fin and Grebe 2003), the *nervous system* (Liang and Liu 2006) the *lymphatic system* (Margaris and Black 2012) and growth and remodelling of the tissue (Humphrey and Rajagopal 2002). For some of them (*e.g.* the venous and respiratory systems) research has made remarkable progress in recent years. Nonetheless, the mathematical investigation of these systems is still in its infancy; in particular, their coupling with the cardiovascular system is almost absent. Many research avenues are open to the contribution of both pure and applied mathematicians, with the dream of enabling mathematical achievements to play a decisive role in everyday clinical practice.

*Acknowledgements.* The authors would like to thank P. Masci, J. Schwitter, P. Tozzi (CHUV – Centre Hospitalier Universitaire Vaudois, Lausanne,

[1] By slightly rephrasing Blaise Pascal's quotation, we can state that '*we were not good enough* to make it shorter.'

Switzerland), P. Biondetti, M. Domanin, L. Forzenigo (Fondazione IRCSS Ca' Granda, Ospedale Maggiore Policlinico, Milan, Italy), S. Ippolito, (Ospedale S. Maria del Carmine, Rovereto (TN), Italy), for providing the radiological images; G. Aloe (Politecnico di Milano) for his help in preparing the figures; L. Azzolin, D. Bonomi, S. Fresca, B. Guerciotti, R.M. Lancellotti, S. Pagani, S. Palamara (Politecnico di Milano), D. Forti, A. Gerbi, F. Negri, L. Pegolotti, A. Tagliabue (EPFL, Lausanne, Switzerland), L. Barbarotta (Technische Universiteit Eindhoven), E. Faggiano (University of Pavia) for their help in preparing the plots of some numerical results; E. Faggiano and A. Gerbi for the fruitful suggestions.

AQ acknowledges the project 'Integrative HPC Framework for Coupled Cardiac Simulations' (IFCCS) within the PASC (Platform for Advanced Scientific Computing) network 'Life Sciences Across Scales' and the Swiss National Supercomputing Centre (CSCS), project ID s635. CV was partially supported by the Italian MIUR PRIN12 project 201289 A4XL and by the H2020-MSCA-ITN-2017, EU project 765374 "ROMSOC – Reduced Order Modelling, Simulation and Optimization of Coupled systems".

The authors acknowledge the ERC Advanced Grant iHEART, "An Integrated Heart Model for the simulation of the cardiac function", 2017–2022, P.I. A. Quarteroni (ERC2016ADG, project ID: 740132).

Last but not least, the authors warmly thank Glennis Starling for her fantastic editorial job.

# PART ONE

# ARTERIAL CIRCULATION

# 1

# Basic facts about quantitative physiology

The cardiovascular system is a closed circuit that carries oxygenated blood to all the tissues and organs of the body. Functionally, it can be regarded as made up of three compartments: the *heart*, the *systemic* and *pulmonary circulations*, and the *microvasculature*. In this chapter we will recall the most important features of the physiology of the systemic circulation characterizing the mathematical models that will be introduced later on. We will also highlight the main peculiarities of the pulmonary circulation. Heart physiology will be addressed in Chapter 4.

The systemic circulation is made up of the arteries, which carry oxygenated blood ejected by the left part of the heart to the living tissues, and the veins, which allow non-oxygenated blood to return to the right part. The exchange of oxygen between blood and the body tissues occurs in the microvasculature, which in fact separates the systemic arterial tree from the venous systems. In the pulmonary circulation, non-oxygenated blood ejected by the right part of the heart flows in the pulmonary arteries towards the lungs where it becomes oxygenated and goes back to the left part through the pulmonary veins.

Blood is composed of *plasma* (about 55% of its total volume), which consists of water (about 92% of plasma volume), proteins and ions. The remainder corresponds to the blood cells, of which 97% of the volume is made up of *erythrocytes* (red blood cells), which carry the oxygen in oxygenated blood. The other cells are *leucocytes* (white blood cells) and *platelets*. The diameter of blood cells is approximately $10^{-3}$ cm, whereas that of the smallest arteries and veins is about $10^{-1}$ cm. This is why blood in the systemic and pulmonary circulations is often considered to be Newtonian, that is, characterized by a linear relationship between internal forces and velocity gradients (Perktold and Hilbert 1986, Formaggia *et al.* 2009*a*). However, in the smallest arteries, such as coronary arteries (the arteries perfusing the

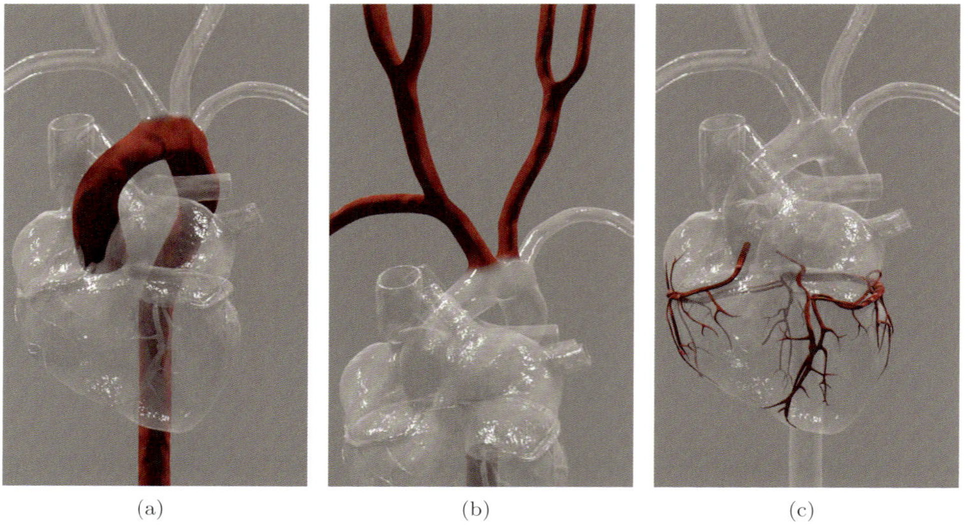

Figure 1.1 The aorta (a), the carotid arteries (b) and (a subset of) the coronary arteries (c).

heart and the corresponding veins; see Figure 1.1(c)), in the aortic root (where the blood flow reaches its peak velocity) or in the presence of vessel narrowing (stenosis), non-Newtonian blood rheology is more appropriate: see *e.g.* Chen, Lu and Wang (2006), Fasano and Sequeira (2017) and references therein.

Thanks to the synchronous heart contraction, blood flow is pulsatile, and blood is pumped into the two circulations by means of discrete pulses with a pressure usually varying during a heartbeat in the ranges 70–130 mmHg and 20–30 mmHg for the systemic and pulmonary networks, respectively (1 mmHg $\simeq$ 133.3 Pa $=$ 1333 g cm$^{-1}$ s$^{-2}$).

In the systemic circulation, blood first enters the *aorta* (the largest artery with diameter equal to about 2.5 cm in adults: see Figure 1.1(a)) and then flows through a network of hundreds of branching arteries of decreasing size, reaching all the regions of the body. Dimensions and numbers of veins are comparable with those of arteries. The waveform of the flow rate as a function of time is characterized by different peak values when moving downstream towards the smallest arteries. In particular, the flow rate peak value is about 200 cm$^3$ s$^{-1}$ in the aorta, 80 cm$^3$ s$^{-1}$ in the abdominal aorta, 15 cm$^3$ s$^{-1}$ in the carotid arteries (the arteries supplying blood to the brain: see Figure 1.1(b)), and 1 cm$^3$ s$^{-1}$ in the coronary arteries (corresponding to a maximum blood velocity of about 150 cm s$^{-1}$ in the aorta, 100 cm s$^{-1}$

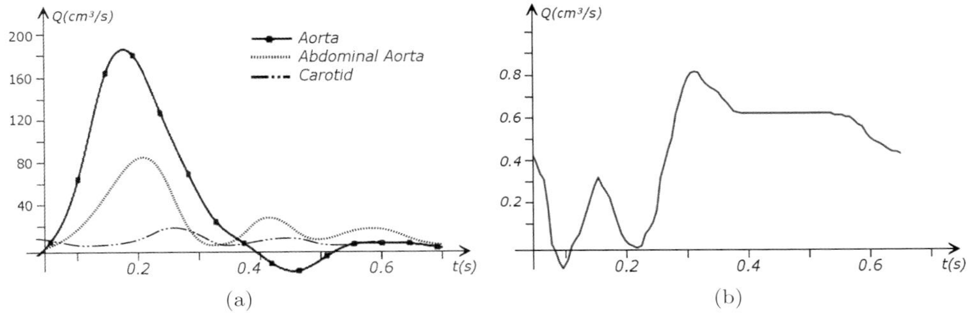


Figure 1.2 Typical flow rate waveforms in the ascending aorta, abdominal aorta and carotid arteries (a), and in the coronary arteries (b).

in the abdominal aorta, 80 cm $s^{-1}$ in the carotid arteries and 40 cm $s^{-1}$ in the coronary arteries). Further, the shape of the waveforms changes while moving downstream: see Figure 1.2(a). In particular, in the ascending aorta, after the systolic peak, the flow rate decelerates assuming null or even negative values, whereas in the abdominal aorta and in carotid arteries it is more spread out and always positive. In any case, we can distinguish the *systolic phase* – the interval of acceleration and deceleration of blood flow – and the *diastolic phase* – the interval of almost constant or possibly reverse flow.[1] A different situation occurs in coronary arteries, where the peak flow rate is reached during diastole: see Figure 1.2(b). The coronary arteries are not directly fed by the heart; indeed, blood in the proximal part of the aorta (the sinuses of Valsalva from which the coronary arteries originate) during diastole is allowed to enter the coronary arteries thanks to the elastic response of the aorta and isovolumic ventricle relaxation (see below for more details). The systemic circulation also comprises the venous system which returns the de-oxygenated blood to the right part of heart.

In the pulmonary circulation blood first enters the *pulmonary artery* (diameter equal to about 3.0 cm in adults) and then flows into another network of branching arteries of decreasing size reaching the lungs. The waveforms and peak intensities are similar to those of the systemic arteries. After oxygenation in the lungs, the blood returns to the left heart through the pulmonary veins.

The different characteristics of blood flow in the arteries of the systemic

[1] The above definition of systole and diastole is formulated from the perspective of the arteries. An almost equivalent definition could be given from the perspective of the heart and possibly for each of its chambers: see Chapter 4.

circulation result in different values of the *Reynolds number*,

$$Re = \frac{\rho_f D U}{\mu},$$

(where $\rho_f$ is the blood density, $D$ and $U$ are the characteristic vessel dimension and blood velocity, respectively, and $\mu$ is the fluid viscosity), a dimensionless number which quantifies the importance of inertial forces over the viscous forces. In the cardiovascular system this variability is mainly due to the size of the vessel and blood velocity. In particular, $Re \simeq 4000$ in the aorta and $Re \simeq 400$ in coronary arteries, with intermediate values found when moving downstream along the aorta. Thus, blood covers a range of Reynolds numbers where both the inertial and the viscous components of the flow are relevant. Although in the aorta $Re$ is higher than the critical value of 2000 above which the flow would no longer be laminar in a straight pipe, the pulsatile nature of blood flow does not allow transition to full turbulence in physiological conditions. It is debatable whether transition to turbulence effects occur in the aorta. Some authors speculate that the helicoidal velocity pattern in the aorta, induced by the torsion of the heart's contraction, inhibits any transition to turbulence, thus supporting the thesis that in healthy conditions fully developed turbulence is never observed in the cardiovascular system (Morbiducci *et al.* 2009). This is not necessarily the case for some pathological conditions, such as carotid stenosis, yielding a narrowing of the vessel lumen and increased complexity of the geometry together with higher Reynolds numbers: see *e.g.* Ahmed and Giddens (1984), Lee *et al.* (2008), Kefayati, Holdsworth and Poepping (2014) and Lancellotti *et al.* (2017). The *Womersley number*,

$$W = \sqrt{\frac{2 A f}{\mu}},$$

(where $A$ and $f$ are the characteristic cross-section vessel area and time frequency of the flow rate signal, respectively) is a dimensionless number quantifying the pulsatility of flow. We find decreasing values in the systemic circulation moving downstream: $W \simeq 10$ in the aorta, $W \simeq 3$ in the carotid arteries. Similar values of $Re$ and $W$ are found in the pulmonary arteries.

In the veins of the systemic circulation, we find values of the flow rate, Reynolds and Womersley numbers comparable to the arteries, the only difference being that the blood flow waveform is more spread out than for the corresponding arteries. Another major difference is given by blood pressure values. In the arteries the range of pressure is almost the same, independent of the location in the tree (70–130 mmHg), whereas in the veins it reduces, assuming an average value of about 10 mmHg. This is due to the high resistance experienced by blood flow in the microvasculature. The latter is composed of thousands of *arterioles* and *venules* and billions of *capillaries*. The blood velocity and vessel dimensions are here greatly reduced (about $10^{-1}$ cm $s^{-1}$ in the former and $10^{-2}$ cm in the latter). This means that $Re$ is very small (typically much smaller than one) in comparison with the systemic circulation since viscous forces completely dominate the inertial forces. As a result, the highest resistance to flow is found in the microvasculature, thus provoking a big decrease in the blood pressure. Since the typical dimension of capillaries is comparable to that of erythrocytes, a multiphase (multicomponent) model seems appropriate for their mathematical description (Enden and Popel 1992). Finally, we observe that most veins are supplied with valves that prevent backflow of blood, and venous flow is highly sensitive to muscle contraction and respiratory effects.

As observed, blood pressure assumes the same range of values along the entire systemic arterial tree, 70–130 mmHg. More precisely, negligible dissipation is experienced by the pressure signal in large and medium sized vessels before reaching the small vessels and microvasculature. Of course, at a given instant the pressure is not constant in space along the tree. Indeed, a time shift characterizes the pressure waveforms at different locations which generate gradient pressures between proximal and distal regions facilitating blood movement. These spatial gradients are due to the propagating nature of the pressure, which is in fact a wave travelling along the arterial network. The pressure wave speed ranges from about 500 cm $s^{-1}$ in the aorta to 1200 cm $s^{-1}$ in the coronary arteries. The presence of bifurcations or high-resistance regions, such as the microvasculature, produces wave reflections that propagate back towards the heart.

The propagation of a pressure wave along the vascular tree is due to vessel *compliance*, that is, the ability of the vessel to distend under the forces exerted by blood pressure. Vessel wall displacements are quite large, reaching up to 10% of the lumen diameter. This is possible thanks to the structure of the vessel walls: their total thickness is about 10% of the lumen diameter and they are composed of three layers: the *intima*, the *media* and the *adventitia*. The inner part of the intima is the *endothelium* (facing the blood), whereas the remaining part is made up of connective tissue. The media and the adventitia play a major role in characterizing the mechanical response of the vessel wall. Their main structural components are *elastin* and *collagen*. The media is also formed of *smooth muscle cells* which provide tone to the vessel wall. Elastin forms complex networks that are very distensible, providing the elasticity of the vessel wall at small strain. In contrast, collagen forms stiff fibres oriented in a helical form providing tensile strength at large strain; see *e.g.* Tricerri, Dede', Deparis, Quarteroni, Robertson and Sequeira (2015) and Tricerri, Dede', Gambaruto, Quarteroni and Sequeira (2016) for cerebral arteries. Thus, the artery vessel wall is characterized by highly non-linear elastic properties. The quantity of elastin and collagen progressively decreases moving downstream along the arterial network, whereas the quantity of smooth muscle cells increases. This allows the proximal arteries (those close to the heart), in particular the aorta, to be very extensible and, thanks to the high peripheral resistances due to the elevated tone of the distal arteries and to the microvasculature, to store about 50% of the blood entering during systole. This blood reserve is then discharged during diastole owing to the vessel wall elastic response (the so-called *windkessel effect*). This effect is responsible for the smoothing of the blood flow waveform discussed above, going downstream along the arterial network, which guarantees nearly continuous peripheral blood flow and thus an almost continuous exchange of oxygen with the tissues. Further, pulmonary artery walls are extensible too (with muscular tone increasing downstream), even though their thickness is only about 1% of the lumen diameter.

As already observed, there is mutual exchange of energy between blood and extensible vessel walls: the latter accumulate elastic potential energy under the forces exerted by the blood pressure, which is then transferred to the blood as kinetic energy (from the mathematical point of view, this gives rise to the *fluid–structure interaction* problem). This process occurs at short time scales, proportional to the duration of a heartbeat ($\sim 1$ s). Other interaction mechanisms may take place at larger time scales yielding wall modifications of vessel properties; these are usually referred to as growth and remodelling problems. This occurs in the case of several arterial diseases, such as *atherosclerosis* and *aneurysm* formation. In the first case, an increased permeability of vessel wall to lipoprotein provokes a cascade of events at the cellular level which leads to the accumulation of fatty material in the intima, just below the endothelium, and then to plaque formation in the media. Preferential sites of atherosclerotic plaque formation are the carotid arteries and the coronary arteries. The main complications are partial occlusion of the lumen with consequent (cerebral or cardiac) ischaemia, or even total occlusion resulting in (cerebral or cardiac) infarction. An aneurysm consists in the dilatation of the vessel wall with formation of a (possibly huge) bulge, mainly in the aorta and cerebral arteries, due to a loss of elastin and to the consequent remodelling of collagen, resulting in a weakening of the arterial wall; 80–90% of ruptured abdominal aortic aneurysms and 45% of ruptured cerebral aneurysms result in death. The role of blood fluid dynamics has been recognized as crucial for the development of both of these diseases (Glagov, Zarins, Giddens and Ku 1988, Bagci *et al.* 2008). In particular, *wall shear stresses*, that is, the viscous/friction forces exerted by the blood on the endothelium, despite being 100 times smaller in magnitude than pressure, regulate the permeability of the wall to lipoprotein and determine the loss of elastin, thus playing an important role in atherosclerosis and aneurysm development. Other than the wall shear stresses, their spatial distribution and gradient play a major role. For both these arterial diseases, this supplementary interaction between fluid and structure occurs at time scales of several years.

More on the physiology of the systemic and pulmonary circulations and microvasculature in view of mathematical modelling is available in Nichols and O'Rourke (2005), Quarteroni, Tuveri and Veneziani (2000*c*) and Formaggia *et al.* (2009*a*), just to name a few.

# 2
# An insight into vascular data

The ultimate ambition of mathematical models in medicine and clinical applications is to provide quantitative results to enhance the understanding of biophysical processes and hence to support clinicians in their diagnostic and therapeutic procedures. To this end, we must consider data that are *patient-specific*, to use the bioengineering jargon – that is, related to real patients. Obtaining and processing patient-specific data is a major issue which deserves a specific book in its own right. Here, we provide a brief overview of the most common techniques for acquisition and analysis of 'clinical' data. This data *preprocessing* is essential for feeding the mathematical models prior to the set-up of a numerical simulation.

In this chapter we address the case of data related to the arterial (or venous) circulation, whereas in Chapter 5 we will discuss cardiac data. In arteries we have two interacting processes: the blood flow in the *vessel lumen* (the region occupied by the blood, which is referred to as the *fluid domain* for the corresponding mathematical problem) and the displacement of the *vessel wall* (referred to as *structure*). As we anticipated, mathematical models need *geometric*, *boundary* and *biological* data, which are discussed below.

## 2.1 Geometric vascular data

Geometric data are necessary for building the geometry of the computational domains wherein the differential problems are numerically solved. At the end of the geometric preprocessing step, we obtain the fluid computational domain for the blood fluid dynamics problem and the structure computational domain for the vessel wall displacement problem. The construction of the computational domain is an essential step as our typical mathematical model, very often constituted by systems of partial differential equations (PDEs), is defined *in* a bounded subset of the three-dimensional space $\mathbb{R}^3$; in

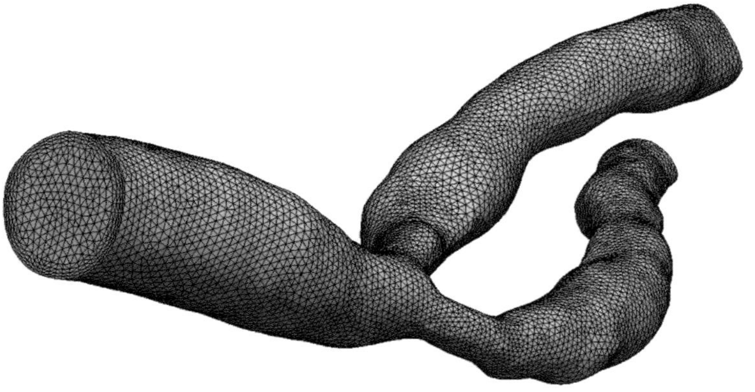

Figure 2.1 Computational mesh of a carotid bifurcation: unstructured volumetric mesh comprised of tetrahedrons.

the case of the fluid problem, this is *e.g.* the artery lumen, while for the solid problem this is the vessel wall. However, mathematical models described by PDEs are almost never endowed with solutions in closed form. Hence, numerical methods are nowadays well established for looking for approximate solutions of such models. Among these, the most widespread is the *Finite Element method* which carries the spatial approximation of the PDEs; see *e.g.* Brenner and Scott (2008), Ciarlet (1978), Ern and Guermond (2004), Hughes (2000) and Quarteroni and Valli (1994). The Finite Element method – as well as other families of methods – is based on the approximation of the computational domain wherein the PDEs are defined, thus requiring the construction of the so-called *computational mesh*; an example of volumetric mesh comprised of tetrahedrons is depicted in Figure 2.1.

The processing of geometric data for blood flow simulations is a major task since vessels exhibit high morphological variability due, for example, to the evident tortuousness of vessels and the presence of several bifurcations. Moreover, in unhealthy cases, this variability is further emphasized, because of the possible presence of calcifications, stenoses, aneurysms or even prostheses (such as stents).

Geometric preprocessing consists of the following steps, which are usually performed in sequence (Antiga *et al.* 2008, Antiga, Peiró and Steinman 2009):

(i) acquisition of clinical images,
(ii) image enhancement,
(iii) image segmentation,
(iv) generation of the computational mesh.

These items are addressed below.

### *2.1.1 Acquisition of clinical images*

*Angiography* is an imaging technique successfully used to 'identify' the vessel lumen. It exploits the property that a liquid inside the vessel appears brighter than the vessel wall and the surrounding tissue. Angiographies are usually acquired as two-dimensional (2D) images,corresponding to different slices of the domain of interest, but three-dimensional (3D) acquisitions of volumes are also possible.

One of the most common techniques for obtaining an angiography is *X-ray imaging*, based on the projection of X-ray beams through the body onto suitable screens, and on the contrast produced in the 2D image by the different absorption properties of body structures. To highlight the vessel lumen, a radio-opaque dye is inserted into the bloodstream through the arterial system. To reconstruct tortuous geometries, a *rotational angiography* (RA) is performed, where X-ray sources and detectors are rapidly rotated around the patient, allowing one to acquire many projections within a few seconds. The excellent spatial resolution of projection angiography (about 0.2 mm, 0.4 mm for RA) makes this technique the gold standard for most vascular imaging applications. Another X-ray angiography technique, widely used for blood flow simulation, is based on *computed tomography* (CT) technology, where multiple X-ray sources and detectors are rotated rapidly around the patient, allowing one to acquire 3D images with excellent spatial resolution (less than 1 mm in *computed tomography angiography*, CTA). Unlike projection angiography, another advantage of CTA is the possibility of using intravenous rather than arterial injections. Recently, temporally resolved CTA (4D-CTA) has become feasible. This allows one to obtain several (15–20) 3D images during a heartbeat.

Difficulties may arise in the presence of metal artifacts in subjects bearing metallic prostheses such as pacemakers, resulting in streaks on the images obscuring anatomical details; see Robertson, Yuan, Wang and Vannier (1997) and Faggiano, Lorenzi and Quarteroni (2014) for possible mathematical treatments.

Another widely used technique to obtain angiographies is *magnetic resonance imaging* (MRI), based on the different decay rates exhibited by body structures on exposure to radio frequency (RF) energy. This is called *magnetic resonance angiography* (MRA). The generated contrast in the images can be tuned by selecting different RF stimuli. This allows MRA to be suitably tuned to detect soft tissues. Another advantage of MRA is that angiography can be generated without using exogenous agents. However, usually an intravenous injection of a paramagnetic contrast agent is used to improve the blood signal and reduce the acquisition time (*contrast-enhanced* (CE)-MRA).

Finally, we mention *ultrasound* (US) imaging, based on the reflections of high-frequency sound waves (a few MHz) transmitted into the body. Ultrasound is the least expensive and invasive of the techniques discussed here and allows real-time acquisition of 2D images. In contrast, its spatial resolution is the poorest. Recently it has even been possible to acquire 3D images (3D US) by reconstructing a 3D volume from 2D slices.

On the other hand, only a few techniques currently allow us to obtain images of vessel walls. Among these we cite *black blood* (BB)-MRA, by which the vessel wall and the surrounding tissue can also be viewed, and *intravascular ultrasound* (IVUS), which is however very invasive since the transducer is placed directly into the artery (typically a coronary artery) via a catheter.

Independently of which technique is used, we can assume that, from a mathematical standpoint, we are able to obtain a vector $\boldsymbol{I}^{\text{clin}}$, whose $j$th component, $I_j^{\text{clin}}$, corresponds to the intensity of the image at the point $\boldsymbol{x}_j$ in grey-scale representing the contrast generated by the imaging technique. The collection of the points $\boldsymbol{x}_j$, $j = 1, \ldots, N^{\text{clin}}$, forms the lattice $\mathcal{L}^{\text{clin}}$,where $N^{\text{clin}}$ is the total number of acquisition points (pixels or voxels) where the image contrast has been evaluated. Here and below, a lattice is a simple collection of points determined by the point coordinates. It can be useful to associate a corresponding image intensity (scalar) function with the image intensity vector $\boldsymbol{I}^{\text{clin}}$, which is typically obtained by interpolation, and will be denoted by $I^{\text{clin}}(\boldsymbol{x})$.

### 2.1.2 Image enhancement

Medical images are often affected by noise and artifacts that may interfere with the quality of the final results of the preprocessing step. Thus, prior to the reconstruction of the 3D geometry, an image enhancement procedure is usually performed.

One popular enhancement technique is *resampling*, which consists in suitably changing the resolution of the images in one or more directions. In practice, an interpolation of image intensity values $\boldsymbol{I}^{\text{clin}}$ onto a more refined lattice is performed. The most commonly used methods are piecewise constant interpolation, first-order composite Lagrangian interpolation, B-spline (Unser 1999), and windowed sinc interpolation (Crochiere and Rabiner 1983).

The noise in the medical images may be due to thermal effects in the signal processing electronics or to other undesired sources. Reduction of noise could be obtained by means of a *smoothing filter*, which does not require any prior knowledge about the nature of the noise and has a regularizing effect on the image. This technique is the most commonly used both for CT and MRI images. A very popular filter is the *Gaussian* filter, consisting in performing a discrete convolution with a Gaussian kernel over the lattice $\mathcal{L}^{\text{clin}}$ of the image intensity $\boldsymbol{I}^{\text{clin}}$. Unfortunately, together with the noise, smoothing could also cut off significant high-frequency image contents when performing the filtering procedure. Moreover, since the image is separated from the background by sharp boundaries, characterized by high-frequency content, the smoothing filter could blur and displace the boundaries. To prevent this, *anisotropic diffusion filtering* has been introduced (Perona and Malik 1990): the parabolic diffusion equation (often known the heat equation) is solved for a new image intensity function, with diffusion coefficient decreasing for increasing values of the gradient magnitude of intensity. By so doing, the filtering is not performed at the boundaries where the gradient is large.

Another technique, called *multiscale vessel enhancement* (Frangi *et al.* 1999), exploits the specific tubular shape of vascular geometries, and therefore assumes that the minimum modulus eigenvalue of the Hessian matrix of the image intensity function $I^{\text{clin}}$ is small, while the other two are large and of equal sign.

At the end of this substep we obtain a new image intensity vector $\boldsymbol{I}^{\text{en}}$ whose $j$th component, $I_j^{\text{en}}$, denotes the intensity of the enhanced image in grey-scale at the point $\boldsymbol{x}_j$, $j = 1, \dots, N^{\text{en}}$, in the lattice $\mathcal{L}^{\text{en}}$ (and correspondingly an associated enhanced image intensity function $I^{\text{en}}(\boldsymbol{x})$ via interpolation). Here, $N^{\text{en}}$ is the total number of points in the enhanced image intensity vector. Usually, $N^{\text{en}} > N^{\text{clin}}$.

### *2.1.3 Image segmentation*

Image segmentation is the cornerstone of the preprocessing step. It consists in the construction of the shape of a vascular district from the image obtained after the enhancement substep. In particular, the segmentation allows one to detect those points of the lattice $\mathcal{L}^{\text{en}}$ which – presumably – belong to the boundary of the vessel lumen. The precise definition of the boundary of the lumen is a challenging task which generally requires considerable experience on the part of the user.

The first technique we describe is *thresholding*, which consists in selecting a threshold value $k \in \mathbb{R}$ to identify the points $\boldsymbol{x}_j \in \mathcal{L}^{\text{en}}$ such that $I_j^{\text{en}} > k$. This is motivated by the assumption that $k$ separates different anatomical structures, in our case the vessel lumen (characterized by intensity values larger than $k$) and the background, obtained by the collection of points for which $I_j^{\mathrm{en}} \leq k$. The value of $k$ is determined either manually or via a suitable algorithm. In the latter case, one commonly used strategy is *full width at half maximum* (FWHM), which consists in setting the threshold halfway between the peak intensity within the lumen and the intensity of the background. For the segmentation of special structures, such as calcifications or stents, higher-bound thresholds are used (Boldak, Rolland and Toumoulin 2003).

A more sophisticated class of segmentation methods than thresholding is given by *front propagation methods*, where the propagation of a suitable wavefront is tracked. The speed of the wave is small in regions where $\boldsymbol{I}^{\mathrm{en}}$ changes rapidly and high for other regions, so that the wavefront slows down when approaching the boundary. The most popular front propagation method is the *fast marching method*, which provides an efficient solution to the eikonal problem:

$$\|\nabla T(\boldsymbol{x})\| = \frac{1}{V(I^{\mathrm{en}}(\boldsymbol{x}))}, \quad \boldsymbol{x} \in \mathcal{D}^{\mathrm{en}},$$

where $\mathcal{D}^{\mathrm{en}} \subset \mathbb{R}^3$ is a region that contains all the points $\boldsymbol{x}_j \in \mathcal{L}^{\mathrm{en}}$, and where suitable boundary conditions are prescribed on a selected boundary where the propagation starts (Zhu and Tian 2003). In the above equation, $V$ is the wavefront velocity and $T(\boldsymbol{x})$ is the first arrival time at point $\boldsymbol{x}$. In fact, $T$ is exploited through isocontours, denoting a collection of surfaces describing the shape of the waveform. The vessel boundary is then represented by the points $\boldsymbol{x}_j \in \mathcal{L}^{\mathrm{en}}$ such that $T(\boldsymbol{x}_j) = T^b$ (up to a given tolerance), where $T^b$ is a suitable value selected by the user.

Another class of segmentation methods is that of *deformable models*, where a suitable energy functional is minimized, allowing the deformation of the body (in our case the boundary of the vessel lumen) to reach a final state with the smallest energy, accounting for external terms derived from the image and internal terms constraining the boundary to be regular. The most widely used class of deformable models is the *level-set method*, where a deformable surface is represented implicitly as the zero level of a higher-dimensional embedding function (Sethian 1999). Deformable models, for example those based on cylindrically parametrized surface meshes, incorporate anatomical knowledge of the vessel shape (Frangi *et al.* 1999, Yim *et al.* 2001).

For the segmentation of the vessel wall, Steinman *et al.* (2001), starting from BB-MRA images, segmented the vessel wall outer boundary using the same deformable model as used for the vessel lumen segmentation. Usually,

BB-MRA or other images detecting the vessel wall are not routinely acquired in clinical practice. In this case, a reasonable approach to obtaining the vessel wall is to 'extrude' the reconstructed boundary lumen along the outward unit vector by using a suitable function specifying the vessel wall thickness in the different regions of the district of interest.

In those cases where the image intensity vectors $\boldsymbol{I}^{\text{clin}}$ and $\boldsymbol{I}^{\text{en}}$ refer to 2D slices, application of the above segmentation strategies leads to identification of several vessel boundaries (contours), one for each slice, which now need to be connected to obtain the 3D boundary surface. This operation is called *surface reconstruction*. A simple procedure is to connect successive contours with straight lines defining surface triangle edges. This strategy is not suitable in the presence of changes of shape such as in bifurcations. Better surface reconstruction is provided by least-squares fitting of polynomial surfaces to the contour set (Wang, Dutton and Taylor 1999). This strategy is suited to managing bifurcations whose branches are fitted separately with a successive extension into the parent vessel. A variant of this approach has been proposed in Geiger (1993), where contours are first filled with triangles which are then connected to the triangles of the adjacent contours by means of tetrahedra. The final lumen surface is then represented by the boundary of this tetrahedral mesh (formed by triangles). We also mention *shape-based interpolation* where, for each contour, a characteristic function with positive (resp. negative) values for points located inside (resp. outside) the contour is constructed. The final lumen boundary surface is then represented by the zero level-set of the interpolation of all these characteristic functions (Raya and Udupa 1990). Finally, we briefly describe interpolation by means of *radial basis functions* (RBFs), which provide a flexible way of interpolating data in multi-dimensional spaces, even for unstructured data where interpolation nodes are scattered and/or do not form a regular grid, and for which it is often impossible to apply polynomial or spline interpolation (Carr, Fright and Beatson 1997, Fornefett, Rohr and Stiehl 2001). The coefficients (weights) in the linear combination with respect to the RBF basis are determined by solving a suitable linear system, which is in fact invertible under very mild conditions (Peiró *et al.* 2007).

A special mention must go to *centreline* reconstruction. The centreline is a curve (a one-dimensional manifold) centred inside the vessel lumen. Many segmentation tools use the centreline as the starting point, making the assumption that the shape of the section around each centreline location is known (O'Donnell, Jolly and Gupta 1998). Centreline reconstruction allows complete reconstruction of the computational domain when using *one-dimensional modelling* of blood flow: see Section 3.5.1.

In any case, at the end of the segmentation step we obtain the lattice $\mathcal{L}^{\text{surf}}$ which collects the points $\boldsymbol{x}_j$, $j = 1, \ldots, N^{\text{surf}}$, classified as belonging to the lumen vessel surface or to the outer wall, where $N^{\text{surf}}$ denotes the total number of points of the surface lattice.

### *2.1.4 Building the computational mesh*

Once the final boundary lattice $\mathcal{L}^{\text{surf}}$ (made up of points on the lumen boundary) is made available, we are ready to build the volumetric mesh $\mathcal{T}^{\text{vol}}$ in the lumen. This mesh usually consists of unstructured tetrahedra, because of their flexibility in filling volumes of complex shape.

Unstructured volumetric meshes are constructed starting from an analytical expression, say $\mathcal{S}(\boldsymbol{x})$, representing the surface associated with the boundary lattice $\mathcal{L}^{\text{surf}}$. This expression can derive from an explicit representation, for instance a bivariate parametric function built as a collection of adjacent polygons. The latter are typically triangles, generated by Lagrangian shape functions, or patches, generated by high-degree piecewise polynomials such as NURBS (Sun, Starly, Nam and Darling 2005). Alternatively, the surface is represented implicitly as the isosurface of an embedding function. Note that some of the segmentation strategies described above, such as deformable models and those used for the surface reconstruction, directly provide an analytical expression $\mathcal{S}(\boldsymbol{x})$ of the lumen boundary surface.

For the construction of unstructured volumetric meshes $\mathcal{T}^{\text{vol}}$, we mention two possible approaches. In the first, a boundary surface mesh $\mathcal{T}^{\text{surf}}$ is generated. To this end, we start from a lattice $\widetilde{\mathcal{L}}^{\text{surf}}$ (in principle different to $\mathcal{L}^{\text{surf}}$) composed of points of $\mathcal{S}$. Then, the *Voronoi diagram* for $\widetilde{\mathcal{L}}^{\text{surf}}$ is constructed. This is a partition of $\mathcal{S}$ into non-overlapping regions, each one containing exactly one point (node) of $\widetilde{\mathcal{L}}^{\text{surf}}$ and composed of all the points of $\mathcal{S}$ that are closer to that node than to any other node. Starting from the Voronoi diagram, it is possible to generate a *Delaunay mesh* $\mathcal{T}^{\text{surf}}$: see Thompson, Soni and Weatherill (1999). We emphasize that the vertices of the mesh $\mathcal{T}^{\text{surf}}$ do not necessarily coincide with the points of the lattice $\widetilde{\mathcal{L}}^{\text{surf}}$. Popular algorithms for generating a Delaunay mesh have been proposed by Watson (1981) and Weatherill and Hassan (1994). Once a surface mesh $\mathcal{T}^{\text{surf}}$ is made available, the volumetric mesh $\mathcal{T}^{\text{vol}}$ is generated. The latter could be obtained by *advancing front* methods, where, starting from the triangles of the surface mesh, a front composed of internal nodes is generated. These new nodes allow us to identify tetrahedra, whose validity is verified by checking that they do not intersect the front (Bentley and Friedman 1979).

The second approach relies on directly generating the volumetric mesh

$\mathcal{T}^{\mathrm{vol}}$, for example by means of Delaunay 3D mesh generation, where a starting volumetric lattice $\widetilde{\mathcal{L}}^{\mathrm{vol}}$ is obtained by locating the nodes in the volume $\mathcal{V}(\boldsymbol{x})$ contained in $\mathcal{S}(\boldsymbol{x})$. One of the main problems related to this approach is that boundary meshing is often difficult, since the related surface triangulation could not be of Delaunay type. An alternative approach is given by *octree mesh generation*, where $\mathcal{V}(\boldsymbol{x})$ is embedded in a box and successive subdivisions are performed until the smallest cells permitaccurate description of the boundary. Despite being faster, this strategy generates meshes with poor quality near the boundary.

When a volumetric mesh $\mathcal{T}^{\mathrm{vol}}$ is obtained, a further step (*mesh optimization*) could be introduced prior to the generation of the final mesh, in order to improve its quality. Mesh optimization helps controlling mesh distortion, for example in presence of very large angles in the mesh elements, which could harm the convergence of the algorithms used for the numerical solution of the PDE of interest and thus their accuracy. Mesh optimization is incorporated in the strategies described above; it leads to an *optimal mesh*, providing the best accuracy for a given number of nodes.

A mesh is deemed valid for blood flow simulations if it allows recovery of outputs of physical interest. Even if the latter concerns the postprocessing stage of the computational pipeline, the accuracy of the results and the quality of the outputs evaluation strongly depend on the properties and quality of the mesh. In arteries, the mesh should be fine enough to capture wall shear stress (WSS) (Celik *et al.* 2008) and, to this end, the construction of a boundary layer mesh is essential, even at low Reynolds numbers (Bevan *et al.* 2010). Here *WSS* expresses the magnitude of tangential viscous forces exerted by the fluid on the lumen boundary $\Sigma^t$, defined by

$$WSS = \mu \sqrt{\sum_{j=1}^{2} \big( (\nabla \boldsymbol{v}\, \boldsymbol{n}) \cdot \boldsymbol{\tau}^{(j)} \big)^2} \quad \text{on } \Sigma^t,$$

where $\boldsymbol{v}$ is the fluid velocity, $\boldsymbol{n}$ is the outward directed unit vector normal to $\Sigma^t$ and $\boldsymbol{\tau}^{(j)}$, $j = 1, 2$, represent the tangential unit vectors. Note that *WSS* is a scalar function of $\boldsymbol{x} \in \Sigma^t$ and $t > 0$. In componentwise notation,

$$WSS = \mu \left( \sum_{j=1}^{2} \left( \sum_{i,k=1}^{3} \left( \frac{\partial v_i}{\partial x_k} n_k \right) \tau_i^{(j)} \right)^2 \right)^{1/2} \quad \text{on } \Sigma^t.$$

For the structure domain, hexahedral meshing is preferable in order to prevent the locking phenomenon, whereas tetrahedral meshes are used when conforming meshes at the boundary lumen interface are needed, in view of fluid–structure interaction problems (see Section 3.3). Usually, three or four layers of mesh elements are enough to obtain an accurate result (Younis *et al.* 2004).

For recent reviews on geometric reconstruction for blood flow simulation, see Antiga *et al.* (2009), Sazonov *et al.* (2011) and Lesage, Angelini, Bloch and Funka-Lea (2009).

## 2.2 Boundary vascular data

The differential problems – namely systems of PDEs – we will treat in the following chapters need appropriate boundary conditions. In the case of models like the incompressible Navier–Stokes equations for the fluid problem and finite elasticity for the structure problem, we anticipate the kind of boundary conditions that should ideally be prescribed. These are

$$\boldsymbol{v} = \boldsymbol{g}_f \quad \text{on } \Gamma_f^{D,t}, \qquad -p\boldsymbol{n} + \mu(\nabla\boldsymbol{v} + (\nabla\boldsymbol{v})^{\mathrm{T}})\boldsymbol{n} = \boldsymbol{h}_f \quad \text{on } \Gamma_f^{N,t}$$

for the fluid problem and

$$\boldsymbol{d} = \boldsymbol{g}_s \quad \text{on } \Gamma_s^{D,t}, \qquad \boldsymbol{T}_s\boldsymbol{n} = \boldsymbol{h}_s \quad \text{on } \Gamma_s^{N,t}$$

for the structure problem. In the above equations, the Dirichlet and Neumann boundaries, $\Gamma_j^{D,t}$ and $\Gamma_j^{N,t}$, respectively, are such that $\Gamma_j^{D,t} \cap \Gamma_j^{N,t} = \emptyset$, $\Gamma_j^{D,t} \cup \Gamma_j^{N,t} = \partial\Omega_j^t$, $j = f, s$, where $\Omega_f^t$ and $\Omega_s^t$ are the fluid and structure domains at time $t$: see Figure 2.2(a). Moreover, $p$ denotes the fluid pressure, $-p\boldsymbol{n} + \mu(\nabla\boldsymbol{v} + (\nabla\boldsymbol{v})^{\mathrm{T}})\boldsymbol{n}$ is the fluid normal Cauchy stress at the boundary, $\boldsymbol{d}$ is the structure displacement, $\boldsymbol{T}_s$ is the Cauchy stress tensor of the wall material, and $\boldsymbol{g}_f$, $\boldsymbol{g}_s$, $\boldsymbol{h}_f$, $\boldsymbol{h}_s$ are data: see Chapter 3. We use the superscript $^t$ to indicate time-dependence of the computational domain, its boundary, and their subsets.

As we will see below, the boundary of the computational domain (for either the fluid or the structure) will be composed of two parts, namely the *physical boundary* and the *artificial boundary*. On the physical boundary, suitable conditions are often suggested by physical principles. For example, for the fluid problem, *no-slip* Dirichlet conditions should be prescribed at the lumen boundary, since it is assumed that the fluid particles perfectly adhere to the vessel wall. This leads to a homogeneous Dirichlet condition ($\boldsymbol{v} = \boldsymbol{0}$) in the case of rigid walls, and instead to a kinematic interface condition ($\boldsymbol{v} = \dot{\boldsymbol{d}}$) for fluid–structure interaction problems (see Section 3.3). As for the structure problem, at the internal physical boundary (*i.e.* at the lumen boundary) the fluid pressure is often prescribed. This leads to a Neumann boundary condition ($\boldsymbol{T}_s\boldsymbol{n} = -P\boldsymbol{n}$, where $P$ is a measurement of

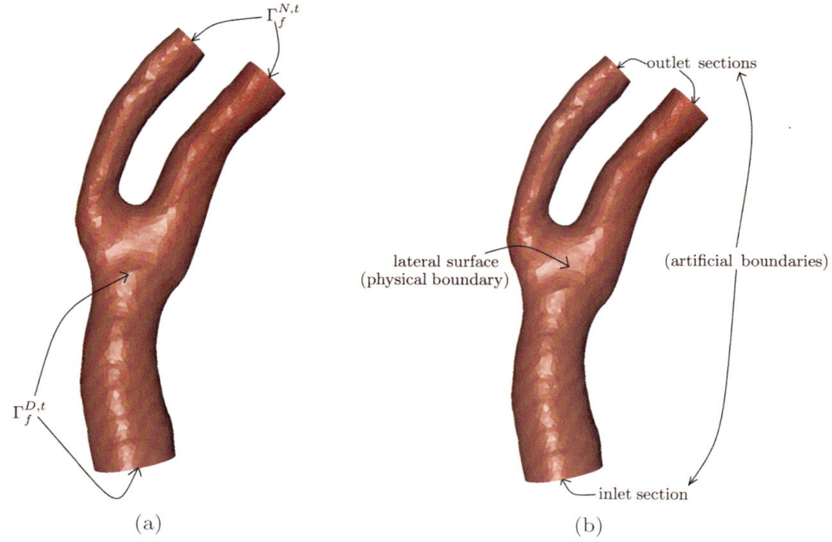


Figure 2.2 Possible choices of the Dirichlet and Neumann boundaries (a) and physical and artificial boundaries (b) for a carotid domain in the fluid stand-alone problem (reconstructed from MRA images).

the fluid pressure) for a pure structure problem, while to a dynamic interface condition ($\boldsymbol{T}_s\boldsymbol{n} = -p\boldsymbol{n} + \mu(\nabla\boldsymbol{v} + (\nabla\boldsymbol{v})^{\mathrm{T}})\boldsymbol{n}$) for fluid–structure interaction. On the outer wall boundary $\Gamma_{\text{ext}}$, the interaction with the surrounding tissue should be considered. This is often modelled by means of a Robin boundary condition of the form

$$\alpha_{ST}\boldsymbol{d} + \boldsymbol{T}_s\boldsymbol{n} = P_{\text{ext}}\boldsymbol{n} \quad \text{on } \Gamma_{\text{ext}}, \tag{2.1}$$

which assimilates the surrounding tissue to a sequence of elastic springs with rigidity $\alpha_{ST} > 0$ and where $P_{\text{ext}}$ is the external pressure (Moireau *et al.* 2012).

In contrast, the artificial sections are those introduced by the truncation of the computational domains: see Figure 2.2(b). Truncation is done in order to focus on a specific domain of interest. Ideally, the boundary conditions to be used on artificial sections should derive from clinical measurements.

The technique mainly used to obtain boundary data on artificial boundaries is ultrasound. This is because of its non-invasiveness and the fact that it is used on a daily basis in clinical practice. If the ultrasound beam is swept through a plane or sector (unlike in geometric acquisitions where it is kept fixed), it is possible to measure the blood velocity at a single point of a cross-section, let say $\Gamma^t$, in the direction of the ultrasound beam by exploiting the Doppler effect. The velocity is then converted into a flow rate measure $Q$ across $\Gamma^t$ for each time (this is the principle of the so-called *echo-colour-Doppler* technique: Savader, Lund and Osterman 1997) and can then be used to prescribe a *flow rate condition*

$$\rho_f \int_{\Gamma^t} \boldsymbol{v} \cdot \boldsymbol{n} \, \mathrm{d}\gamma = Q. \tag{2.2}$$

Condition (2.2) is *defective* since it is not rich enough to ensure well-posedness of the fluid problem. The treatment of defective conditions will be addressed in Section 3.4. Another technique allowing measurement of cross-sectional flow rates is based on the acquisition of thermal images (Mahmoud *et al.* 2013). Another quantity easily measurable by means of ultrasound is the lumen area $\int_{\Gamma^t} \mathrm{d}\gamma$. This information could be used to prescribe a defective condition for the vessel wall if $\Gamma^t$ coincides with a subset $\Gamma_f^t$ of the boundary of the fluid domain.

More sophisticated techniques could acquire velocity measurements in several points on the same cross-section, thus in principle leading to a Dirichlet boundary condition (possibly after suitable regularization). This is the case for *phase contrast* (PC)-MRA, where the blood velocities are encoded into images taken at several instants during a heartbeat (Morbiducci *et al.* 2009). The spatial resolution of modern PC-MRA is of the order of 1–2 mm on each cross-section $\Gamma^t$ of the vessel and 4 mm along the longitudinal axis. The required mesh size is often less than 1 mm, however, such interpolation is needed to obtain a usable Dirichlet condition. The temporal resolution is about 0.03 s.

If the lumen artificial cross-section is orthogonal to the axial direction, then the viscous terms in the fluid normal Cauchy stress are very small (Heywood, Rannacher and Turek 1996). In this case, a measurement of the pressure $P(t)$ could be used to prescribe a Neumann boundary condition. This could be obtained for the arterial system non-invasively by means of a *sphygmomanometer*, which usually measures the pressure at the level of the radial aorta (remember that the pressure peak could be considered constant along the arterial tree, at least until the capillary net: see Section 1). To have continuous monitoring of the pressure (e.g. during hospital recovery) or to take a measurement in the venous system (where the pressure reduces), a catheter with a transducer could be placed in the region of interest. In any case, the average pressure over the cross-section is measured. This leads at each time to the following defective boundary condition for the normal component of the normal Cauchy stress of the fluid:

$$\frac{1}{|\Gamma^t|}\int_{\Gamma^t}\left(p\boldsymbol{n}-\mu(\nabla\boldsymbol{v}+(\nabla\boldsymbol{v})^{\mathrm{T}})\boldsymbol{n}\right)\cdot\boldsymbol{n}\,\mathrm{d}\gamma=P. \tag{2.3}$$

Unfortunately, measurements are not available at the artificial sections of the structure, so 'empirical' and 'practical' choices are very often made (see Section 3.4).

Finally, we observe that measurements acquired at several instants along the heartbeat could be applied in principle for physical boundaries as well. For example, from 4D-CTA imaging the boundary lumen displacement could be used as the Dirichlet condition for the structure problem, whereas from PC-MRA the blood velocity at the boundary lumen could be used to prescribe a Dirichlet condition for the fluid problem. Since, at the physical boundaries, physical principles are used to prescribe boundary conditions, these 'extra' data could be used for validation of the numerical results or in a *parameter estimation* fashion, as described in Chapter 9. PC-MRA also allows us to acquire internal measurements of blood velocity. This could also be used for validation or parameter estimation.

## 2.3 Biological vascular data

Finally, we need to know the values of physical parameters appearing in the differential equations. For the fluid problem, two parameters characterize it, namely blood *density* $\rho_f$ and blood *viscosity* $\mu_f$. Although density is easily measurable in principle, patient-specific acquisition is generally not made because its value never significantly departs from an average value of 1.06 g cm$^{-3}$. In contrast, the variability range of viscosity is larger. Indeed, its value depends on the shear rate (non-Newtonian behaviour) and on the physical state of the patient. When the assumption of Newtonian fluid (holding for medium and large healthy vessels) is made, typical values of the viscosity range in the interval 0.03–0.04 P (the poise, symbol P, is the unit of dynamic viscosity, *i.e.* 1 P = 1 g cm$^{-1}$ s$^{-1}$). Again, no patient-specific viscosity measurements are usually made and, except for pathological situations, a value in the previous range is selected.

The parameters characterizing the vessel wall depend (also in number) on the constitutive law used to represent its behaviour. More typically, these are the density, the *elasticity* (or compliance) and the amount of compressibility allowed or, very often, *incompressibility*. For linear elastic models, the latter two are quantified by *Young's modulus* and the *Poisson ratio*, respectively. For the non-linear elastic laws typically used to characterize the arterial tissue, compliance and compressibility properties are quantified by suitable parameters and coefficients typical of the constitutive model at hand. The tissue density value is very similar to that of blood, the upper limit of the range most commonly used being close to 1.2 g $cm^{-3}$. The compliance of the vessel could be qualitatively seen as the ratio between the volume and pressure variations (Nichols and O'Rourke 2005). Patient-specific acquisitions could be obtained from simultaneous (invasive) measurement of pressure and cross-sectional area at different locations, by measuring the rate of propagation of flow waves (Boese, Bock, Schoenberg and Schad 2000), or by *elastography*, where the elasticity properties are analyzed by images before and after a deformation (Oberai, Gokhale and Feijóo 2003). The range of variability of vessel compliance is quite wide (200–800 kPa in normal conditions), with large dependence on the location and on the possible presence of aneurysms or calcifications. As for the Poisson ratio, only *ex vivo* measurements are possible. An acceptable value used by the community is 0.49, meaning that vessels could be considered as quasi-incompressible. Finally, let us mention that the coefficient $\alpha_{ST}$ in (2.1) can be regarded as representative of the Young's modulus of the surrounding tissue. As such, it could thus be measured, though this is a difficult endeavour. Estimates have been provided in Liu *et al.* (2007), for example.

When not available from measurements, patient-specific values of biological data could alternatively be obtained by means of parameter estimation mathematical techniques. This will be the topic of Chapter 9.

Figure 2.3 provides a sketch of the computational pipeline; this can be defined as the sequence of procedures making available clinically meaningful quantities of interest starting from clinical data (images, boundary and biological), and passing through geometry handling, mesh generation and Finite Element approximation of the partial differential equations describing the physical problem.

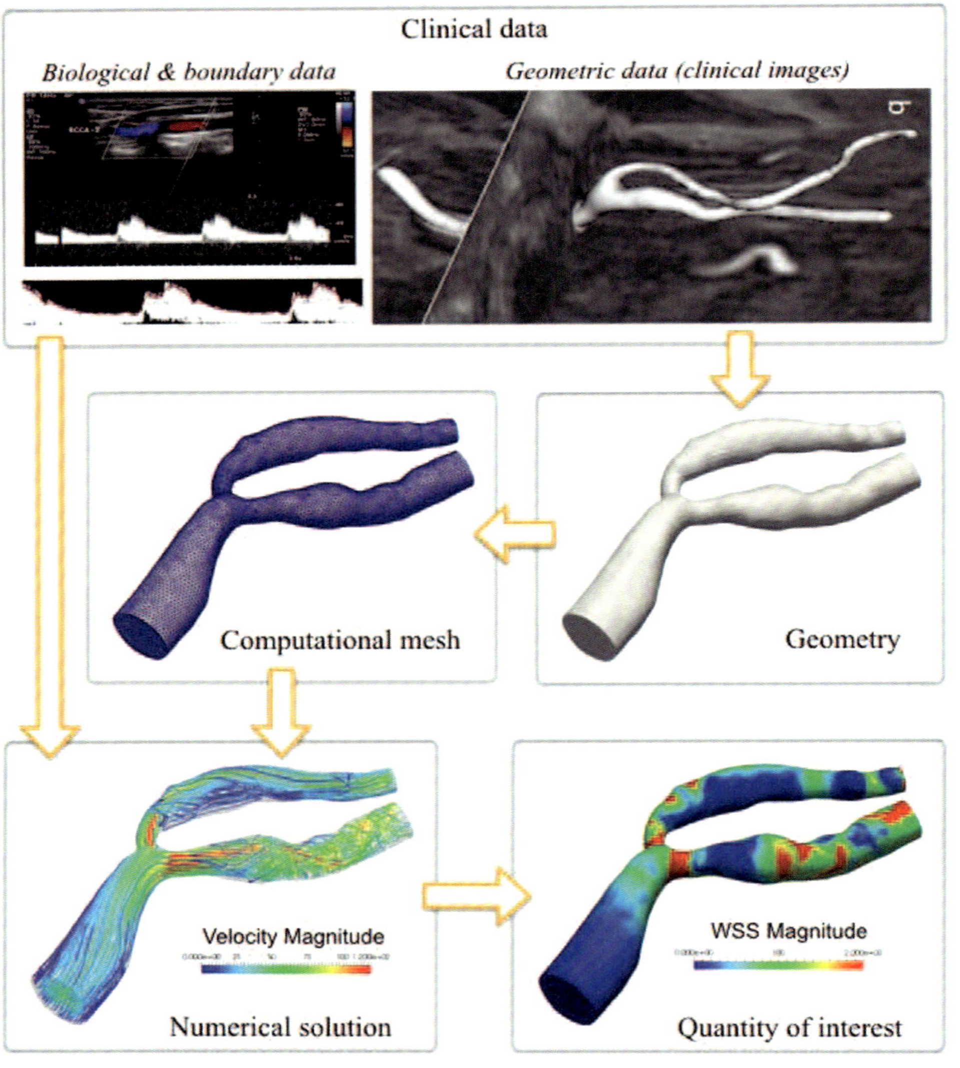


Figure 2.3 Sketch of the computational pipeline applied to the blood flow dynamics in carotid bifurcation; images at top generated by data and CT images provided by the Vascular Surgery and Radiology Divisions at Fondazione IRCSS Ca Granda, Ospedale Maggiore Policlinico, Milan, Italy.

# 3
# Modelling blood flow

We review in this chapter the mathematical and numerical models related to blood flows in the vascular system and the mechanical deformation of wall arteries. We address the fluid and solid problems, their interaction – which yields the fluid–structure interaction problem – as well as geometric reduced models, the issue of boundary conditions and the geometric multi-scale approach. Finally, we outline commonly used numerical strategies for the solution of these problems.

## 3.1 The fluid problem

In large and medium sized arteries – those more typically affected by vascular diseases – blood can be modelled by means of the Navier–Stokes (NS) equations for incompressible homogeneous Newtonian fluids (Perktold, Thurner and Kenner 1994, Taylor, Hughes and Zarins 1996, Taylor, Hughes and Zarins 1998, Formaggia *et al.* 2009*a*). Non-Newtonian rheological models are necessary for describing some specific flow processes, such as clotting or sickle cell diseases, or more generally flow in capillaries, and for them we refer to Robertson, Sequeira and Owens (2009) and Fasano, Santos and Sequeira (2012), for example.

For the mathematical formulation of the problem, we write the fluid equations with respect to an Eulerian frame of reference, and we let $\Omega_f^t = \Omega_f(t) \subset \mathbb{R}^3$ denote the time-varying arterial lumen, at time $t > 0$ (see Figure 3.1(a)).

Then, at each time $t > 0$, we look for the fluid velocity $\boldsymbol{v}$ and pressure $p$ such that

$$\rho_f\left(\frac{\partial \boldsymbol{v}}{\partial t} + (\boldsymbol{v}\cdot\nabla)\boldsymbol{v}\right) - \nabla\cdot\boldsymbol{T}_f(\boldsymbol{v},p) = \boldsymbol{0} \quad \text{in } \Omega_f^t, \tag{3.1a}$$

$$\nabla\cdot\boldsymbol{v} = 0 \quad \text{in } \Omega_f^t. \tag{3.1b}$$

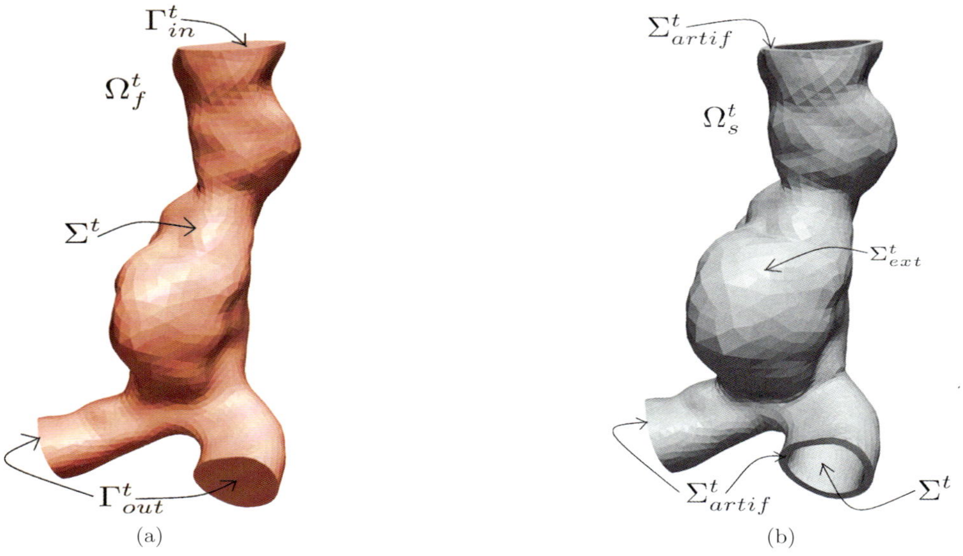


Figure 3.1 Representation of the fluid domain (a) and structure domain (b). The fluid domain illustrated is that of an abdominal aorta in the presence of an aneurysm, reconstructed from CTA images. The structure domain was obtained via extrusion of the fluid domain.

Note that volumetric forces acting in the fluid domain (*e.g.* due to gravity) have been set to zero since they are quite often negligible. Moreover,

$$\boldsymbol{T}_f(\boldsymbol{v}, p) = -p\boldsymbol{I} + \mu(\nabla \boldsymbol{v} + (\nabla \boldsymbol{v})^{\mathrm{T}}) \tag{3.2}$$

is the fluid Cauchy stress tensor already mentioned in Section 2.2, where $\mu$ is the blood viscosity. As we consider only Newtonian rheology here, $\mu$ is assumed to be constant.

Finally, problem (3.1) is completed by the initial condition

$$\boldsymbol{v}|_{t=0} = \boldsymbol{v}_0 \quad \text{in } \Omega_f,$$

where $\Omega_f = \Omega_f^0$, and boundary conditions. The latter typically prescribe no-slip conditions on the physical boundary $\Sigma^t$,

$$\boldsymbol{v} = \boldsymbol{\phi} \quad \text{on } \Sigma^t, \tag{3.3}$$

the upstream velocity on the proximal boundaries, say $\Gamma^t_{\mathrm{in}}$,

$$\boldsymbol{v} = \boldsymbol{v}_{\mathrm{up}} \quad \text{on } \Gamma^t_{\mathrm{in}}, \tag{3.4}$$

and traction conditions on the distal boundaries, say $\Gamma^t_{\mathrm{out}}$,

$$\boldsymbol{T}_f\, \boldsymbol{n} = \boldsymbol{h}_f \quad \text{on } \Gamma^t_{\mathrm{out}}. \tag{3.5}$$

Here, $\boldsymbol{v}_0$, $\boldsymbol{v}_{\rm up}$, $\boldsymbol{\phi}$ and $\boldsymbol{h}_f$ are suitable functions with the required regularity (Quarteroni and Valli 1994). Note that the lumen boundary displacement $\boldsymbol{\phi}$ at this level is a known function of space and time. For rigid boundaries, we have $\boldsymbol{\phi} = \boldsymbol{0}$.

When patient-specific measurements are available, other conditions might be prescribed as discussed in Section 2.2. However, measurements seldom provide a complete dataset to be used in the computation: see our discussion in Section 2.2.This prompts the issue of solvability of Navier–Stokes equations, which we address in Section 3.4.

For each $t > 0$ (a.e. $t > 0$), the weak formulation of (3.1) together with the boundary conditions (3.3, 3.4, 3.5) reads as follows: find $\boldsymbol{v} = \boldsymbol{v}(t) \in [H^1(\Omega_f^t)]^3$, with $\boldsymbol{v} = \boldsymbol{v}_{\rm up}$ on $\Gamma_{\rm in}^t$, $\boldsymbol{v} = \boldsymbol{\phi}$ on $\Sigma^t$, $\boldsymbol{v} = \boldsymbol{v}_0$ for $t = 0$ in $\Omega_f$, and $p = p(t) \in L^2(\Omega_f^t)$ such that

$$\rho_f \int_{\Omega_f^t} \frac{\partial \boldsymbol{v}}{\partial t} \cdot \boldsymbol{w} \, {\rm d}\omega + \mathcal{A}_f^t(\boldsymbol{v}, \boldsymbol{v}, \boldsymbol{w}) + \mathcal{B}^t(p, \boldsymbol{w}) = \int_{\Gamma_{\rm out}^t} \boldsymbol{h}_f \cdot \boldsymbol{n} \, {\rm d}\gamma, \qquad (3.6a)$$

$$\mathcal{B}^t(q, \boldsymbol{v}) = 0, \qquad (3.6b)$$

for all

$$\boldsymbol{w} \in \boldsymbol{V}^t = \{[H^1(\Omega_f^t)]^3 : \boldsymbol{w} = \boldsymbol{0} \text{ on } \partial\Omega \setminus \Gamma_{\rm out}^t\}$$

and $q \in L^2(\Omega_f^t)$, and where we have set

$$\mathcal{A}_f^t(\boldsymbol{z}, \boldsymbol{v}, \boldsymbol{w}) = \rho_f \int_{\Omega_f^t} (\boldsymbol{z} \cdot \nabla)\boldsymbol{v} \cdot \boldsymbol{w} \, {\rm d}\omega + \mu \int_{\Omega_f^t} (\nabla \boldsymbol{v} + (\nabla \boldsymbol{v})^{\rm T}) : \nabla \boldsymbol{w} \, {\rm d}\omega$$

and

$$\mathcal{B}^t(q, \boldsymbol{w}) = -\int_{\Omega_f^t} q \nabla \cdot \boldsymbol{w} \, {\rm d}\omega.$$

The existence of a global-in-time weak solution of the above problem was proved by Leray (1934) for the case $\Omega_f = \mathbb{R}^3$ and by Hopf (1951) for the case of a bounded domain. The uniqueness has been proved only for the two-dimensional case (Lions and Prodi 1959); for the three-dimensional case, only local-in-time uniqueness results are available (Prodi 1962). See also Temam (1984).

## 3.2 Mechanical wall models

The problem that models the deformation of vessel walls is given by the elastodynamics equation, which is usually written in a reference domain $\Omega_s = \Omega_s(0) \subset \mathbb{R}^3$ using a Lagrangian framework. For any $t > 0$, the material domain $\Omega_s^t = \Omega_s(t)$ (depicted in Figure 3.1(b)) is the image of $\Omega_s$ by a proper Lagrangian map $\mathcal{L} : \Omega_s \to \Omega_s^t$. We use the notation $\widehat{g} = g \circ \mathcal{L}$ to denote the function $\widehat{g}$ induced on $\Omega_s$ by the function $g$ defined in the current solid configuration $\Omega_s^t$.

For simplicity, we assume that the arterial wall obeys a (possibly non-linear) finite elastic law relating stress to strain in the arterial tissue; for more complex behaviours of arterial walls see Holzapfel, Gasser and Ogden (2000) and Holzapfel and Ogden (2010), for example. In more realistic settings, stress is a function of the strain but also of the past loading history (Fung, Fronek and Patitucci 1979).

The problem we consider is as follows: find, at each time $t > 0$, the structure displacement $\widehat{\boldsymbol{d}}$ such that

$$\rho_s \frac{\partial^2 \widehat{\boldsymbol{d}}}{\partial t^2} - \nabla \cdot \widehat{\boldsymbol{T}}_s(\widehat{\boldsymbol{d}}) = \mathbf{0} \quad \text{in } \Omega_s, \tag{3.7}$$

where $\rho_s$ is the structure density. Note that volumetric forces acting in the solid domain (*e.g.* due to muscle forces) have been set to zero since they are quite often negligible.

The above equation is stated in terms of the first Piola–Kirchhoff tensor $\widehat{\boldsymbol{T}}_s(\widehat{\boldsymbol{d}})$, which is related to the Cauchy tensor $\boldsymbol{T}_s(\boldsymbol{d})$ via the relation $\widehat{\boldsymbol{T}}_s = J\boldsymbol{T}_s\boldsymbol{F}^{-T}$. Here, $\boldsymbol{F} = \nabla \boldsymbol{x}$ is the deformation gradient tensor, where the gradient is taken with respect to the reference space coordinates and $\boldsymbol{x}$ denotes point coordinates in the current configuration. Correspondingly, $J = \det(\boldsymbol{F})$ denotes the change of volume between the reference and the current configurations; note that $\boldsymbol{F}$ (and thus $J$) depends on the current configuration $\Omega_s^t$.

For a *hyperelastic* material, the first Piola–Kirchhoff stress tensor is obtained by differentiating a suitable strain energy density function $\Theta$:

$$\widehat{\boldsymbol{T}}_s = \frac{\partial \Theta}{\partial \boldsymbol{F}}. \tag{3.8}$$

Several non-linear elastic energy functions have been proposed for arteries. For the *Saint Venant–Kirchhoff* material,

$$\begin{aligned} \Theta(\boldsymbol{C}) = {} & \frac{E\nu}{2(1+\nu)(1-2\nu)} \left( \operatorname{tr}\left( \frac{1}{2}(\boldsymbol{C}^{\mathrm{T}} - \boldsymbol{I}) \right) \right)^2 \\ & + \frac{E}{2(1+\nu)} \operatorname{tr}\left( \left( \frac{1}{2}(\boldsymbol{C}^{\mathrm{T}} - \boldsymbol{I}) \right)^2 \right), \end{aligned} \tag{3.9}$$

where $\boldsymbol{C} = \boldsymbol{F}^{\mathrm{T}}\boldsymbol{F}$, $E$ is *Young's modulus* and $\nu$ is the *Poisson ratio* of the vessel wall. More complex and accurate functions widely used for arteries are based on separating the isotropic elastic behaviour due to the *elastin* and the anisotropic behaviour accounting for the stiffening increment at large displacements due to the *collagen* distributed along preferred directions called *fibre*:

$$\Theta = \Theta^{\text{iso}} + \Theta^{\text{aniso}}. \tag{3.10}$$

A common choice for the isotropic part is the *neo-Hookean* law

$$\Theta^{\text{iso}}(\boldsymbol{C}) = \frac{G}{2}(\text{tr}(\boldsymbol{C}) - 3), \tag{3.11}$$

whereas for the anisotropic part, an exponential law is often considered,

$$\Theta^{\text{aniso}}(\boldsymbol{C}) = \frac{k_1}{2k_2}\left(\mathrm{e}^{(k_2(\boldsymbol{a}\cdot(\boldsymbol{C}\boldsymbol{a})-1)^2)} - 1\right), \tag{3.12}$$

where $\boldsymbol{a}$ is the unit vector identifying the preferred direction of the collagen fibres, $G$ is the *shear modulus*, and $k_1, k_2$ are material parameters, where $k_2$ characterizes the stiffness of the material for large displacements (Fung 1993, Holzapfel *et al.* 2000, Raghavan and Vorp 2000). More complete laws also account for the symmetrical helical arrangement of the collagen fibres, introducing a second predominant direction of fibres (Holzapfel and Ogden 2010). When not available from medical images, the fibre directions are computed by means of suitable algorithms under the assumption that their orientation is mainly governed by the principal stresses: see *e.g.* Hariton, de Botton, Gasser and Holzapfel (2006) and Kuhl and Holzapfel (2006). For distal arteries of muscular type, viscoelastic and pseudoelastic terms are also considered (Holzapfel and Gasser 2001). Multi-layer constitutive models, *i.e.* models taking into account separately the mechanical properties of the intima, media and adventitia, are also considered in literature for different arteries (Balzani, Neff, Schroder and Holzapfel 2006, Dalong, Robertson, Lin and Lovell 2012, Holzapfel and Gasser 2000). Even if experimental measurements of the properties of the vessel wall layers (including orientation and density of collagen fibres) are not often available – as highlighted in Dalong *et al.* (2012) for cerebral arteries – multi-layer models represent a significant enhancement toward the understanding of vascular diseases as cerebral aneurysms (Tricerri *et al.* 2015, Tricerri *et al.* 2016).

Sometimes the arterial tissue is modelled as being (strictly) incompressible by imposing the incompressibility constraint $J = 1$ on the strain energy function via Lagrange multipliers (Holzapfel 2000), that is,

$$\Theta^{\text{inc}} = \Theta + p_s(J - 1). \tag{3.13}$$

Here $p_s$ is the hydrostatic pressure related to the vessel wall displacement, which plays the role of the Lagrange multiplier for the incompressibility constraint. Correspondingly, the Cauchy stress tensor is augmented as follows:

$$\boldsymbol{T}_s^{\mathrm{inc}}(\boldsymbol{d}, p_s) = \boldsymbol{T}_s(\boldsymbol{d}) + p_s \boldsymbol{I},$$

where $\boldsymbol{T}_s$ is the component arising from the energy $\Theta$. However, experimental studies have shown that the arterial tissue in fact exhibits *nearly incompressible* behaviour (Carew, Vaishnav and Patel 1968). This means that the strain energy function could be decomposed into two terms

$$\Theta(\boldsymbol{C}) = \Theta_{\mathrm{vol}}(J) + \Theta_{\mathrm{isoc}}(\bar{\boldsymbol{C}}),$$

where $\bar{\boldsymbol{C}} = J^{-2/3}\boldsymbol{C}$, $\det \bar{\boldsymbol{C}} = 1$. The *isochoric* part $\Theta_{\mathrm{isoc}}$ is given by the general function (3.10) provided that $\boldsymbol{C}$ is replaced by $\bar{\boldsymbol{C}}$ and characterizes the mechanical response of the material to incompressible deformations. The *volumetric* part is usually given by

$$\Theta_{\mathrm{vol}}(J) = \frac{\kappa}{2}(J-1)^2,$$

where $\kappa$ (*bulk modulus*) is a penalty parameter to enforce the incompressibility constraint $J = 1$ (Li and Robertson 2013). In this case, the related Cauchy stress tensor is the same as in the compressible case. For a review of arterial vessel wall models we refer the reader to Holzapfel and Ogden (2010).

Problem (3.7) has to be completed by the initial conditions

$$\widehat{\boldsymbol{d}}|_{t=0} = \boldsymbol{d}_0, \quad \left.\frac{\partial \widehat{\boldsymbol{d}}}{\partial t}\right|_{t=0} = \boldsymbol{d}_1 \quad \text{in } \Omega_s,$$

and boundary conditions. The latter typically prescribe on the artificial sections $\Gamma^t_{\mathrm{artif}}$ either

$$\widehat{\boldsymbol{d}} = \boldsymbol{0} \quad \text{on } \Gamma_{\mathrm{artif}} \tag{3.14}$$

(fixed boundary) or $\widehat{\boldsymbol{d}} \cdot \boldsymbol{n} = 0$ together with $(\widehat{\boldsymbol{T}}_s \boldsymbol{n}) \cdot \boldsymbol{\tau}^{(j)} = \boldsymbol{0}$, $j = 1, 2$, where $\boldsymbol{\tau}^{(j)}$ are the unit tangential directions (displacement allowed in the tangential direction), whereas at the internal physical boundary $\Sigma^t$ they prescribe the solid traction

$$\widehat{\boldsymbol{T}}_s \boldsymbol{n} = \boldsymbol{h}_s \quad \text{on } \Sigma. \tag{3.15}$$

Here $\boldsymbol{d}_0$, $\boldsymbol{d}_1$ and $\boldsymbol{h}_s$ are suitable given functions. When considering the fluid–structure (FS) coupling, $\boldsymbol{h}_s$ is of course provided by the normal Cauchy stress from the fluid side: see Section 3.3. To account for the effect of the tissues surrounding the artery, the algebraic law (2.1) is often prescribed at the external lateral surface $\Gamma_{\text{ext}}$ of $\Omega_s$, to mimic the elastic behaviour of this tissue (Moireau *et al.* 2012).

For each time $t > 0$, the weak form of (3.7) together with the boundary conditions (2.1), (3.14) and (3.15), in the case for fixed boundaries, reads as follows: find $\widehat{\boldsymbol{d}} = \widehat{\boldsymbol{d}}(t) \in \boldsymbol{D}$, $\widehat{\boldsymbol{d}} = \boldsymbol{0}$ on $\Gamma_{\text{artif}}$, $\widehat{\boldsymbol{d}} = \boldsymbol{d}_0$ and $\partial\widehat{\boldsymbol{d}}/\partial t = \boldsymbol{d}_1$ for $t = 0$ in $\Omega_s$, such that

$$\begin{aligned}\rho_s \int_{\Omega_s} \frac{\partial^2 \widehat{\boldsymbol{d}}}{\partial t^2} \cdot \widehat{\boldsymbol{e}}\,\mathrm{d}\omega + \int_{\Omega_s} \widehat{\boldsymbol{T}}_s(\widehat{\boldsymbol{d}}) : \nabla \widehat{\boldsymbol{e}}\,\mathrm{d}\omega + \int_{\Gamma_{\text{ext}}} \alpha_{ST}\widehat{\boldsymbol{d}} \cdot \widehat{\boldsymbol{e}}\,\mathrm{d}\sigma \\ = \int_{\Gamma_{\text{ext}}} P_{\text{ext}}\widehat{\boldsymbol{n}} \cdot \widehat{\boldsymbol{e}}\,\mathrm{d}\sigma + \int_{\Sigma} \widehat{\boldsymbol{h}}_s \cdot \widehat{\boldsymbol{e}}\,\mathrm{d}\sigma, \end{aligned} \tag{3.16}$$

for all $\widehat{\boldsymbol{e}} \in \boldsymbol{D} = \boldsymbol{D}^0$, where

$$\boldsymbol{D}^t = \{\boldsymbol{e} \in [H^1(\Omega_s^t)]^3 : \boldsymbol{e} = \boldsymbol{0} \text{ on } \Gamma_{\text{artif}}^t\}.$$

The existence of strong (steady) solutions of the above problems could be proved using the theory developed in Ball (1976). For example, this is the case for the Saint Venant–Kirchhoff constitutive law given in (3.9) (Ciarlet and Necas 1985). The existence and uniqueness of weak solutions are guaranteed by the coercivity and convexity of the energy $\Theta$ (Ciarlet 1988, Dacorogna 2000). However, a convex strain energy function is not generally able to describe instabilities such as buckling (Ball 1977). Thus, to avoid the use of convex functions, the property of *polyconvexity* was introduced (Ball 1976). Its fulfilment guarantees physically admissible solutions (Dacorogna 2000). Both the neo-Hookean law (3.11) and the exponential law (3.12) satisfy the polyconvexity property (Balzani *et al.* 2006).

### 3.2.1 Modelling the structure as a 2D membrane

In some circumstances, because of the thinness of the vessel wall, a non-linear shell model has been proposed: see *e.g.* Leuprecht *et al.* (2002) and Zhao *et al.* (2000). In this case, the structure problem is described by two-dimensional equations defined with respect to the middle surface, consisting of the computation of the deformation of this surface.

A simpler equation may be obtained if the structure is modelled as a 2D *membrane* whose position in space at any time exactly coincides with internal boundary $\Sigma^t$, yielding the so-called *generalized string model*

$$\rho_s H_s \frac{\partial^2 \widehat{d}_r}{\partial t^2} - \nabla \cdot (\boldsymbol{P} \nabla \widehat{d}_r) + \chi H_s \widehat{d}_r = \widehat{f}_s \quad \text{in } \Sigma \tag{3.17}$$

(Quarteroni *et al.* 2000*c*). Here $\Sigma$ denotes the reference membrane configuration, $d_r$ is the radial displacement and $H_s$ is the structure thickness. The tensor $\boldsymbol{P}$ accounts for *shear deformations* and, possibly, for *pre-stress*,

$$\chi = \frac{E}{1-\nu^2}(4\rho_1^2 - 2(1-\nu)\rho_2),$$

where $\rho_1(\boldsymbol{x})$ and $\rho_2(\boldsymbol{x})$ are the *mean* and *Gaussian curvatures* of $\Sigma$, respectively (Nobile and Vergara 2008), and $f_s$ is the forcing term, given by a measurement of the fluid pressure. Equation (3.17) is derived from *Hooke's law* for linear elasticity under the assumptions of small thickness, *plane stresses*, and negligible *elastic bending terms* (Zienkiewicz and Taylor 2005). To account for the effect of the surrounding tissue, the term $\chi$ in (3.17) needs to be augmented by the elastic coefficient of the tissue $\alpha_{ST}$ (Formaggia, Quarteroni and Vergara 2013).

Denoting by $\Sigma$ the lateral surface of a cylinder, then a further simplification occurs if we discard any dependence on the circumferential coordinate, in which case model (3.17) reduces to

$$\rho_s H_s \frac{\partial^2 \widehat{d}_r}{\partial t^2} - kGH_s \frac{\partial^2 \widehat{d}_r}{\partial z^2} + \frac{EH_s}{(1-\nu^2)R_0^2} H_s \widehat{d}_r = \widehat{f}_s \quad \text{in } \Sigma, \tag{3.18}$$

where $k$ is the *Timoshenko correction factor*, $G$ is the *shear modulus*, $R_0$ is the initial cylinder radius and $z$ is the axial coordinate. Often, in the latter case, a *viscoelastic term* of the form $\gamma_v(\partial^3 d_r/\partial^2 z \partial t)$ is also added, with $\gamma_v$ denoting a suitable viscoelastic parameter (Quarteroni *et al.* 2000*c*).

## 3.3 The coupled fluid–structure interaction problem

Blood flow in the vessel lumen and deformation of the vessel wall are intimately connected via a fluid–structure interaction (FSI). In particular, fluid and structure interact via the fluid–structure (FS) interface $\Sigma^t$ which coincides with the physical fluid boundary and the internal vessel wall boundary introduced in the previous sections. The coupled problem is obtained by combining (3.1) and (3.7) at each $t > 0$, as follows:

$$\rho_f\left(\frac{\partial \boldsymbol{v}}{\partial t} + (\boldsymbol{v}\cdot\nabla)\boldsymbol{v}\right) - \nabla\cdot \boldsymbol{T}_f(\boldsymbol{v}, p) = \boldsymbol{0} \quad \text{in } \Omega_f^t, \tag{3.19a}$$

$$\nabla\cdot\boldsymbol{v} = 0 \quad \text{in } \Omega_f^t, \tag{3.19b}$$

$$\boldsymbol{v} = \frac{\partial \boldsymbol{d}}{\partial t} \quad \text{at } \Sigma^t, \tag{3.19c}$$

$$\boldsymbol{T}_s(\boldsymbol{d})\,\boldsymbol{n} = \boldsymbol{T}_f(\boldsymbol{v},p)\,\boldsymbol{n} \qquad \text{at } \Sigma^t, \tag{3.19d}$$

$$\rho_s \frac{\partial^2 \widehat{\boldsymbol{d}}}{\partial t^2} - \nabla \cdot \widehat{\boldsymbol{T}}_s(\widehat{\boldsymbol{d}}) = \boldsymbol{0} \qquad \text{in } \Omega_s, \tag{3.19e}$$

$$\boldsymbol{d}_f = \boldsymbol{d} \qquad \text{at } \Sigma^t, \tag{3.19f}$$

together with the boundary conditions (2.1), (3.4), (3.5), (3.14), and where $\boldsymbol{d}_f$ is the displacement of the fluid domain $\Omega_f^t$ at the FS interface and we have used the convention that $\boldsymbol{n}$ is the structure outward unit normal. The matching conditions (3.19c, 3.19d) enforced at the FS interface express the *continuity of velocities* (kinematic condition) and the *continuity of normal stresses* (dynamic condition), respectively, whereas condition (3.19f) guarantees the geometry adherence between the fluid and structure domains (geometric condition). The well-posedness analysis of the coupled problem (3.19) (supplemented by the relevant boundary conditions) has been carried out under several regularity assumptions. For a comprehensive description of this topic we refer to Beirão da Veiga (2004), Grandmont (1998), Bodnár, Galdi and Nečasová (2014) and Maday (2009), for example.

For each time $t > 0$, the weak formulation of the FSI problem (3.19) together with its boundary conditions (for simplicity we set $\boldsymbol{v}_{\text{up}} = \boldsymbol{0}$ in (3.4)) reads as follows: find

$$(\boldsymbol{v}(t), \widehat{\boldsymbol{d}}(t)) \in \boldsymbol{W}^t = \{(\boldsymbol{w}, \widehat{\boldsymbol{e}}) \in [H^1(\Omega_f^t)]^3 \times [H^1(\Omega_s)]^3 : \\ (\boldsymbol{w}, \widehat{\boldsymbol{e}}) = (\boldsymbol{0}, \boldsymbol{0}) \text{ on } \Gamma_{\text{in}}^t \times \Gamma_{\text{artif}} \text{ and } \boldsymbol{w} = \dot{\boldsymbol{e}} \text{ on } \Sigma^t\},$$

$\boldsymbol{v} = \boldsymbol{v}_0$ for $t = 0$ in $\Omega_f$, $\widehat{\boldsymbol{d}} = \boldsymbol{d}_0$ and $\partial\widehat{\boldsymbol{d}}/\partial t = \boldsymbol{d}_1$ for $t = 0$ in $\Omega_s$, and $p(t) \in L^2(\Omega_f^t)$, such that

$$\begin{aligned}
\rho_f \int_{\Omega_f^t} \frac{\partial \boldsymbol{v}}{\partial t} \cdot \boldsymbol{w} \,\mathrm{d}\omega + \mathcal{A}_f^t(\boldsymbol{v}, \boldsymbol{v}, \boldsymbol{w}) + \mathcal{B}^t(p, \boldsymbol{w}) + \rho_s \int_{\Omega_s} \frac{\partial^2 \widehat{\boldsymbol{d}}}{\partial t^2} \cdot \widehat{\boldsymbol{e}} \,\mathrm{d}\omega \\
+ \int_{\Omega_s} \widehat{\boldsymbol{T}}_s(\widehat{\boldsymbol{d}}) : \nabla \widehat{\boldsymbol{e}} \,\mathrm{d}\omega + \int_{\Gamma_{\text{ext}}} \alpha_{ST} \widehat{\boldsymbol{d}} \cdot \widehat{\boldsymbol{e}} \,\mathrm{d}\sigma \\
= \int_{\Gamma_{\text{out}}^t} \boldsymbol{h}_f \cdot \boldsymbol{n} \,\mathrm{d}\gamma + \int_{\Gamma_{\text{ext}}} P_{\text{ext}} \widehat{\boldsymbol{n}} \cdot \widehat{\boldsymbol{e}} \,\mathrm{d}\sigma, \\
\mathcal{B}^t(q, \boldsymbol{v}) = 0, \\
\boldsymbol{d}_f = \boldsymbol{d} \quad \text{at } \Sigma^t,
\end{aligned} \tag{3.20}$$

for all $(\boldsymbol{w}, \widehat{\boldsymbol{e}}) \in \boldsymbol{W}^t$ and $q \in L^2(\Omega_f^t)$. Note that in the above weak formulation, the two terms arising after integration by parts and involving the normal Cauchy stresses $\boldsymbol{T}_f\boldsymbol{n}$ and $\boldsymbol{T}_s\boldsymbol{n}$ at the interface $\Sigma^t$ cancel out, thanks to (3.19d) and to the special choice of the test functions in $\boldsymbol{W}^t$.

After introducing the total energy for the FSI problem, that is,

$$\mathcal{E}_{3D}(t) = \frac{\rho_f}{2}\int_{\Omega_f^t} |\boldsymbol{v}|^2 \,\mathrm{d}\omega + \int_{\Omega_s} \frac{\rho_s}{2}|\dot{\widehat{\boldsymbol{d}}}|^2 \,\mathrm{d}\omega + \int_{\Omega_s} \Theta(\widehat{\boldsymbol{d}}) \,\mathrm{d}\omega + \int_{\Gamma_{\text{ext}}} \alpha_{ST}|\widehat{\boldsymbol{d}}|^2 \,\mathrm{d}\gamma, \tag{3.21}$$

the following conservation property holds true for the case of homogeneous boundary conditions:

$$\frac{\mathrm{d}}{\mathrm{d}t}\mathcal{E}_{3D}(t) + \frac{\mu}{2}\int_{\Omega_f^t} (\nabla \boldsymbol{v} + (\nabla \boldsymbol{v})^t)^2 \,\mathrm{d}\omega = 0$$

(Formaggia, Gerbeau, Nobile and Quarteroni 2001, Formaggia *et al.* 2013).

When the membrane model (3.17) is used instead of (3.19e), the matching conditions (3.19c, 3.19d) are replaced by

$$\begin{aligned} \boldsymbol{v}\cdot\boldsymbol{n} &= \frac{\partial d_r}{\partial t} && \text{at } \Sigma^t, \\ \boldsymbol{T}_f(\boldsymbol{v},p)\boldsymbol{n}\cdot\boldsymbol{n} &= -f_s && \text{at } \Sigma^t, \end{aligned}$$

where $d_r$ is the membrane displacement written in the current configuration and $f_s$ is the forcing term of the membrane equation (see (3.17)), acting only at the FS interface; in this case it also plays the role of structure stress exerted at the FS interface. Owing to (3.17) itself, we can rewrite the above interface conditions as follows:

$$\boldsymbol{v}\cdot\boldsymbol{n} = \frac{\partial d_r}{\partial t} \qquad \text{at } \Sigma^t, \tag{3.23a}$$

$$\boldsymbol{T}_f(\boldsymbol{v},p)\boldsymbol{n}\cdot\boldsymbol{n} = -\left(\rho_s H_s \frac{\partial^2 d_r}{\partial t^2} - \nabla\cdot(\boldsymbol{P}\nabla d_r) + \chi H_s d_r\right) \qquad \text{at } \Sigma^t. \tag{3.23b}$$

Since the coupling only occurs in the radial direction, we have to complete the conditions at $\Sigma^t$ for the fluid problem in the tangential directions by prescribing further equations on the fluid variables, for example homogeneous Dirichlet or Neumann conditions (Nobile 2001).

Figueroa *et al.* (2006) propose an effective formulation to solve the FSI problem with a membrane structure, while Colciago, Deparis and Quarteroni (2014) discuss the accuracy of the FSI-membrane problem in comparison to a full 3D/3D simulation. In particular, for Hooke's law, the wall shear stresses computed with these two FSI models are in good quantitative agreement for a distal arterial tract such as a femoropopliteal bypass. In contrast, when larger displacements are considered such as in the ascending aorta, the discrepancies between the two FSI models increase.

## 3.4 The boundary issue

According to the mathematical theory of the incompressible Navier–Stokes equations, three scalar conditions need to be prescribed at each point of the boundary. This, however, is seldom realistic in clinical practice. For instance, PC-MRA provides velocity data, but this technique is not routinely used and *ad hoc* studies are required (Morbiducci *et al.* 2009). Alternatively, the flow rate $Q = Q(t)$ can be obtained across a boundary cross-section $\Gamma^t$, by suitable postprocessing of data retrieved by echo-colour-Doppler or by thermal images: see Section 2.2. This yields the flow rate condition (2.2). In other situations, at both the inlet and outlet cross-sections, pressure measurements $P = P(t)$ may be considered as representative of an average estimate, leading to condition (2.3).

From a mathematical perspective, (2.2) and (2.3) are *defective* conditions as they prescribe only one scalar function over the entire section $\Gamma^t$ (Formaggia, Gerbeau, Nobile and Quarteroni 2002). Several strategies have been proposed so far to supplement (2.2) or (2.3) with other conditions that allow us to 'close' the system. For clarity, we can classify them according to three different strategies, which are reported below.

### *3.4.1 Conjecturing velocity and pressure profiles*

A common trick to effectively prescribe the flow rate condition (2.2) consists in prescribing a velocity profile

$$\boldsymbol{v}(t) = \boldsymbol{g}(t) \quad \text{on } \Gamma^t, \tag{3.24}$$

where $\boldsymbol{g} = \boldsymbol{g}(t, \boldsymbol{x})$ is chosen in such a way as to satisfy (2.2); that is,

$$\rho_f \int_{\Gamma^t} \boldsymbol{g}(t) \cdot \boldsymbol{n} \, \mathrm{d}\gamma = Q(t). \tag{3.25}$$

The flow rate condition (2.2) is therefore replaced with the standard (vectorial) Dirichlet condition (3.24). A classical choice for $\boldsymbol{g}$ is a parabolic profile (*e.g.* for flow simulations in the carotid arteries: Campbell *et al.* 2012), a constant profile (often used for the ascending aorta: Moireau *et al.* 2012), or that obtained from the Womersley solution (He, Ku and Moore 1993). Both the parabolic and Womersley profiles require a circular section to be prescribed, while non-circular sections require an appropriate morphing (He *et al.* 1993).

In spite of its straightforward implementation, this choice has a major impact on the solution, particularly in the neighbourhood of the section $\Gamma^t$ and for elevated values of the Reynolds number (Veneziani and Vergara

2007). To reduce the sensitivity to the arbitrary choice of the profile, the computational domain can be artificially elongated by operating what is called a *flow extension* (Moore, Steinman and Ethier 1997).

A similar approach could be applied to the mean normal Cauchy stress condition (2.3) as well. In the case at hand, we can postulate that the pressure on $\Gamma^t$ is constant and that the viscous stress can be neglected; that is, we can prescribe

$$p\boldsymbol{n} - \mu(\nabla\boldsymbol{v} + (\nabla\boldsymbol{v})^{\mathrm{T}})\,\boldsymbol{n} = P\boldsymbol{n} \quad \text{on } \Gamma^t. \tag{3.26}$$

Note that the above condition in particular satisfies the defective condition (2.3). Condition (3.26) is generally acceptable because the pressure changes in arteries mainly occur along the axial direction and the viscous stresses are negligible on orthogonal cross-sections.

Since $P\boldsymbol{n}$ plays the role of boundary normal Cauchy stress in the weak formulation of the fluid problem (3.6), no further action is required beyond assembling the vector for Neumann conditions. For this reason, the treatment has been called the '*do-nothing*' approach (Heywood *et al.* 1996). As pointed out by Veneziani (1998*a*, 1998*b*), this procedure is in fact not completely 'innocent'. The do-nothing approach corresponds to the following weak formulation (for simplicity we assume homogeneous Dirichlet conditions, $\boldsymbol{v}_{\mathrm{up}} = \boldsymbol{0}$): for each $t > 0$, find $\boldsymbol{v} \in \widetilde{\boldsymbol{V}}^t$, $\boldsymbol{v} = \boldsymbol{v}_0$ for $t = 0$ in $\Omega_f$, and $p \in L^2(\Omega_f^t)$ such that

$$\begin{aligned}
&\rho_f \int_{\Omega_f^t} \frac{\partial \boldsymbol{v}}{\partial t} \cdot \boldsymbol{w}\,\mathrm{d}\omega + \mathcal{A}_f^t(\boldsymbol{v},\boldsymbol{v},\boldsymbol{w}) + \mathcal{B}^t(p,\boldsymbol{w}) \\
&\qquad = \int_{\Gamma_{\mathrm{out}}^t} \boldsymbol{h}_f \cdot \boldsymbol{n}\,\mathrm{d}\gamma - P\int_{\Gamma^t} \boldsymbol{w}\cdot\boldsymbol{n}\,\mathrm{d}\gamma, \\
&\mathcal{B}^t(q,\boldsymbol{v}) = 0,
\end{aligned}$$

for all

$$\boldsymbol{w} \in \widetilde{\boldsymbol{V}}^t = \{[H^1(\Omega_f^t)]^3 : \boldsymbol{w} = \boldsymbol{0} \quad \text{on } \partial\Omega \setminus (\Gamma_{\mathrm{out}}^t \cup \Gamma^t)\}$$

and $q \in L^2(\Omega_f^t)$.

A do-nothing formulation for the flow rate conditions is possible too: see Heywood *et al.* (1996) and Veneziani (1998*b*).

Note that as an alternative to (2.3), other defective conditions involving the fluid pressure could be considered as well. This is the case for *mean pressure conditions* (Heywood *et al.* 1996), or conditions involving the total pressure (Formaggia *et al.* 2013), defined by $p_{\mathrm{tot}} = p + (\rho_f/2)|\boldsymbol{v}|^2$. For a comprehensive review of these conditions, we refer the interested reader to Quarteroni *et al.* (2016*c*).

### 3.4.2 Augmented formulation

An alternative approach is to regard the flow rate boundary condition (2.2) as a constraint for the solution of the fluid problem and then enforce it via a Lagrange multiplier approach. Since this is a scalar constraint, we need a scalar multiplier $\lambda = \lambda(t)$ at each time, resulting in the following weak formulation (we again consider the case of homogeneous Dirichlet conditions): for each $t > 0$, find $\boldsymbol{v} \in \widetilde{\boldsymbol{V}}^t$, $\boldsymbol{v} = \boldsymbol{v}_0$ for $t = 0$ in $\Omega_f$, $p \in L^2(\Omega_f^t)$, and $\lambda \in \mathbb{R}$ such that

$$\begin{aligned}
&\rho_f \int_{\Omega_f^t} \frac{\partial \boldsymbol{v}}{\partial t} \cdot \boldsymbol{w}\,\mathrm{d}\omega + \mathcal{A}_f^t(\boldsymbol{v}, \boldsymbol{v}, \boldsymbol{w}) + \mathcal{B}^t(p, \boldsymbol{w}) + \mathcal{C}^t(\lambda, \boldsymbol{w}) = \int_{\Gamma_{\text{out}}^t} \boldsymbol{h}_f \cdot \boldsymbol{w}\,\mathrm{d}\gamma,\\
&\mathcal{B}^t(q, \boldsymbol{v}) = 0,\\
&\mathcal{C}^t(\psi, \boldsymbol{v}) = \psi \frac{Q}{\rho_f},
\end{aligned} \tag{3.27}$$

for all $\boldsymbol{w} \in \widetilde{\boldsymbol{V}}^t$, $q \in L^2(\Omega_f^t)$, and $\psi \in \mathbb{R}$, and where we have set

$$\mathcal{C}^t(\psi, \boldsymbol{w}) = \psi \int_{\Gamma^t} \boldsymbol{w} \cdot \boldsymbol{n}\,\mathrm{d}\gamma.$$

See Formaggia *et al.* (2002) and Veneziani and Vergara (2005), who also analyze the well-posedness of this problem.

Besides prescribing the flow rate condition (2.2), the above augmented formulation enforces at each time a constant-in-space normal Cauchy stress on $\Gamma^t$ aligned with its normal direction, which precisely coincides with the Lagrange multiplier $\lambda$; that is,

$$-p\boldsymbol{n} + \mu(\nabla \boldsymbol{u} + (\nabla \boldsymbol{v})^{\mathrm{T}})\,\boldsymbol{n} = \lambda \boldsymbol{n} \quad \text{on } \Gamma^t.$$

This method is particularly suitable when the artificial cross-section is orthogonal to the longitudinal axis, so that vector $\boldsymbol{n}$ is truly aligned along the axial direction.

Since the velocity spatial profile is not prescribed *a priori*, this technique has been used to improve the parabolic-based law implemented in the Doppler technology for the estimation of the flow rate starting from the peak velocity (Ponzini, Vergara, Redaelli and Veneziani 2006, Vergara *et al.* 2010, Ponzini *et al.* 2010).

Extension of the augmented formulation to the case of compliant walls is addressed in Formaggia, Veneziani and Vergara (2009*b*) and to the quasi-Newtonian case in Ervin and Lee (2007).

An augmented formulation has been proposed by Formaggia *et al.* (2002) to prescribe condition (2.3) as well. However, as noticed by Formaggia *et al.* (2002), in this case it yields at each time the condition

$$\boldsymbol{v} = \lambda \boldsymbol{n} \quad \text{at } \Gamma^t,$$

where $\lambda = \lambda(t)$ is again the constant-in-space Lagrange multiplier. This is a non-homogeneous Dirichlet boundary condition for the fluid velocity, which is generally incompatible with the no-slip condition $\boldsymbol{v} = \boldsymbol{\phi}$ prescribed at the physical boundary $\Sigma^t$. For this reason, the approach is no longer popular.

### *3.4.3 A control-based approach*

A different strategy for the fulfilment of condition (2.2) is based on the minimization of the mismatch functional

$$J(\boldsymbol{v}) = \frac{1}{2}\left(\int_{\Gamma^t} \boldsymbol{v} \cdot \boldsymbol{n} \, \mathrm{d}\gamma - Q\right)^2, \tag{3.28}$$

constrained by the fact that $\boldsymbol{v}$ satisfies the incompressible Navier–Stokes equations (Formaggia, Veneziani and Vergara 2008). This PDE-constrained optimization – which can be regarded as the dual of the above augmented strategy – yields a system of optimality conditions to be fulfilled (also referred to as the Karush–Kuhn–Tucker (KKT) system): see Section 8.1.2 for further details. In particular, Formaggia *et al.* (2008) used the normal component of the normal Cauchy stress on $\Gamma^t$ as the control variable for the minimization of the mismatch functional. This approach was considered by Formaggia *et al.* (2009*b*) for the compliant case, whereas Lee (2011), Galvin and Lee (2013) and Galvin, Lee and Rebholz (2012) address the non-Newtonian, quasi-Newtonian and viscoelastic cases.

The same approach can also be used to fulfil the defective condition (2.3) provided that a suitable functional to be minimized is introduced (Formaggia *et al.* 2008). This allows us to prescribe (2.3) on a section oblique with respect to the longitudinal axis too. In this case the control variable is the full normal Cauchy stress vector; that is, the direction of the normal Cauchy stress is also *a priori* unknown.

Boundary data may also be lacking for the cross-section of the vessel wall. In this case we end up with defective boundary conditions for the vessel wall and related issues: see *e.g.* Quarteroni *et al.* (2016*c*).

## 3.5 Geometric reduced models and the geometric multiscale approach

### 3.5.1 The 1D and 0D models

Numerical modelling of the entire cardiovascular system by means of 3D models is currently not affordable because of the complexity of the computational domain, which is composed of thousands of arteries and veins and billions of arterioles, capillaries and venules (Nichols and O'Rourke 2005). In many applications, reduced-dimensional models are used instead, either as stand-alone models or coupled with the 3D ones.

The first one-dimensional (1D) model was introduced almost 250 years ago by Euler (1775). Subsequently this approach was brought into the engineering environment by Barnard, Hunt, Timlake and Varley (1966), Hughes (1974) and Hughes and Lubliner (1973). These models allow the description of blood flow in a compliant vessel where the unique space coordinate is the centreline of the vessel.

One-dimensional models may be derived from 3D models by making simplifying assumptions on the behaviour of the flow, the structure, and their interaction (Quarteroni and Formaggia 2004, Peiró and Veneziani 2009). The starting fluid domain is a truncated cone: see Figure 3.2. Referring to cylindrical coordinates $(r, \varphi, z)$, we make the following simplifying assumptions:

(i) the axis of the cylinder is fixed;

(ii) for any $z$, the cross-section $\mathcal{S}(t, z)$ is a circle with radius $R(t, z)$;

(iii) the solution of both fluid and structure problems does not depend on $\varphi$;

(iv) the pressure is constant over each section $\mathcal{S}(t, z)$;

(v) the axial fluid velocity $v_z$ dominates the other velocity components;

(vi) only radial displacements are allowed, so the structure deformation takes the form $\boldsymbol{d} = d\boldsymbol{e}_r$, where $\boldsymbol{e}_r$ is the unit vector in the radial direction, and $d(t, z) = R(t, z) - R_0(z)$, where $R_0(z)$ is the reference radius at the equilibrium;

(vii) the fluid is assumed to obey Poiseuille's law, so that the viscous effects are modelled by a linear term proportional to the flow rate;

(viii) the vessel structure is modelled as a membrane with constant thickness.

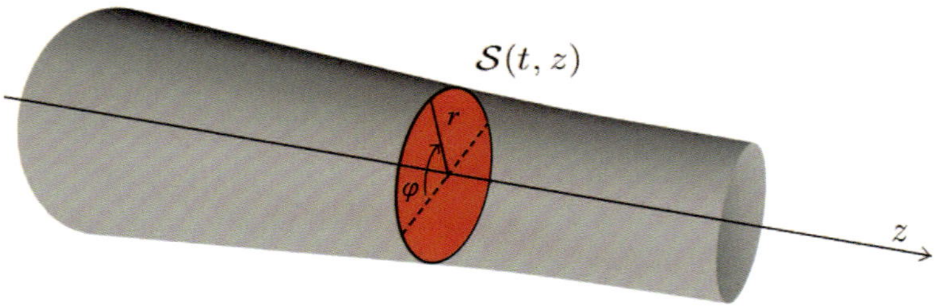


Figure 3.2 Fluid domain for the derivation of the 1D model.

We introduce the following quantities:

$$
\begin{aligned}
&A(t,z) = |\mathcal{S}(t,z)| = \pi R(t,z)^2 && \text{lumen section area,}\\
&\bar{v}(t,z) = A^{-1}\int_{\mathcal{S}(t,z)} v_z(t,z)\,\mathrm{d}S && \text{mean velocity,}\\
&s(r/R) \quad \text{such that } v_z(t,r,z) = \bar{v}(t,z)s(r/R(t,z)) && \text{velocity profile,}\\
&Q(t,z) = \rho_f\int_{\mathcal{S}(t,z)} v_z\,\mathrm{d}S = \rho_f A(t,z)\bar{v}(t,z) && \text{flow rate,}\\
&P(t,z) = A^{-1}\int_{\mathcal{S}(t,z)} p(t,z)\,\mathrm{d}S && \text{mean pressure.}
\end{aligned}
$$

As for the structure and its interaction with the fluid, we need to introduce a membrane law, which in fact prescribes a relation between the pressure and the lumen area (which is determined by $d_r$) of the form

$$P(t,z) = P_{\mathrm{ext}} + \psi(A(t,z), A_0(z), \boldsymbol{\beta}(z)), \tag{3.29}$$

where $\psi$ is a given function satisfying $\partial\psi/\partial A > 0$, $\psi(A_0) = 0$. Here $\boldsymbol{\beta}$ is a vector of parameters describing the mechanical properties of the membrane.

By integrating over the sections $\mathcal{S}$ the momentum fluid equation (3.19a) in the $z$-direction and the mass conservation law (3.19b), we obtain the system

$$\frac{\partial \boldsymbol{U}}{\partial t} + \mathrm{H}(\boldsymbol{U})\frac{\partial \boldsymbol{U}}{\partial z} + \boldsymbol{B}(\boldsymbol{U}) = \mathbf{0} \quad z \in (0,L),\ t > 0, \tag{3.30}$$

where $\boldsymbol{U} = (A\ Q)^{\mathrm{T}}$ is the vector of the unknowns,

$$\alpha = \frac{\int_S u_z^2}{A\bar{v}^2} = \frac{1}{A}\int_0^1 s^2(y)\,\mathrm{d}y$$

is the *Coriolis coefficient*, $K_r = -2\pi\mu s'(1)$ is the *friction parameter*,

$$c_1 = \sqrt{\frac{A}{\rho_f}\frac{\partial\psi}{\partial A}},$$

while

$$\mathrm{H}(\boldsymbol{U}) = \begin{bmatrix} 0 & 1 \\ c_1^2 - \alpha\left(\dfrac{Q}{A}\right)^2 & 2\alpha\dfrac{Q}{A} \end{bmatrix}, \tag{3.31a}$$

$$\boldsymbol{B}(\boldsymbol{U}) = \begin{bmatrix} 0 \\ K_r\frac{Q}{A} + \dfrac{A}{\rho_f}\dfrac{\partial\psi}{\partial A_0}\dfrac{\partial A_0}{\partial z} + \dfrac{A}{\rho_f}\dfrac{\partial\psi}{\partial\boldsymbol{\beta}}\dfrac{\partial\boldsymbol{\beta}}{\partial z} \end{bmatrix} \tag{3.31b}$$

represent the flux matrix and the dissipation vector term, respectively. A complete derivation of the model can be found in Pedley (1980), Hughes (1974) and Peiró and Veneziani (2009), for example. Classical choices of the velocity profile $s$ are flat ($\alpha = 1$) and parabolic ($\alpha = 4/3$).

The term $\partial A_0/\partial z$ in $\boldsymbol{B}$ is typically non-positive, accounting for vessel 'tapering', that is, reduction of the area of the lumen when proceeding from proximal to distal arteries. The term $\partial\boldsymbol{\beta}/\partial z$ originates from possibly different mechanical properties along the vessel, to describe, for example, the presence of atherosclerotic plaques or vascular prostheses.

If $A > 0$, system (3.30) has two real distinct eigenvalues,

$$\lambda_{1,2} = \alpha\bar{v} \pm \sqrt{c_1^2 + \bar{v}^2\alpha(\alpha-1)} \tag{3.32}$$

(see *e.g.* Quarteroni and Formaggia 2004), so it is *strictly hyperbolic* (see *e.g.* LeVeque 1992). Under physiological conditions, $c_1 \gg \alpha\bar{v}$, yielding $\lambda_1 > 0$ and $\lambda_2 < 0$, we thus have two waves travelling in opposite directions, associated with corresponding characteristic variables. An explicit expression of these variables as a function of the physical variables could, in general, be derived; that is,

$$W_i = \zeta_i(A, Q), \quad i = 1, 2. \tag{3.33}$$

A simple membrane law (3.29) can be obtained by the algebraic relation

$$\psi(A, A_0, \eta) = \eta\frac{\sqrt{A} - \sqrt{A_0}}{A_0}, \quad \text{with } \eta = \frac{\sqrt{\pi}H_s E}{1-\nu^2} \tag{3.34}$$

(Formaggia, Lamponi and Quarteroni 2003, Formaggia *et al.* 2013), where $\nu$ is the Poisson ratio of the membrane, $E$ is its Young's modulus, and $H_s$

is its thickness, yielding

$$c_1 = \sqrt{\frac{\eta\sqrt{A}}{2\rho_f A_0}}.$$

This simple law, stating that the membrane radial displacement $d_r$ is linearly proportional to the fluid pressure, has been considered successfully in many applications: see *e.g.* Steele *et al.* (2003), Matthys *et al.* (2007) and Grinberg *et al.* (2010). Other laws have been proposed to account for additional features of arterial walls, such as viscoelasticity, wall-inertia and longitudinal pre-stress (Quarteroni *et al.* 2000*c*, Formaggia *et al.* 2003).

**Remark 3.1** One-dimensional models do not allow us to describe secondary flows, such as vortices or recirculation regions. However, they provide average quantities about the axial component of the velocity, the radial vessel wall displacements and the pressure of a complex network at computational costs that are orders of magnitude lower than those of the corresponding three-dimensional FSI models (Kufahl and Clark 1985, Hillen, Hoogstraten and Post 1986, Blanco *et al.* 2015, Boileau *et al.* 2015, Malossi *et al.* 2013).

The accuracy of the solution provided by 1D models was addressed by Avolio (1980), Steele *et al.* (2003) and Reymond *et al.* (2009), who successfully compared the numerical results of different networks with clinical measurements, and by Matthys *et al.* (2007) and Muller and Toro (2013), who performed a comparison with *in vitro* measurements for a complete network of the cardiovascular system.

A further geometric reduction is represented by the so-called *lumped parameter models*, which are zero-dimensional (0D) models obtained by integrating the 1D problem over the axial direction. These are typically used to describe the peripheral part of the arterial and venous tree, such as the capillaries and the arterioles.

In this case only dependence on time is allowed, and nominal values of the unknowns are used as representative of the entire compartment. To this end, we introduce the *average* flow rate and pressure in the district at hand, defined by

$$\begin{aligned}
\widehat{Q}(t) &= \frac{1}{l}\int_{z_p}^{z_d} Q(t,z)\,\mathrm{d}z = \frac{\rho_f}{l}\int_{z_p}^{z_d}\int_{\mathcal{S}(t,z)} v_z(t,z)\,\mathrm{d}S\,\mathrm{d}z,\\
\widehat{P}(t) &= \frac{1}{l}\int_{z_p}^{z_d} P(t,z)\,\mathrm{d}z = \frac{1}{V}\int_{z_p}^{z_d}\int_{\mathcal{S}(t,z)} p(t,z)\,\mathrm{d}S\,\mathrm{d}z
\end{aligned}$$

respectively, where $z_p$ and $z_d$ are the proximal and longitudinal abscissas of the segment, respectively, $l$ is its length and $V$ its volume. The convective term is dropped since in the peripheral sites the velocity is small.

If we take the longitudinal average of the momentum equation given by the first of (3.30) and combine it with (3.34), we obtain the ordinary differential equation (ODE)

$$\frac{\rho_f l}{A_0}\frac{\mathrm{d}\widehat{Q}}{\mathrm{d}t} + \frac{\rho_f K_R l}{A_0^2}\widehat{Q} + \widehat{P}_d - \widehat{P}_p = 0, \tag{3.35}$$

where $\widehat{P}_d$ and $\widehat{P}_p$ are the distal and proximal pressure, respectively. When taking the longitudinal average of the mass conservation law given by the second of (3.30) and using (3.34), we obtain

$$\frac{\sqrt{A_0}l}{\eta}\frac{\mathrm{d}\widehat{P}}{\mathrm{d}t} + \widehat{Q}_d - \widehat{Q}_p = 0, \tag{3.36}$$

where $\widehat{Q}_d$ and $\widehat{Q}_p$ are the distal and proximal flow rate, respectively. See Peiró and Veneziani (2009).

The two ODEs (3.35, 3.36) can be regarded as the starting point for a 0D description of a compartment model of an arterial tract. In fact, the term $L(\mathrm{d}\widehat{Q}/\mathrm{d}t)$, with $L = \rho_f l/A_0$, corresponds to the blood acceleration, $R\widehat{Q}$, with $R = \rho_f K_R l/A_0^2$, stems from the blood resistance due to the viscosity, while $C(\mathrm{d}\widehat{P}/\mathrm{d}t)$, with $C = \sqrt{A_0}l/\eta$, is due to the compliance of the vessel wall. Usually an electrical analogy is used to easily interpret 0D models. In particular, the flow rate plays the role of the current whereas the pressure is the potential. Accordingly, the acceleration term is represented by an inductance, the viscosity term by a resistance, and the compliance term by a capacitance.

To close the system (3.35, 3.36) (featuring four unknowns) we also need to include the boundary conditions originally prescribed on the 1D model. For instance, we can assume a Dirichlet condition at the inlet and a Neumann condition at the outlet. Thus, we may localize the unknown pressure $\widehat{P}$ at the proximal section ($\widehat{P} \approx \widehat{P}_p$), assuming that the distal pressure $\widehat{P}_d$ is given. Similarly we assume that the flow rate $\widehat{Q}$ is approximated by $\widehat{Q}_d$ and that the proximal flow rate $\widehat{Q}_p$ is given. Then, from (3.35, 3.36), we obtain

$$\begin{aligned} \widehat{P} - L\frac{\mathrm{d}\widehat{Q}}{\mathrm{d}t} - R\widehat{Q} &= \widehat{P}_d, \\ C\frac{\mathrm{d}\widehat{P}}{\mathrm{d}t} + \widehat{Q} &= \widehat{Q}_p, \end{aligned} \tag{3.37}$$

corresponding to the electrical circuit drawn in Figure 3.3. Other sequences corresponding to different boundary conditions and then to different state

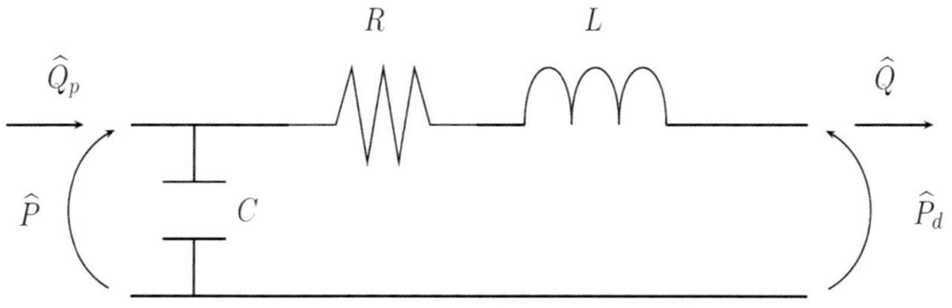


Figure 3.3 Example of lumped parameter scheme for an arterial tract.

variables are also possible (see *e.g.* Quarteroni *et al.* 2016*c*). Even though these schemes are equivalent in terms of functionality, they play a different role when coupled with higher-dimensional models (see *e.g.* Quarteroni *et al.* 2016*c*).

For modelling more complex vascular districts, we may combine several 0D elementary tracts, by gluing them via classical continuity arguments. However, the lumped parameter models have mainly been used to provide suitable boundary conditions at the distal artificial sections of 3D and 1D models. In this case, one simple compartment is enough to describe the entire arterial system downstream of the region of interest. Examples are provided by the *windkessel model* (Westerhof, Lankhaar and Westerhof 2009), featuring an average resistance and capacitance, the 3-*element windkessel model* (Westerhof *et al.* 2009), where a second resistance is added before the windkessel compartment, and the 4-*elements windkessel model* (Stergiopulos, Westerhof, Meister and Westerhof 1996, Stergiopulos, Westerhof and Westerhof 1999), where an inductance element is added to the 3-elements windkessel model. A 0D model given simply by a resistance is used to provide absorbing boundary conditions at the outlets of the fluid domain in FSI simulations: see *e.g.* Nobile and Vergara (2008). Instead, more sophisticated approaches account for the propagative dynamics associated with the peripheral circulation, such as the *structured tree* model (Olufsen *et al.* 2000), which assumes an asymmetric self-similar structure for the peripheral network.

### *3.5.2 Geometric multiscale coupling*

The geometric multiscale approach, first introduced in Quarteroni and Veneziani (1997), consists in the coupling among the 3D, 1D and 0D models. The idea is to use higher-dimensional models in those regions where a very detailed description is required, and lower-dimensional models in the remain-

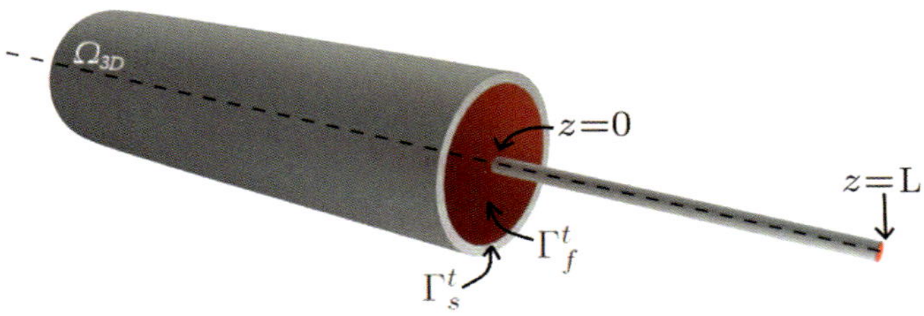


Figure 3.4 Schematic representation of the reference 3D/1D coupled model.

ing parts of the region of interest. This allows us to describe much of the circulatory system.

As discussed earlier, 0D models are typically used to provide boundary conditions for 3D and 1D models. For this reason, the coupling between 3D or 1D models with an extended 0D network has rarely been considered in applications. Instead, the 3D/1D coupling has received a great deal of attention. For this reason, we will detail only the latter case, while referring to Quarteroni, Ragni and Veneziani (2001), Quarteroni and Veneziani (2003), Vignon-Clementel, Figueroa, Jansen and Taylor (2006), Kim *et al.* (2009), Migliavacca *et al.* (2006) and Haggerty *et al.* (2013) for the 3D/0D coupling, and Formaggia, Nobile, Quarteroni and Veneziani (1999) and Fernández, Milisic and Quarteroni (2005) for the 1D/0D coupling.

As shown in Figure 3.4, we consider a 3D/FSI problem (3.19) in a 3D cylindrical domain together with initial conditions and boundary conditions at the proximal boundaries and at the external structure.

At the distal boundaries, the 3D problem is coupled with the 1D model (3.30) written in the domain $z \in [0, L]$, together with initial conditions and a boundary condition at the distal boundary. We let $\Gamma^t = \Gamma^t_f \cup \Gamma^t_s$ be the coupling interface from the 3D side, which corresponds to the point $z = 0$ from the 1D side (see Figure 3.4).

A major mathematical issue is how to couple 3D and 1D models at the common interface. Several strategies can be pursued, yielding many (alternative) sets of interface conditions. For a rigorous derivation of the 3D/1D problem and a detailed discussion of the interface conditions, we refer the interested reader to the recent review article by Quarteroni *et al.* (2016*c*).

Here we will follow the guiding principle described in Formaggia *et al.* (2013), where suitable interface conditions are derived from a global energy estimate. In particular, we introduce, together with the 3D energy (3.21), the 1D energy

$$\mathcal{E}_{1D}(t) = \frac{\rho_f}{2} \int_0^L A\,\bar{v}^2 \,\mathrm{d}x + \int_0^L \chi(A)\,\mathrm{d}x$$

(Formaggia *et al.* 2001), where $\chi(A) = \int_{A_0}^{A} \psi(\tau)\,\mathrm{d}\tau$ and $\psi$ is the vessel law (see (3.29)). Note that the stand-alone 1D problem satisfies bounds for this energy functional as proved in Formaggia *et al.* (2001).

Let

$$P_{\mathrm{tot}} = \psi(A) + (\rho_f/2)\bar{v}^2$$

be the total pressure for the 1D model, and let

$$p_{\mathrm{tot}} = p + (\rho_f/2)|\boldsymbol{v}|^2$$

be that of the 3D model. For the interface coupling conditions holding at $\Gamma^t$, let us assume that the following inequality holds:

$$\int_{\Gamma_f^t} \boldsymbol{T}_f(\boldsymbol{v}, p_{\mathrm{tot}})\boldsymbol{n} \cdot \boldsymbol{v}\,\mathrm{d}\gamma + \int_{\Gamma_s^t} \boldsymbol{T}_s(\boldsymbol{d})\boldsymbol{n} \cdot \dot{\boldsymbol{d}}\,\mathrm{d}\gamma + Q|_{z=0}\,P_{\mathrm{tot}}|_{z=0} \leq 0. \quad (3.38)$$

Then, for all $t > 0$, the coupled 3D/1D problem (3.19, 3.30) with homogeneous boundary conditions satisfies the energy decay property

$$\frac{\mathrm{d}}{\mathrm{d}t}(\mathcal{E}^{3D}(t) + \mathcal{E}^{1D}(t)) \leq 0.$$

For the proof see Formaggia *et al.* (2013).

The above result provides an indication of how to find suitable interface conditions for the 3D/1D coupled problem. In particular, for inequality (3.38) to be fulfilled it is sufficient that the interface conditions

$$\rho_f \int_{\Gamma_f^t} \boldsymbol{v} \cdot \boldsymbol{n}\,\mathrm{d}\gamma = Q|_{z=0}, \quad (3.39a)$$

$$(\boldsymbol{T}_f(\boldsymbol{v}, p_{\mathrm{tot}})\boldsymbol{n})|_{\Gamma_f^t} = -P_{\mathrm{tot}}|_{z=0}\boldsymbol{n} \quad (3.39b)$$

hold for the fluid, together with

$$\boldsymbol{T}_s(\boldsymbol{d})\boldsymbol{n} = \boldsymbol{0} \quad \text{on } \Gamma_s^t \quad (3.40)$$

for the structure (Formaggia, Moura and Nobile 2007, Formaggia *et al.* 2013). Similarly, inequality (3.38) holds if relation (3.40) is replaced by

$$\boldsymbol{d} \cdot \boldsymbol{n} = \boldsymbol{0} \quad \text{on } \Gamma_s^t, \quad (3.41a)$$

$$(\boldsymbol{T}_s(\boldsymbol{d})\boldsymbol{n}) \times \boldsymbol{n} = \boldsymbol{0} \quad \text{on } \Gamma_s^t. \quad (3.41b)$$

The interface conditions (3.39) prescribe the continuity of the flow rate (kinematic condition) and a dynamic condition involving the total pressures. Note that (3.40) and (3.41) are in fact independent of the 1D model, resulting in boundary conditions for the 3D structure problems only. This allows a discontinuity to manifest in the displacement between the 3D and 1D models.

Usually, dynamic interface conditions involving the pressure (instead of the total pressure) are considered in place of (3.39b), such as

$$\frac{1}{|\Gamma_f^t|}\int_{\Gamma_f^t} \boldsymbol{T}_f(\boldsymbol{v},p)\boldsymbol{n}\,\mathrm{d}\gamma = -\psi(A|_{z=0})\boldsymbol{n}. \tag{3.42}$$

However, the above condition does not satisfy the compatibility condition (3.38). More precisely, in this case we have

$$\frac{\mathrm{d}}{\mathrm{d}t}(\mathcal{E}^{3D}(t)+\mathcal{E}^{1D}(t)) = \frac{\rho_f}{2}\left(\frac{(Q(t)|_{z=0})^3}{(A(t)|_{z=0})^2} - \int_{\Gamma_f^t} |\boldsymbol{v}(t)|^2\boldsymbol{v}(t)\cdot\boldsymbol{n}\,\mathrm{d}\gamma\right).$$

Even though the right-hand side is not necessarily (always) negative, numerical evidence indicates that condition (3.42) leads to stable results for several haemodynamic applications: see Malossi *et al.* (2013). This interface condition is indeed the most commonly used among dynamic ones.

## 3.6 Numerical strategies

In this section we comment on the numerical solution of the problems presented in the previous subsections. Because of the complexity of the problem, we do not seek to be exhaustive. Instead, we review some of most suitable methods for computational haemodynamics. In particular, for space discretization, we will focus on Galerkin methods, such as finite elements, spectral elements and discontinuous Galerkin methods.

We will use the following notation. Let $\Delta t$ and $h$ be the time and space discretization parameters. In our examples $\Delta t$ is assumed to be fixed, but adaptive strategies could be considered as well: see *e.g.* Veneziani and Villa (2013). Correspondingly, the discrete times are $t^n = n\Delta t$. As usual, $h$ is instead defined as a representative value of the mesh size, for example $h = \min\{h_K : K \in \mathcal{K}\}$, where $\mathcal{K}$ is the set of all tetrahedra in the mesh and $h_K$ is the radius of the sphere inscribed in $K \in \mathcal{K}$. Given the functions $w(t)$ and $z(\boldsymbol{x})$, we let $w^n$ denote the approximation of $w(t^n)$ and let $z_h(\boldsymbol{x})$ be the Galerkin approximation of $z(\boldsymbol{x})$.

### 3.6.1 Numerical methods for the fluid problem

We start by reviewing some numerical methods for the fluid problem (3.1) together with its initial and boundary conditions.

As for the time discretization, we usually consider implicit methods with a semi-implicit treatment of the convective term and (for a moving domain) of the fluid domain. The problem is solved at discrete time $t^{n+1}$ in the domain $\Omega_f^*$ and with convective term $\rho_f(\boldsymbol{v}^* \cdot \nabla)\boldsymbol{v}^{n+1}$, where $\Omega_f^*$ and $\boldsymbol{v}^*$ are suitable extrapolations of $\Omega_f^{n+1}$ and $\boldsymbol{v}^{n+1}$ of the same order as the time discretization. This choice introduces a CFL-like (Courant–Friedrichs–Lewy) restriction on the time step to preserve absolute stability (Quarteroni and Valli 1994). However, this condition is not strict in haemodynamic applications, since, for accuracy purposes, the pulsatility of the blood signal and the quick dynamics around systole can only be accommodated by choosing a small $\Delta t$. Usually, a second-order approximation is considered a good choice in haemodynamics; in this respect, the second-order backward difference formula (BDF2) and Crank–Nicolson are the most widely used methods (Quarteroni, Sacco and Saleri 2000*a*).

The first class of methods we present is based on a decomposition of the semi-discrete problem at the spatial continuous level (*differential splitting* or *projection* methods). The basic idea underlying these methods is to split the computation of velocity and pressure, with a final step aiming to recover the incompressibility constraint. In what follows we detail the Chorin–Teman method (Chorin 1968, Temam 1969), originally proposed for homogeneous Dirichlet conditions and fixed domain, which is the progenitor of these methods. We only detail the case of the backward Euler discretization.

*Chorin–Temam method*

For $n \geq 0$, at time $t^{n+1}$:

(1) Solve in $\Omega_f$ the vectorial advection–reaction–diffusion problem with homogeneous Dirichlet condition for the intermediate unknown velocity $\widetilde{\boldsymbol{v}}^{n+1}$:

$$\rho_f \frac{\widetilde{\boldsymbol{v}}^{n+1} - \boldsymbol{v}^n}{\Delta t} - \mu(\nabla \widetilde{\boldsymbol{v}}^{n+1} + (\nabla \widetilde{\boldsymbol{v}}^{n+1})^{\mathrm{T}}) + \rho_f(\boldsymbol{v}^n \cdot \nabla)\widetilde{\boldsymbol{v}}^{n+1} = \mathbf{0}.$$

(2) Solve in $\Omega_f$ the pressure problem with homogeneous Neumann conditions:

$$\triangle p^{n+1} = \frac{\rho_f}{\Delta t} \nabla \cdot \widetilde{\boldsymbol{v}}^{n+1}.$$

(3) Correct the velocity:

$$\boldsymbol{v}^{n+1} = \widetilde{\boldsymbol{v}}^{n+1} - \frac{\Delta t}{\rho_f} \nabla p^{n+1}.$$

This splitting method is based on the *Ladyzhenskaya theorem* (see, *e.g.* Girault and Raviart (1986)), which states that a vector function belonging to $[L^2(\Omega_f)]^3$ can always be decomposed as the sum of a solenoidal part and a gradient term. In fact, the correction step (3) corresponds to projecting the intermediate velocity $\widetilde{\boldsymbol{v}}^{n+1}$ onto

$$\boldsymbol{H} = \{\boldsymbol{w} \in [L^2(\Omega_f)]^3 : \nabla \cdot \boldsymbol{w} = 0, \, \boldsymbol{w} \cdot \boldsymbol{n}|_{\partial\Omega_f} = 0\}.$$

Thus, it is possible to show that $\boldsymbol{v}^{n+1}$ and $p^{n+1}$ are in fact solutions of the original semi-discrete problem. The Chorin–Temam method is very effective since it overcomes the saddle-point nature of the problem and solves two standard uncoupled elliptic problems. However, it suffers from inaccuracies at the boundary. In particular, the tangential velocity cannot be controlled (see the definition of $\boldsymbol{H}$) and spurious pressure values appear as a consequence of the artificial Neumann condition for the pressure problem (Rannacher 1992). This has an effect on the accuracy of the semi-discrete solution. In particular, the following error estimate holds true (Rannacher 1992):

$$\|\boldsymbol{v}(t^n, \boldsymbol{x}) - \boldsymbol{v}^n(\boldsymbol{x})\|_{[H^1]^3} + \|p(t^n, \boldsymbol{x}) - p^n(\boldsymbol{x})\|_{L^2} \lesssim \sqrt{\Delta t}.$$

The use of higher-order time approximations leads to the same accuracy.

An improvement of the above method is given by the *rotational incremental* variant of the Chorin–Temam scheme (Timmermans, Minev and van de Vosse 1996). Below we detail the case of BDF2 and second-order extrapolation of the convective term, since the first-order approximation does not lead to any improvement with respect to the previous method.

*Rotational–incremental Chorin–Temam method*

For $n \geq 0$, at time $t^{n+1}$:

(1) Solve in $\Omega_f$ the advection-reaction-diffusion problem with homogeneous Dirichlet condition in the intermediate unknown velocity $\widetilde{\boldsymbol{v}}^{n+1}$:

$$\rho_f \frac{3\widetilde{\boldsymbol{v}}^{n+1} - 4\boldsymbol{v}^n + \boldsymbol{v}^{n-1}}{2\Delta t} - \mu(\nabla \widetilde{\boldsymbol{v}}^{n+1} + (\nabla \widetilde{\boldsymbol{v}}^{n+1})^{\mathrm{T}}) \\ + \rho_f((2\boldsymbol{v}^n - \boldsymbol{v}^{n-1}) \cdot \nabla)\widetilde{\boldsymbol{v}}^{n+1} + \nabla p^n = \boldsymbol{0}.$$

(2) Solve the pressure problem:

$$\begin{aligned}
\triangle p^{n+1} &= \triangle p^n + \left(\frac{3\rho_f}{2\Delta t} - \mu\right)\nabla\cdot\widetilde{\boldsymbol{v}}^{n+1}, && \boldsymbol{x}\in\Omega_f,\\
\frac{\partial p^{n+1}}{\partial \boldsymbol{n}} &= \mu(\nabla\times\nabla\times\widetilde{\boldsymbol{v}}^{n+1})\cdot\boldsymbol{n}, && \boldsymbol{x}\in\partial\Omega_f.
\end{aligned}$$

(3) Correct the velocity:

$$\boldsymbol{v}^{n+1} = \widetilde{\boldsymbol{v}}^{n+1} - \frac{2}{3}\frac{\Delta t}{\rho_f}\nabla(p^{n+1} - p^n + \mu\nabla\cdot\widetilde{\boldsymbol{v}}^{n+1}).$$

Unlike the classical Chorin–Temam scheme, in the above method the boundary conditions for the pressure problem are consistent, and numerical boundary layers for the pressure are not observed. This is confirmed by the improved error estimate

$$\|\boldsymbol{v}(t^n,\boldsymbol{x}) - \boldsymbol{v}^n(\boldsymbol{x})\|_{[H^1]^3} + \|p(t^n,\boldsymbol{x}) - p^n(\boldsymbol{x})\|_{L^2} \lesssim \Delta t^{3/2}$$

(Guermond and Shen 2006).

The above two methods belong to the general class of *pressure-correction* methods; see also Codina and Badia (2006), Guermond, Minev and Shen (2006) and Guermond and Quartapelle (1998), for example. A different class is obtained by switching the role of velocity and pressure in the splitting; that is, the viscous term is now ignored or treated explicitly in the first step and the velocity is then corrected accordingly (*velocity-correction* schemes: Orszag, Israeli and Deville 1986, Karniadakis, Israeli and Orszag 1991). These schemes are characterized by the same non-optimal error estimates as the pressure-correction schemes due to artificial Neumann conditions for the pressure problem. Again, an improvement could be obtained by considering a rotational-incremental variant (Guermond and Shen 2003).

In haemodynamics it is often the case that Neumann boundary conditions are prescribed at some artificial section. The extension of the differential splitting methods to this case is addressed in Guermond, Minev and Shen (2005): on the Neumann boundary we have an artificial Dirichlet condition for the pressure, which again diminishes the optimal rate of convergence with respect to $\Delta t$.

Given the next methods we are going to review, it is convenient to introduce the algebraic problem arising from the application of a Galerkin-like method to the semi-discrete-in-time problem. First of all we notice that the solvability of the discretized-in-space problem is guaranteed by a suitable compatible choice of the approximation spaces for the velocity and the pressure in order to satisfy the discrete *inf–sup stability condition* (Quarteroni and Valli 1994). As is well known, an example of finite elements for a tetrahedral mesh is provided by piecewise polynomials of order 2 for the velocity approximation and of order 1 for the pressure approximation. This choice guarantees the existence and uniqueness of the solution to the linearized fully discrete problem and is often used to provide a stable solution in haemodynamics. In this case, we have the optimal error estimate

$$\|\boldsymbol{v}^n(\boldsymbol{x}) - \boldsymbol{v}_h^n(\boldsymbol{x})\|_{[H^1]^3} + \|p^n(\boldsymbol{x}) - p_h^n(\boldsymbol{x})\|_{L^2} \lesssim h^2,$$

provided that $\boldsymbol{v}^n$ and $p^n$ are sufficiently regular. (For other stable choices see Quarteroni and Valli 1994 and Boffi, Brezzi and Fortin 2013.) Alternatively, suitable stabilization terms could be added to the problem, circumventing the inf–sup condition and allowing the use of polynomials of equal order. In this case, additional terms are added to the mass conservation equation and, if needed, to the momentum conservation equation. Usually, these techniques also stabilize convected-dominated problems arising when the Reynolds number is high, for example in the aorta or in stenotic carotid arteries. One stabilization technique is *streamline upwind/Petrov–Galerkin* (SUPG) method (Brooks and Hughes 1982, Muller *et al.* 2005). A generalization of SUPG and other residual-based stabilization methods is the *variational multiscale* (VMS) method (Hughes 1995, Hughes, Mazzei and Jansen 2000), which is based on a decomposition of the unknown into two terms, one accounting for the large scales and the other for the small scales of the unknown field. The same decomposition is used for the test functions, so that a system of two coupled problems is obtained. Suitable assumptions are made to express the fine scale solution in terms of the coarse scale residual of the PDE so that a closure rule is determined for the coarse scale problem. Thanks to this strategy, the VMS method only amounts to solving the coarse scale problem by taking into account the contribution of the fine scale solution without directly solving the corresponding problem, and therefore at no additional computational cost. Further generalizations of the VMS method have been proposed to account for turbulence modelling when solving the incompressible Navier–Stokes equations according to the *Large Eddy Simulation* (LES) framework in Bazilevs, Calo, Cottrell, Hughes, Reali and Scovazzi (2007) and later *e.g.* in Forti and Dede' (2015); the corresponding VMS method allows modelling the transition to turbulence effects, which may occur in some pathological conditions such as stenoses (Akkerman *et al.* 2008).

Here we introduce the algebraic problem related to the fully discretized linearized problem. For the sake of exposition, we limit ourselves to the cases without stabilization terms. For the more general case, we refer the interested reader to Elman, Silvester and Wathen (2005) and Benzi, Golub and Liesen (2005), for example. At each time step we have to solve a linear system in the saddle point form

$$\begin{bmatrix} A & B^{\mathrm{T}} \\ B & 0 \end{bmatrix} \begin{bmatrix} \boldsymbol{V} \\ \boldsymbol{P} \end{bmatrix} = \begin{bmatrix} \boldsymbol{F}_f \\ \boldsymbol{0} \end{bmatrix},$$

where $\boldsymbol{V}$ and $\boldsymbol{P}$ are the vectors collecting the velocity and pressure unknowns,

$$A = \rho_f(\alpha/\Delta t)M_f + \rho_f N(\boldsymbol{V}^*) + \mu K$$

($M_f$ is the mass matrix, $N$ is the matrix related to the linearized convective term, $K$ is the stiffness matrix), $\boldsymbol{F}_f$ accounts for non-homogeneous Dirichlet and Neumann conditions and the terms coming from time discretization, $\alpha$ depends on the time discretization scheme, and where we have omitted the current temporal index $^{n+1}$.

The above non-symmetric linear system can be solved by means of a Krylov method, for example the GMRES method (Saad 1996). Suitable preconditioners are required. A classical choice is given by block preconditioners – see *e.g.* (Quarteroni and Valli 1999) and (Toselli and Widlund 2005) – which again split the solution of the velocity and of the pressure:

$$P = \begin{bmatrix} P_A & B^{\mathrm{T}} \\ 0 & -P_\Sigma \end{bmatrix}.$$

If $P_A = A$ and $P_\Sigma = \Sigma = BA^{-1}B^{\mathrm{T}}$ (the *Schur complement*), then the solution is achieved in three GMRES iterations (Elman *et al.* 2005). In fact, this choice is equivalent to formally solving the momentum equation for the velocity and substituting its expression in the mass equation. However, in practice this preconditioner is not efficient, since the linear system involving the Schur complement is too onerous, $\Sigma$ being a full matrix whose explicit construction requires knowledge of $A^{-1}$. Efficient preconditioners can be obtained by approximating $\Sigma$ (and, if needed, $A$). For low Reynolds numbers (less than 10, say), an effective choice is given by $P_\Sigma = \mu^{-1}M_{\mathrm{P}}$, where $M_{\mathrm{P}}$ is the *pressure mass matrix*, (or even its diagonal: Elman and Silvester 1996). Therefore this is a good choice in haemodynamics for small vessels. For increasing Reynolds numbers, the convergence properties of this preconditioner deteriorates since it does not account for the convective term. A better choice for medium and large vessels is given by $P_\Sigma = A_{\mathrm{P}}F_{\mathrm{P}}^{-1}M_{\mathrm{P}}$, where $A_{\mathrm{P}}$ is the pressure stiffness matrix, and $F_{\mathrm{P}} = \mu A_{\mathrm{P}} + \rho_f N_{\mathrm{P}}(\boldsymbol{V}^*)$, where $N_{\mathrm{P}}$ is the matrix related to the convective term defined on the pressure space (*pressure convection–diffusion* preconditioner: Elman *et al.* 2005,

Benzi *et al.* 2005). For the solution of the velocity problem, suitable preconditioners for the advection–reaction–diffusion problem could be introduced. Alternatively, fast solutions such as V-cycle multigrid can be considered (Turek 1999).

Another class of preconditioners is obtained by an inexact block LU factorization of the fluid matrix. The starting point is the exact factorization

$$\begin{bmatrix} A & B^{\mathrm{T}} \\ B & 0 \end{bmatrix} = \begin{bmatrix} A & 0 \\ B & -\Sigma \end{bmatrix} \begin{bmatrix} I & A^{-1}B^{\mathrm{T}} \\ 0 & I \end{bmatrix}.$$

Again, different preconditioners are obtained by suitable approximations $\widehat{A}_1$ and $\widehat{A}_2$ of $A$ and $\widehat{\Sigma}$ of $\Sigma$, leading to

$$P = \begin{bmatrix} \widehat{A}_1 & 0 \\ B & -\widehat{\Sigma} \end{bmatrix} \begin{bmatrix} I & \widehat{A}_2^{-1}B^{\mathrm{T}} \\ 0 & I \end{bmatrix}.$$

A convenient choice is $\widehat{A}_1 = \widehat{A}_2 = D_A$ and $\widehat{\Sigma} = BD_A^{-1}B^{\mathrm{T}}$, where $D_A$ is the diagonal of $A$ (*SIMPLE* preconditioner: Patankar and Spalding 1972, Li and Vuik 2004). Note that in this case $\widehat{\Sigma}$ is sparse and could be explicitly assembled. This is an effective choice when the fluid matrix is diagonally dominant; that is, when small values of $\Delta t$ are used. Another choice is the *Yosida* preconditioner, where

$$\widehat{\Sigma} = \frac{\Delta t}{\rho_f \alpha} BM_f^{-1}B^{\mathrm{T}}, \quad \widehat{A}_1 = A \quad \text{and} \quad \widehat{A}_2 = \frac{\rho_f \alpha}{\Delta t} M_f$$

(Veneziani 2003). Again, the efficiency deteriorates for increasing $\Delta t$. The Yosida preconditioner was originally introduced as a solver in Veneziani (1998*b*); see also Quarteroni, Saleri and Veneziani (1999, 2000*b*). This led to a splitting of the velocity and of the pressure computation, which could be seen as the algebraic counterpart of the Chorin–Temam method (*algebraic pressure-correction* methods). In particular, we have the following steps:

$$\begin{aligned} & A\widetilde{\boldsymbol{V}} = \boldsymbol{F}_f && \text{computation of the velocity,} \\ & \Delta t BM_f^{-1}B^{\mathrm{T}}\boldsymbol{P} = B\widetilde{\boldsymbol{V}} && \text{computation of the pressure,} \\ & \boldsymbol{V} = \widetilde{\boldsymbol{V}} - \frac{\Delta t}{\rho_f \alpha} M_f^{-1}B^{\mathrm{T}}\boldsymbol{P} && \text{correction of the velocity.} \end{aligned}$$

Again, an incremental version of the algebraic pressure-correction methods can also be considered (Quarteroni, Saleri and Veneziani 2000*b*). An extension to spectral methods is provided in Gervasio, Saleri and Veneziani (2006).

For a comparison of the performance of different preconditioners (all described above) used for haemodynamic applications, see Deparis, Grandperrin and Quarteroni (2014).

In healthy conditions, blood flow is mainly laminar. Transitional flow may develop in some pathological instances, or with the assistance of devices. In these circumstances, suitable mesh refinement is often employed, possibly accompanied by the use of turbulence models. We mention the case of stenotic carotid arteries, for which Stroud, Berger and Saloner (2002) and Grinberg, Yakhot and Karniadakis (2009) use Reynolds-averaged Navier–Stokes (RANS) models, Lee *et al.* (2008), Fischer *et al.* (2007) and Cheung *et al.* (2010) use *direct numerical simulation* (DNS), and Rayz, Berger and Saloner (2007) and Lancellotti *et al.* (2017) use LES models. Bazilevs *et al.* (2009) use the VMS-LES formulation previously mentioned for describing describe transitional effects in the ascending aorta under the influence of the left ventricular assist device (LVAD).

In Figure 3.5 we show some examples of numerical results obtained in four real geometries reconstructed from radiological images (see the caption for details). These results highlight the complex pattern of blood flow induced by the geometry and by the heart pulsatility. To highlight the vortex structures in stenotic carotid arteries, Figure 3.5(c) plots the $Q$ criterion, defined by

$$Q = -\frac{1}{2}\sum_{i,j} S_{ij}^2 - \Omega_{ij}^2,$$

where $\boldsymbol{S} = \nabla \boldsymbol{u} + (\nabla \boldsymbol{u})^{\mathrm{T}}$ and $\boldsymbol{\Omega} = \nabla \boldsymbol{u} - (\nabla \boldsymbol{u})^{\mathrm{T}}$ (Lee *et al.* 2008). Positive values of $Q$ indicate locations where rotations dominate strain and shear; hence isosurfaces of positive values of $Q$ are used to identify vortex structures.

### *3.6.2 Numerical methods for the vessel wall problem*

In this section we review some of the most commonly used numerical approaches for the solution of problem (3.7), endowed with its initial and boundary conditions.

For the time discretization, a popular family of schemes is that of *Newmark*, which is characterized by two parameters $\theta$ and $\zeta$ (Newmark 1959). The special combination $\theta = 1/2$ and $\zeta = 1/4$ yields the following semi-

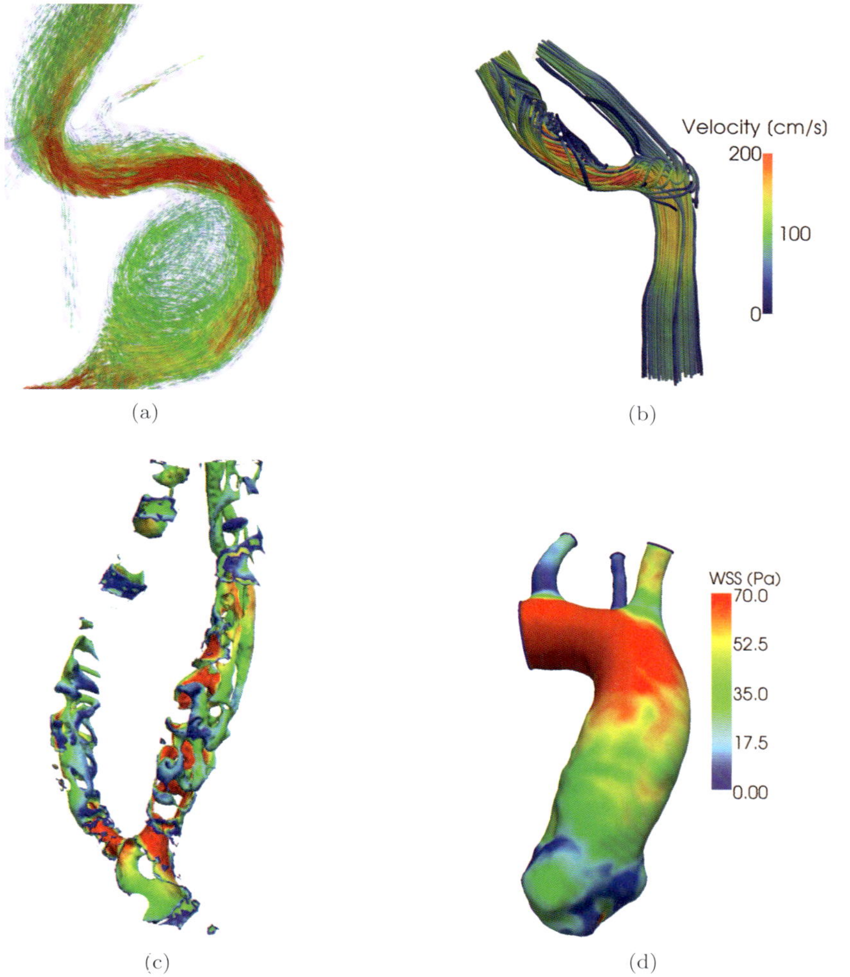


Figure 3.5 (a) Velocity vectors in the aneurysm of an abdominal aorta (data from CT images provided by the Vascular Surgery and Radiology Divisions at Fondazione IRCSS Cà Granda, Ospedale Maggiore Policlinico, Milan, Italy). (b) Velocity streamlines in a stenotic carotid artery (data from MRI images provided by the Vascular Surgery and Radiology Divisions at Ospedale Maggiore Policlinico, Milan). (c) Coherent vortical structures by $Q$ criterion in a stenotic carotid artery (we show only the regions with $Q > 50\,000$ shaded by the velocity magnitude; data from CT images provided by Vascular Surgery and Radiology Divisions at Ospedale Maggiore Policlinico, Milan). (d) Wall shear stress in an ascending aorta (data from MRI images provided by the Cardio Surgery and Radiology Divisions at Ospedale Borgo Trento, Verona, Italy). Numerical results were obtained using the finite element library LifeV, P2/P1 finite elements, the backward Euler scheme for the time discretization with a semi-implicit treatment of the non-linear term, and the Yosida preconditioner. For the stenotic carotid arteries an LES model has been used.

discrete form of (3.16) (for simplicity we set $P_{\mathrm{ext}} = 0$ and $\boldsymbol{h}_s = \boldsymbol{0}$):

$$\rho_s \int_{\Omega_s} \frac{4\widehat{\boldsymbol{d}}^{n+1} - 4\widehat{\boldsymbol{d}}^{n}}{\Delta t^2} \cdot \widehat{\boldsymbol{e}} \,\mathrm{d}\omega + \int_{\Omega_s} \widehat{\boldsymbol{T}}_s(\widehat{\boldsymbol{d}}^{n+1}) : \nabla \widehat{\boldsymbol{e}} \,\mathrm{d}\omega + \int_{\Gamma_{\mathrm{ext}}} \alpha_{ST} \widehat{\boldsymbol{d}}^{n+1} \cdot \widehat{\boldsymbol{e}} \,\mathrm{d}\sigma$$
$$= \rho_s \int_{\Omega_s} \left( \frac{4\widehat{\boldsymbol{w}}^n}{\Delta t} + \widehat{\boldsymbol{a}}^n \right) \cdot \widehat{\boldsymbol{e}} \,\mathrm{d}\omega, \tag{3.43}$$
$$\widehat{\boldsymbol{w}}^{n+1} = \frac{2}{\Delta t}(\widehat{\boldsymbol{d}}^{n+1} - \widehat{\boldsymbol{d}}^{n}) - \widehat{\boldsymbol{w}}^n, \quad \widehat{\boldsymbol{a}}^{n+1} = \frac{4}{\Delta t^2}(\widehat{\boldsymbol{d}}^{n+1} - \widehat{\boldsymbol{d}}^{n}) - \frac{4}{\Delta t}\widehat{\boldsymbol{w}}^n - \widehat{\boldsymbol{a}}^n,$$

where $\widehat{\boldsymbol{w}}^{n+1}$ and $\widehat{\boldsymbol{a}}^{n+1}$ denote approximations of vessel wall velocity and acceleration, respectively. This method is unconditionally absolutely stable and second-order accurate with respect to $\Delta t$. However the Newmark method does not fully control high-frequency oscillations of the solution for $t \to +\infty$. In order to cope with this numerical issue, an extension of Newmark schemes, namely the *generalized-$\alpha$* method has been purposely introduced in Chung and Hulbert (1993); see *e.g.* Isaksen *et al.* (2008) for an application to haemodynamics.

Space discretization is typically based on finite elements. Whatever the implicit temporal scheme chosen, a system of non-linear algebraic equations is obtained after space and time discretization; that is,

$$\frac{\rho_s \beta}{\Delta t^2} M_s \boldsymbol{D} + \boldsymbol{\Gamma}(\boldsymbol{D}) + \alpha_{ST} M_s^{\mathrm{ext}} \boldsymbol{D} = \boldsymbol{G}_s,$$

where $\beta$ depends on the time discretization (*e.g.* $\beta = 4$ for the Newmark method (3.43)), $\boldsymbol{D}$ is the vector collecting the vessel wall displacement unknowns, $M_s$ is the mass matrix, $M_s^{\mathrm{ext}}$ is the boundary mass matrix related to $\Sigma_{\mathrm{ext}}$, $\boldsymbol{\Gamma}$ is the non-linear operator defined by

$$\Gamma_i = \int_{\Omega_s} \widehat{\boldsymbol{T}}_s(\widehat{\boldsymbol{d}}) : \nabla \widehat{\boldsymbol{e}}_i \,\mathrm{d}\omega,$$

where $\widehat{\boldsymbol{e}}_i$ is the $i$th basis function, and $\boldsymbol{G}_s$ is the vector related to the right-hand side of the time-discretized equation. Notice that we have omitted the temporal index, which is understood. The above system is linearized by means of the Newton method, obtaining at each time step a sequence of linear systems of the form

$$\left( \frac{\rho_s \beta}{\Delta t^2} M_s + T(\boldsymbol{D}_{(k-1)}) + \alpha_{ST} M_s^{\mathrm{ext}} \right) \delta \boldsymbol{D}_{(k)}$$
$$= \boldsymbol{G}_s - \frac{\rho_s \beta}{\Delta t^2} M_s \boldsymbol{D}_{(k-1)} - \boldsymbol{\Gamma}(\boldsymbol{D}_{(k-1)}) - \alpha_{ST} M_s^{\mathrm{ext}} \boldsymbol{D}_{(k-1)},$$

where $k \geq 1$ is the Newton iteration index, to be solved until convergence occurs. Here $\delta \boldsymbol{D}_{(k)} = (\boldsymbol{D}_{(k)} - \boldsymbol{D}_{(k-1)})$, $T$ is the matrix related to the linearization of the first Piola–Kirchhoff tensor; that is,

$$(T)_{ij} = \int_{\Omega_s} (D_F \widehat{\boldsymbol{T}}_s(\widehat{\boldsymbol{d}}_{(k-1)}) : \nabla \widehat{\boldsymbol{e}}_j) : \nabla \widehat{\boldsymbol{e}}_i,$$

where $D_F$ is the Gâteaux derivative with respect to $\boldsymbol{F}$.

For the solution of the above linear system, domain decomposition (DD) methods are often used as efficient preconditioners for iterative Krylov methods. Since the matrix $T$ is symmetric, the conjugate gradient method is usually considered for solving the linear system. Among DD preconditioners, *finite element tearing and interconnect* (FETI) methods (Farhat and Roux 1991) are very often used in structural mechanics. In particular, *all floating* FETI methods have been considered for vessel wall problems, for example in Augustin, Holzapfel and Steinbach (2014). As in classical FETI methods, Lagrange multipliers are introduced to glue the solution together at the subdomain interfaces. In addition, Lagrange multipliers are also used to prescribe Dirichlet boundary conditions. This simplifies the implementation of the FETI method since all the subdomains are treated in the same way. A variant successfully used for arterial vessel walls is the so-called *dual–primal FETI* method: see *e.g.* Balzani *et al.* (2010). Finally, we mention yet another class of DD methods considered for this problem, a two-level overlapping Schwarz method with an energy minimization coarse space: see Dohrmann and Widlund (2009).

In Figure 3.6 we illustrate some examples of numerical results obtained in real geometries reconstructed from radiological images (see the caption for details). These results highlight the anisotropic internal stresses characterizing vascular vessel walls.

### 3.6.3 Numerical methods for the fluid–structure interaction problem

The numerical solution of the coupled FSI problem (3.19) requires us to manage three sources of non-linearities, namely,

(i) the fluid domain is unknown and its deformation is in general non-linear (*geometric non-linearity*),
(ii) the fluid subproblem is non-linear (*fluid constitutive non-linearity*),
(iii) the vessel displacement subproblem is non-linear (*structure constitutive non-linearity*),

together with two different kinds of coupling,

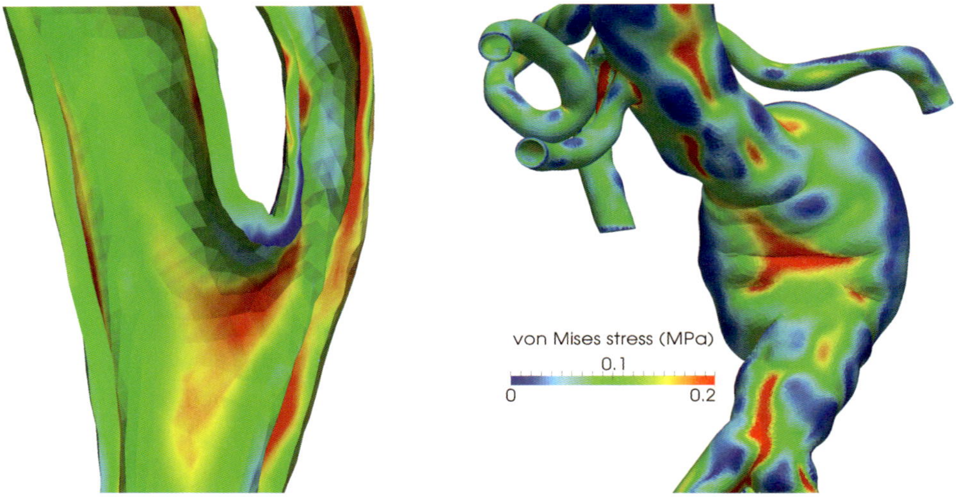


(a) (b)

Figure 3.6 (a) Von Mises internal stresses in a carotid artery (data from MRI images provided by the Vascular Surgery and Radiology Divisions at Ospedale Maggiore Policlinico, Milan, Italy). (b) Von Mises stresses in an abdominal aortic aneurysm (mesh from www.vascularmodel.com/sandbox/doku.php?id=start). Numerical results in (b) were obtained by D. Forti (CMCS-EPFL) using LifeV (carotid artery) and the finite element library redbKIT v2.1 (github.com/redbKIT/redbKIT/releases) (AAA), P2 finite elements, a Newmark unconditionally-stable scheme for the time discretization and an exponential vessel wall law.

(iv) the displacement of the fluid domain at the FS interface needs to match the displacement of the vessel wall (*geometric adherence*: see (3.19f)),

(v) the fluid and vessel displacement subproblems are coupled by means of the kinematic and dynamic conditions (3.19c, 3.19d) (*physical coupling*).

*Arbitrary-Lagrangian formulation.* As for points (i) and (iv), a classical numerical strategy relies on extending the FS interface displacement $\boldsymbol{d}_f = \boldsymbol{d}|_{\Sigma^t}$ to the whole fluid domain, thus associating a displacement with its internal points as well. This is obtained by solving an extra problem for the fluid domain displacement, usually a harmonic extension of the FS interface datum $\boldsymbol{d}_f$, with homogeneous Dirichlet conditions at $\partial\Omega_f^t \setminus \Sigma^t$. The fluid domain displacement is then used to move the points of the fluid mesh accordingly, obtaining the new computational fluid domain. With this aim, the Navier–Stokes equations are reformulated on a frame of reference that moves with the fluid domain. This is neither a Lagrangian description (where the frame moves with the fluid particles) nor an Eulerian description (where a fixed frame would be used). For this reason, it is called the *arbitrary Lagrangian–Eulerian* (ALE) approach (Hirt, Amsden and Cook 1974, Donea 1982). To write the Navier–Stokes equations in an ALE configuration, we use the Reynolds transport formula to express the ALE material time derivative $\delta/\delta t$ of a function $\boldsymbol{z}$ with respect to the Eulerian derivative; that is,

$$\frac{\delta \boldsymbol{z}}{\delta t} = \frac{\partial \boldsymbol{z}}{\partial t} + (\boldsymbol{v}_f \cdot \nabla)\boldsymbol{z},$$

where $\boldsymbol{v}_f = \dot{\boldsymbol{d}}_f$ is the velocity of the points of the fluid domain. Thus, the FSI problem together with its initial and boundary conditions becomes

$$\rho_f\left(\frac{\delta \boldsymbol{v}}{\delta t} + ((\boldsymbol{v} - \boldsymbol{v}_f)\cdot\nabla)\boldsymbol{v}\right) - \nabla\cdot\boldsymbol{T}_f(\boldsymbol{v},p) = \boldsymbol{0} \quad \text{in } \Omega_f^t, \tag{3.44a}$$

$$\nabla\cdot\boldsymbol{v} = 0 \quad \text{in } \Omega_f^t, \tag{3.44b}$$

$$\boldsymbol{v} = \frac{\partial \boldsymbol{d}}{\partial t} \quad \text{on } \Sigma^t, \tag{3.44c}$$

$$\boldsymbol{T}_s(\boldsymbol{d})\boldsymbol{n} = \boldsymbol{T}_f(\boldsymbol{v},p)\boldsymbol{n} \quad \text{on } \Sigma^t, \tag{3.44d}$$

$$\rho_s\frac{\partial^2\widehat{\boldsymbol{d}}}{\partial t^2} - \nabla\cdot\widehat{\boldsymbol{T}}_s(\widehat{\boldsymbol{d}}) = \boldsymbol{0} \quad \text{in } \Omega_s, \tag{3.44e}$$

$$\widehat{\boldsymbol{d}}_f = \widehat{\boldsymbol{d}} \quad \text{at } \Sigma, \tag{3.44f}$$

$$-\triangle\widehat{\boldsymbol{d}}_f = \boldsymbol{0} \quad \text{in } \Omega_f. \tag{3.44g}$$

This choice is particularly suitable when finite elements are considered for the space discretization. Indeed, the terms involving spatial derivatives are as usual expressed with respect to the current configuration, whereas the (material) time derivative term is written in the reference configuration. In particular, given the nodal basis functions $\boldsymbol{\phi}_j$, we write the finite element approximation of $\boldsymbol{v}(t,\boldsymbol{x})$ as $\boldsymbol{v}_h(t,\boldsymbol{x}) = \sum_j v_h^j(t)\boldsymbol{\phi}_j(\boldsymbol{x})$; then, we have

$$\frac{\delta(\boldsymbol{v}_h(t,\boldsymbol{x}))}{\delta t} = \frac{\delta}{\delta t}\left(\sum_j v_h^j(t)\boldsymbol{\phi}_j(\boldsymbol{x}(t))\right) = \sum_j \frac{\mathrm{d}v_h^j(t)}{\mathrm{d}t}\boldsymbol{\phi}_j(\boldsymbol{x}(t)),$$

since the time variations of the basis functions with respect to the reference domain vanish. This makes the computation of the fluid velocity on the nodes of the fluid mesh straightforward: see *e.g.* Nobile (2001).

For time discretization of (3.44), a common choice is to discretize the fluid and the vessel wall problems with two schemes of equal order (of order $p$, say), for example BDF2 or Crank–Nicolson for the fluid and the Newmark scheme (3.43) for the vessel problem.

*Treatment of geometric coupling, geometric adherence and fluid non-linearity.* As for issue (ii) above (constitutive fluid non-linearity), following the approach commonly used for a stand-alone fluid problem, the convective field is usually treated explicitly, by using a suitable extrapolation $\boldsymbol{v}^* - \boldsymbol{v}^*_f$ of order $p$ from previous time steps. This choice introduces a CFL-like condition for $\Delta t$ to preserve absolute stability, which however is always satisfied for the values of $\Delta t$ usually considered in haemodynamics. Another common choice in haemodynamics is the explicit treatment of geometric coupling and adherence (issues (i) and (iv) above). In particular, the fluid problem coupled with the structure problem are solved in a domain $\Omega^*_f$ obtained by a suitable extrapolation from previous time steps of order $p$, and the fluid geometry problem is then solved in sequence (Swim and Seshaiyer 2006, Fernández, Gerbeau and Grandmont 2007, Badia, Quaini and Quarteroni 2008*c*, Nobile and Vergara 2008). Again, a limitation on $\Delta t$ is required to ensure absolute stability. In particular, Fernández *et al.* (2007) prove, for a model problem, that stability is guaranteed under a CFL-like condition. Numerical evidence in real scenarios indicates that this is also a mild condition in the haemodynamics regime: see *e.g.* Moireau *et al.* (2012) and Nobile, Pozzoli and Vergara (2014). Based on the considerations above, the following temporal discretization of the FSI problem (3.44) can be considered.

*Explicit scheme for geometric coupling and adherence*

For $n \geq 1$, at time step $t^n$:

(1) Solve the FSI problem:

$$\frac{\rho_f \alpha}{\Delta t}\boldsymbol{v}^n + \rho_f((\boldsymbol{v}^* - \boldsymbol{v}^*_f)\cdot\nabla)\boldsymbol{v}^n - \nabla\cdot\boldsymbol{T}_f(\boldsymbol{v}^n, p^n) = \boldsymbol{g}^n_f \quad \text{in } \Omega^*_f, \tag{3.45a}$$

$$\nabla\cdot\boldsymbol{v}^n = 0 \quad \text{in } \Omega^*_f, \tag{3.45b}$$

$$\boldsymbol{v}^n = \frac{\alpha}{\Delta t}\boldsymbol{d}^n + \boldsymbol{g}^n_{fs} \quad \text{at } \Sigma^*, \tag{3.45c}$$

$$\boldsymbol{T}_s(\boldsymbol{d}^n)\boldsymbol{n}^* = \boldsymbol{T}_f(\boldsymbol{v}^n, p^n)\boldsymbol{n}^* \quad \text{at } \Sigma^*, \tag{3.45d}$$

$$\frac{\rho_s \beta}{\Delta t^2}\widehat{\boldsymbol{d}}^n - \nabla\cdot\widehat{\boldsymbol{T}}_s(\widehat{\boldsymbol{d}}^n) = \widehat{\boldsymbol{g}}^n_s \quad \text{in } \Omega_s, \tag{3.45e}$$

where $\alpha$ still depends on the time discretization scheme, and

$$\begin{aligned}\boldsymbol{g}_f^n &= \boldsymbol{g}_f^n(\boldsymbol{v}^{n-1}, \boldsymbol{v}^{n-2}, \ldots),\\ \boldsymbol{g}_s^n &= \boldsymbol{g}_s^n(\boldsymbol{d}^{n-1}, \boldsymbol{d}^{n-2}, \ldots),\\ \boldsymbol{g}_{fs}^n &= \boldsymbol{g}_{fs}^n(\boldsymbol{d}^{n-1}, \boldsymbol{d}^{n-2}, \ldots)\end{aligned}$$

account for the terms at previous time steps coming from time discretizations of order $p$ of the corresponding equations (3.44a), (3.44e) and (3.44c), respectively.

(2) Then, solve the fluid geometry problem,

$$-\triangle \widehat{\boldsymbol{d}}_f^n = \mathbf{0} \quad \text{in } \Omega_f, \tag{3.46a}$$

$$\widehat{\boldsymbol{d}}_f^n = \widehat{\boldsymbol{d}}^n \quad \text{at } \Sigma, \tag{3.46b}$$

and build $\Omega_f^*$ accordingly.

In the above substeps, the FSI problem (3.45) is still coupled by means of the physical coupling given by the interface conditions (3.45c, 3.45d): see issue (v) above. For the solution of this problem, both *partitioned* and *monolithic* procedures have been successfully considered so far in haemodynamics. In partitioned schemes, the fluid and vessel wall subproblems are solved separately, one or more times per time step. Each of the two problems is equipped with a suitable boundary condition at the FS interface $\Sigma^*$ derived by splitting the physical interface conditions (3.45c, 3.45d).

*Partitioned algorithms of explicit type*

From the computational point of view, an attractive class of partitioned schemes is that of the *loosely coupled algorithms* where the two subproblems are solved only once per time step. The classic loosely coupled algorithm, widely used in aerodynamics (Piperno and Farhat 2001), is the *explicit Dirichlet–Neumann* scheme, where condition (3.45c) is prescribed explicitly as a Dirichlet condition in the fluid subproblem, whereas condition (3.45d) is prescribed as a Neumann condition on the vessel wall subproblem, leading to the following.

*Explicit Dirichlet–Neumann scheme.* For $n \geq 1$, at time step $t^n$:

(1) Solve the fluid Oseen problem with a Dirichlet condition at the FS interface:

$$\frac{\rho_f \alpha}{\Delta t}\boldsymbol{v}^n + \rho_f((\boldsymbol{v}^* - \boldsymbol{v}_f^*)\cdot\nabla)\boldsymbol{v}^n - \nabla\cdot\boldsymbol{T}_f(\boldsymbol{v}^n, p^n) = \boldsymbol{g}_f^n \quad \text{in } \Omega_f^*, \tag{3.47a}$$

$$\nabla\cdot\boldsymbol{v}^n = 0 \quad \text{in } \Omega_f^*, \tag{3.47b}$$

$$\boldsymbol{v}^n = \frac{\alpha}{\Delta t}\boldsymbol{d}^{n-1} + \boldsymbol{g}_{fs}^{n-1} \quad \text{on } \Sigma^*. \tag{3.47c}$$

(2) Then, solve the non-linear vessel wall problem with a Neumann condition at the FS interface:

$$\frac{\rho_s \beta}{\Delta t^2}\widehat{\boldsymbol{d}}^n - \nabla\cdot\widehat{\boldsymbol{T}}_s(\widehat{\boldsymbol{d}}^n) = \widehat{\boldsymbol{g}}_s^n \quad \text{in } \Omega_s, \tag{3.48a}$$

$$\widehat{\boldsymbol{T}}_s(\widehat{\boldsymbol{d}}^n)\widehat{\boldsymbol{n}} = \widehat{\boldsymbol{T}}_f(\widehat{\boldsymbol{v}}^n, \widehat{p}^n)\widehat{\boldsymbol{n}} \quad \text{on } \Sigma. \tag{3.48b}$$

Note that the time-discretized kinematic condition (3.47c) differs from (3.45c) since now we are considering an explicit Dirichlet condition for the fluid subproblem, so the right-hand side is computed at the previous time step.

A 'parallel' version of this scheme is obtained by replacing $\widehat{\boldsymbol{T}}_f(\widehat{\boldsymbol{v}}^n, \widehat{p}^n)\widehat{\boldsymbol{n}}$ with $\widehat{\boldsymbol{T}}_f(\widehat{\boldsymbol{v}}^{n-1}, \widehat{p}^{n-1})\widehat{\boldsymbol{n}}$ in (3.48b). Notice that in the monolithic FSI problem (3.45), the dynamic continuity condition (3.45d) is written in the current configuration $\Sigma^*$, whereas for the structure subproblem alone (3.48) is written in the reference configuration $\Sigma$. Accordingly, in what follows the structure interface quantities will be written in the current configuration in monolithic FSI problems and in the reference configuration when the structure problem is uncoupledin view of a partitioned scheme.

Unfortunately, the explicit Dirichlet–Neumann scheme can be unstable regardless of the choice of $\Delta t$. In particular, Causin, Gerbeau and Nobile (2005) prove that this happens if the fluid and structure densities are comparable, which is precisely the case for haemodynamics. This is due to the so-called large *added mass effect*. See also Forster, Wall and Ramm (2007) and Nobile and Vergara (2012).

Stable loosely-coupled algorithms have been introduced recently. To this end, in the FSI problem (3.45) the interface conditions (3.45c, 3.45d) are replaced by two linear independent combinations

$$\sigma_f \boldsymbol{v}^n + \boldsymbol{T}_f(\boldsymbol{v}^n, p^n)\boldsymbol{n}^* = \sigma_f\left(\frac{\alpha}{\Delta t}\boldsymbol{d}^n + \boldsymbol{g}_{fs}^n\right) + \boldsymbol{T}_s(\boldsymbol{d}^n)\boldsymbol{n}^* \quad \text{on } \Sigma^*, \tag{3.49a}$$

$$\sigma_s\left(\frac{\alpha}{\Delta t}\boldsymbol{d}^n + \boldsymbol{g}_{fs}^n\right) + \boldsymbol{T}_s(\boldsymbol{d}^n)\boldsymbol{n}^* = \sigma_s \boldsymbol{v}^n + \boldsymbol{T}_f(\boldsymbol{v}^n, p^n)\boldsymbol{n}^* \quad \text{on } \Sigma^*, \tag{3.49b}$$

where $\sigma_f \neq \sigma_s$ are, in general, two functions of space and time. This naturally leads to the following.

*Explicit Robin–Robin scheme.* For $n \geq 1$, at time step $t^n$:

(1) Solve the Oseen problem with a Robin condition at the FS interface:

$$\frac{\rho_f \alpha}{\Delta t}\boldsymbol{v}^n + \rho_f((\boldsymbol{v}^* - \boldsymbol{v}_f^*) \cdot \nabla)\boldsymbol{v}^n - \nabla \cdot \boldsymbol{T}_f(\boldsymbol{v}^n, p^n) = \boldsymbol{g}_f^n \quad \text{in } \Omega_f^*, \tag{3.50a}$$

$$\nabla \cdot \boldsymbol{v}^n = 0 \quad \text{in } \Omega_f^*, \tag{3.50b}$$

$$\sigma_f \boldsymbol{v}^n + \boldsymbol{T}_f(\boldsymbol{v}^n, p^n)\boldsymbol{n}^* = \sigma_f\left(\frac{\alpha}{\Delta t}\boldsymbol{d}^{n-1} + \boldsymbol{g}_{fs}^{n-1}\right) + \boldsymbol{T}_s(\boldsymbol{d}^{n-1})\boldsymbol{n}^* \quad \text{on } \Sigma^*. \tag{3.50c}$$

(2) Then, solve the non-linear vessel wall problem with a Robin condition at the FS interface:

$$\frac{\rho_s \beta}{\Delta t^2}\widehat{\boldsymbol{d}}^n - \nabla \cdot \widehat{\boldsymbol{T}}_s(\widehat{\boldsymbol{d}}^n) = \widehat{\boldsymbol{g}}_s^n \quad \text{in } \Omega_s, \tag{3.51a}$$

$$\frac{\sigma_s \alpha}{\Delta t}\widehat{\boldsymbol{d}}^n + \widehat{\boldsymbol{T}}_s(\widehat{\boldsymbol{d}}^n)\widehat{\boldsymbol{n}} = \sigma_s \widehat{\boldsymbol{v}}^n + \widehat{\boldsymbol{T}}_f(\widehat{\boldsymbol{v}}^n, \widehat{p}^n)\widehat{\boldsymbol{n}} - \sigma_s \widehat{\boldsymbol{g}}_{fs}^n \quad \text{on } \Sigma. \tag{3.51b}$$

Burman and Fernández (2009) propose a discontinuous Galerkin (DG)-like mortaring of the interface coupling conditions (3.45c, 3.45d). The corresponding block Gauss–Seidel explicit algorithm could be reinterpreted as an explicit Dirichlet–Robin scheme, where in (3.50c, 3.51b) we have $\sigma_f = +\infty$, $\sigma_s = -\gamma\mu/h$, where $\gamma$ is the DG penalty parameter. Burman and Fernández show that the DG interface penalty and the viscous dissipation are not able to control the pressure fluctuations at the FS interface appearing in the discrete energy estimate. For this reason, they propose adding to the fluid problem a consistent stabilization term penalizing the pressure fluctuations, which is proved to be absolutely stable under a CFL-like condition. Banks, Henshaw and Schwendeman (2014) have introduced a stable explicit Robin–Robin scheme, setting the parameters in the Robin interface conditions (3.50c, 3.51b) after analyzing the incoming and outgoing characteristic variables of the vessel wall problem. In particular, the above parameters are defined in terms of the outgoing characteristic variable for the fluid subproblem and in terms of the incoming characteristic variable for the vessel wall subproblem. For linear elasticity, the following values are obtained: $\sigma_{f,\mathrm{norm}} = \sqrt{\rho_s(\mu_1 + 2\mu_2)}$ and $\sigma_{f,\mathrm{tang}} = \sqrt{\rho_s \mu_2}$ in the normal and tangential direction, respectively ($\mu_1$ and $\mu_2$ are the Lamé constants), and $\sigma_s = -\sigma_f$.

This choice allows the travelling information contained in the characteristic variables to provide a tighter coupling of the fluid and structure problems than that enforced by (3.45c, 3.45d).

*Partitioned algorithms of semi-implicit type*

Fernández *et al.* (2007) prove that to achieve stability without introducing stabilization terms for the Dirichlet–Neumann scheme, an implicit coupling between the fluid pressure and the vessel wall displacement is required. In particular, a projection scheme is used where the fluid ALE-advection-diffusion step is solved explicitly, whereas the fluid pressure and vessel wall subproblems are coupled and solved in an iterative framework until convergence occurs (see also Astorino and Grandmont 2009 for a convergence analysis).

*Semi-implicit pressure-vessel wall coupled scheme.* For $n \geq 1$, at time step $t^n$:

(1) Solve the ALE-advection-diffusion problem with a Dirichlet condition at the FS interface:

$$\frac{\rho_f \alpha}{\Delta t}\widetilde{\boldsymbol{v}}^n + \rho_f((\boldsymbol{v}^* - \boldsymbol{v}_f^*)\cdot\nabla)\widetilde{\boldsymbol{v}}^n - \nabla\cdot\mu(\nabla\widetilde{\boldsymbol{v}}^n + (\nabla\widetilde{\boldsymbol{v}}^n)^{\mathrm{T}}) = \boldsymbol{g}_f^n \quad \text{in } \Omega_f^*, \tag{3.52a}$$

$$\widetilde{\boldsymbol{v}}^n = \frac{\alpha}{\Delta t}\boldsymbol{d}^{n-1} + \boldsymbol{g}_{fs}^{n-1} \quad \text{on } \Sigma^*. \tag{3.52b}$$

(2) Then, solve the coupled pressure-vessel wall problem. To this end, introduce the following iterations on index $k \geq 1$.

(a) Solve the pressure problem with a Neumann condition at the FS interface:

$$\begin{aligned} \triangle p_{(k)}^n &= \frac{\rho_f \alpha}{\Delta t}\nabla\cdot\widetilde{\boldsymbol{v}}^n && \text{in } \Omega_f^*, \\ \frac{\partial p_{(k)}^n}{\partial \boldsymbol{n}^*} &= \frac{\alpha}{\Delta t}\boldsymbol{d}_{(k-1)}^n + \boldsymbol{g}_{fs}^n && \text{on } \Sigma^*. \end{aligned}$$

(b) Then, solve the non-linear vessel wall problem with a Neumann condition at the FS interface:

$$\begin{aligned} \frac{\rho_s \beta}{\Delta t^2}\widehat{\boldsymbol{d}}_{(k)}^n - \nabla\cdot\widehat{\boldsymbol{T}}_s(\widehat{\boldsymbol{d}}_{(k)}^n) = \widehat{\boldsymbol{g}}_s^n \quad & \text{in } \Omega_s, \\ \widehat{\boldsymbol{T}}_s(\widehat{\boldsymbol{d}}_{(k)}^n)\widehat{\boldsymbol{n}} = \widehat{\boldsymbol{T}}_f(\widehat{\widetilde{\boldsymbol{v}}}^n, \widehat{p}_{(k)}^n)\widehat{\boldsymbol{n}} \quad & \text{on } \Sigma. \end{aligned}$$

Astorino, Chouly and Fernández (2009) apply the DG mortaring approach to this projection scheme, leading to a Robin–Robin-like scheme. An algebraic version of the projection scheme proposed by Fernández *et al.* (2007) is introduced in Badia *et al.* (2008*c*).

*Partitioned algorithms of implicit type*

More generally, a fully implicit treatment of (3.45c, 3.45d) (or (3.49)) by means of partitioned algorithms is often considered. In this case, the fluid and vessel wall subproblems are solved iteratively until the whole interface conditions are satisfied within a prescribed tolerance. A general scheme is given by the following.

*Implicit Robin–Robin scheme.* For $n \geq 1$, $k \geq 1$, at time step $t^n$/iteration $k$:

(1) Solve the Oseen problem with a Robin condition at the FS interface:

$$\frac{\rho_f \alpha}{\Delta t} \boldsymbol{v}^n_{(k)} + \rho_f((\boldsymbol{v}^* - \boldsymbol{v}^*_f) \cdot \nabla)\boldsymbol{v}^n_{(k)} - \nabla \cdot \boldsymbol{T}_f(\boldsymbol{v}^n_{(k)}, p^n_{(k)}) = \boldsymbol{g}^n_f \quad \text{in } \Omega^*_f, \tag{3.55a}$$

$$\nabla \cdot \boldsymbol{v}^n_{(k)} = 0 \quad \text{in } \Omega^*_f, \tag{3.55b}$$

$$\sigma_f \boldsymbol{v}^n_{(k)} + \boldsymbol{T}_f(\boldsymbol{v}^n_{(k)}, p^n_{(k)})\boldsymbol{n}^* = \sigma_f \left( \frac{\alpha}{\Delta t} \boldsymbol{d}^n_{(k-1)} + \boldsymbol{g}^n_{fs} \right) + \boldsymbol{T}_s(\boldsymbol{d}^n_{(k-1)})\boldsymbol{n}^* \quad \text{on } \Sigma^*. \tag{3.55c}$$

(2) Then, solve the non-linear vessel wall problem with a Robin condition at the FS interface:

$$\frac{\rho_s \beta}{\Delta t^2} \widehat{\boldsymbol{d}}^n_{(k)} - \nabla \cdot \widehat{\boldsymbol{T}}_s(\widehat{\boldsymbol{d}}^n_{(k)}) = \widehat{\boldsymbol{g}}^n_s \quad \text{in } \Omega_s, \tag{3.56a}$$

$$\frac{\sigma_s \alpha}{\Delta t} \widehat{\boldsymbol{d}}^n_{(k)} + \widehat{\boldsymbol{T}}_s(\widehat{\boldsymbol{d}}^n_{(k)})\widehat{\boldsymbol{n}} = \sigma_s \widehat{\boldsymbol{v}}^n_{(k)} + \widehat{\boldsymbol{T}}_f(\widehat{\boldsymbol{v}}^n_{(k)}, \widehat{p}^n_{(k)})\widehat{\boldsymbol{n}} - \sigma_s \widehat{\boldsymbol{g}}^n_{fs} \quad \text{on } \Sigma. \tag{3.56b}$$

$\sigma_f$ and $\sigma_s$ in (3.55c, 3.56b)) can be functions of space and time.

As proved in Causin *et al.* (2005), a small relaxation parameter is needed to achieve convergence in the implicit Dirichlet–Neumann scheme (corresponding to setting $\sigma_f = +\infty$, $\sigma_s = 0$ in (3.55c, 3.56b)). In practice, an Aitken relaxation procedure is often used to dynamically estimate an efficient relaxation parameter (Deparis 2004, Kuttler and Wall 2008). A better situation is obtained by properly selecting the parameters in the Robin interface conditions (3.55c, 3.56b). In particular, the choice

$$\sigma_f = \frac{\beta \rho_s H_s}{\alpha \Delta t} + \frac{E H_s \Delta t}{(1 - \nu^2) R^2}, \; \sigma_s = 0$$

(where, as usual, $E$ and $\nu$ are Young's modulus and the Poisson ratio for the vessel material at small deformations, and $H_s$ and $R$ are therepresentative thickness and radius of the vessel) yields fast convergence without any relaxation (*Robin–Neumann* scheme: Badia, Nobile and Vergara 2008*a*, Nobile, Pozzoli and Vergara 2013). Gerardo-Giorda, Nobile and Vergara (2010) and Gigante and Vergara (2015) have characterized the optimal value of $\sigma_s$, leading to further improvement in the convergence history. Yu, Baek and Karniadakis (2013) have derived a Dirichlet–Robin scheme by means of a *generalized fictitious* method, where the coefficients of the fluid pressure and vessel wall acceleration are changed to account for the added mass effect. This again allows one to obtain good convergence properties for haemodynamic parameters without any relaxation. Another class of implicit methods with good convergence properties for high added-mass effect is based on adding a suitable *interface artificial compressibility* (IAC) consistent term to the fluid problem, proportional to the jump of pressure between two successive iterations (Degroote *et al.* 2010). Degroote (2011) showed that for a finite volume approximation, the IAC method based on Dirichlet–Neumann iterations is equivalent to a Robin–Neumann scheme for a suitable choice of the parameter $\sigma_f$.

*Partitioned algorithms for the FSI problem with a membrane structure*

Recently, several papers have analyzed algorithms for FSI problems featuring a reduced membrane model for the vessel wall. In this case, the FSI problem is given by the fluid problem (3.19a), the kinematic continuity condition (3.23a) and the membrane equation (3.23b), which in this case also plays the role of dynamic continuity condition. Moreover, homogeneous Dirichlet or Neumann conditions in the tangential direction need to be prescribed for the fluid problem at the interface $\Sigma$. By considering an implicit time discretization of (3.23b) and an explicit treatment of the geometry coupling, we obtain at each time step the following linearized FSI problem:

$$\frac{\rho_f \alpha}{\Delta t}\boldsymbol{v}^n + \rho_f((\boldsymbol{v}^* - \boldsymbol{v}_f^*)\cdot\nabla)\boldsymbol{v}^n - \nabla\cdot\boldsymbol{T}_f(\boldsymbol{v}^n, p^n) = \boldsymbol{g}_f^n \quad \text{in } \Omega_f^*, \tag{3.57a}$$

$$\nabla\cdot\boldsymbol{v}^n = 0 \quad \text{in } \Omega_f^*, \tag{3.57b}$$

$$\boldsymbol{v}^n\cdot\boldsymbol{n}^* = \frac{\alpha}{\Delta t}{d_r}^n + g_{fs}^n \quad \text{on } \Sigma^*, \tag{3.57c}$$

$$\boldsymbol{v}^n - (\boldsymbol{v}^n\cdot\boldsymbol{n}^*)\boldsymbol{n}^* = \boldsymbol{0} \quad \text{on } \Sigma^*, \tag{3.57d}$$

$$\begin{aligned}\frac{\rho_s H_s \beta}{\Delta t^2}d_r^n - \nabla\cdot(\boldsymbol{P}\nabla d_r^n) + \chi H_s d_r^n \\ = -\boldsymbol{T}_f(\boldsymbol{v}^n, p^n)\boldsymbol{n}^*\cdot\boldsymbol{n}^* + g_s^n\end{aligned} \quad \text{on } \Sigma^*, \tag{3.57e}$$

where, as usual, $\boldsymbol{g}_f^n$, $g_s^n$ and $g_{fs}^n$ account for the terms at previous time steps coming from time discretization.

The explicit Dirichlet–Neumann scheme applied to the previous monolithic problem reads as follows.

*Explicit Dirichlet–Neumann scheme for the FSI problem with membrane structure.* Given the quantities at previous time steps, at time step $t^n$:

(1) Solve the Oseen problem with a Dirichlet condition at the FS interface:

$$\begin{aligned}
&\frac{\rho_f \alpha}{\Delta t}\boldsymbol{v}^n + \rho_f((\boldsymbol{v}^* - \boldsymbol{v}_f^*)\cdot\nabla)\boldsymbol{v}^n - \nabla\cdot\boldsymbol{T}_f(\boldsymbol{v}^n, p^n) = \boldsymbol{g}_f^n && \text{in } \Omega_f^*,\\
&\nabla\cdot\boldsymbol{v}^n = 0 && \text{in } \Omega_f^*,\\
&\boldsymbol{v}^n\cdot\boldsymbol{n}^* = \frac{\alpha}{\Delta t}d_r^{n-1} + g_{fs}^{n-1} && \text{on } \Sigma^*,\\
&\boldsymbol{v}^n - (\boldsymbol{v}^n\cdot\boldsymbol{n}^*)\boldsymbol{n}^* = \boldsymbol{0} && \text{on } \Sigma^*.
\end{aligned}$$

(2) Then, solve the membrane problem:

$$\frac{\rho_s H_s \beta}{\Delta t^2}\widehat{d}_r^n - \nabla\cdot(\boldsymbol{P}\nabla\widehat{d}_r^n) + \chi H_s \widehat{d}_r^n = -\widehat{\boldsymbol{T}}_f(\widehat{\boldsymbol{v}}^n, \widehat{p}^n)\widehat{\boldsymbol{n}}\cdot\widehat{\boldsymbol{n}} + \widehat{g}_s^n \quad \text{on } \Sigma.$$

As in the case of scheme (3.47, 3.48), unfortunately this scheme is unconditionally absolutely unstable in the haemodynamic regime (Causin *et al.* 2005).

Different algorithms are obtained by linearly combining the interface conditions (3.57c) and (3.57e) and by substituting the new condition in (3.57c). In this case, we have to solve a coupled problem consisting of the following.

*Robin–Neumann coupling for the FSI problem with membrane structure.* Given the quantities at previous time steps, at time step $t^n$:

(1) Solve the Oseen problem with a Robin condition at the FS interface:

$$\begin{aligned}
&\frac{\rho_f \alpha}{\Delta t}\boldsymbol{v}^n + \rho_f((\boldsymbol{v}^* - \boldsymbol{v}_f^*)\cdot\nabla)\boldsymbol{v}^n - \nabla\cdot\boldsymbol{T}_f(\boldsymbol{v}^n, p^n) = \boldsymbol{g}_f^n && \text{in } \Omega_f^*, && \text{(3.59a)}\\
&\nabla\cdot\boldsymbol{v}^n = 0 && \text{in } \Omega_f^*, && \text{(3.59b)}\\
&(\sigma_f\boldsymbol{v}^n + \boldsymbol{T}_f(\boldsymbol{v}^n, p^n)\boldsymbol{n}^*)\cdot\boldsymbol{n}^*\sigma_f\left(\frac{\alpha}{\Delta t}d_r^n + g_{fs}^n\right) && &&\\
&\qquad - \left(\frac{\rho_s H_s \beta}{\Delta t^2}d_r^n - \nabla\cdot(\boldsymbol{P}\nabla d_r^n) + \chi H_s d_r^n\right) && \text{on } \Sigma^*, && \text{(3.59c)}\\
&\boldsymbol{v}^n - (\boldsymbol{v}^n\cdot\boldsymbol{n}^*)\boldsymbol{n}^* = \boldsymbol{0} && \text{on } \Sigma^*. && \text{(3.59d)}
\end{aligned}$$

(2) Solve the membrane problem:

$$\frac{\rho_s H_s \beta}{\Delta t^2}\widehat{d}_r^n - \nabla\cdot(\boldsymbol{P}\nabla\widehat{d}_r^n)+\chi H_s\widehat{d}_r^n = -\widehat{\boldsymbol{T}}_f(\widehat{\boldsymbol{v}}^n,\widehat{p}^n)\widehat{\boldsymbol{n}}\cdot\widehat{\boldsymbol{n}}+\widehat{g}_s^n \quad \text{on } \Sigma. \tag{3.60}$$

The above problem could be solved either monolithically or by means of a block Gauss–Seidel method that in fact introduces sub-iterations splitting the solution of (3.59) and (3.60). When $\boldsymbol{P}=\boldsymbol{0}$, the special choice

$$\sigma_f = \widetilde{\sigma}_f = \frac{\rho_s H_s \beta}{\alpha\Delta t} + \frac{\chi H_s \Delta t}{\alpha}, \tag{3.61}$$

introduced in (3.59c), yields

$$(\widetilde{\sigma}_f \boldsymbol{v}^n + \boldsymbol{T}_f(\boldsymbol{v}^n,p^n)\boldsymbol{n}^*)\cdot\boldsymbol{n}^* = \widetilde{\sigma}_f g_{fs}^n \quad \text{on } \Sigma^*. \tag{3.62}$$

At this stage, this is a Robin condition for the fluid problem without any explicit dependence on $d_r^n$. Thus, the monolithic problem given by (3.59–3.61) is equivalent to the stand-alone fluid problem (3.59a, 3.59b, 3.59d, 3.62): see Nobile and Vergara (2008). The solution of this fluid problem can then be used to feed the right-hand side of (3.60) and to get the structure displacement $\widehat{d}_r^n$. In this way, the fluid and structure problems are in fact decoupled, even if the coupling conditions are treated implicitly. This provides a smart and efficient way to solve the monolithic problem (3.57) exactly, at the expense of a single fluid problem solve (note that the membrane problem (3.60) is solved very cheaply).

Starting from this result, Guidoboni, Glowinski, Cavallini and Canic (2009) have proposed a stable Robin–Neumann scheme based on an operator splitting, for a general membrane law ($\boldsymbol{P}\neq\boldsymbol{0}$). The inertial vessel wall term is treated implicitly as in the previous case, leading to a Robin boundary condition for the fluid with $\sigma_f = \rho_s H_s \beta/\alpha\Delta t$, whereas the elastic and algebraic contributions are treated explicitly. Fernández (2013) proposes an incremental version of this scheme, where the elastic and algebraic parts of the membrane law are included in the Robin condition for the fluid problem by means of a suitable extrapolation from previous time steps. Finally, we mention Colciago *et al.* (2014), who treat the whole membrane law implicitly, leading to a generalized Robin condition, which however requires an *ad hoc* implementation.

### *Partitioned algorithms based on the Schur complement*

Here we discuss partitioned schemes arising from an interface equation written for the FSI problem and introduced by Deparis, Discacciati, Fourestey and Quarteroni (2006). For the sake of exposition, we introduce the algebraic counterpart of (3.45) related to a finite element discretization for the case of linear elasticity for the vessel wall problem:

$$\left[\begin{array}{cc:cc} C^{ff} & C^{f\Sigma} & 0 & 0 \\ 0 & M^{\Sigma} & -M^{\Sigma} & 0 \\ \hdashline C^{\Sigma f} & C^{\Sigma\Sigma} & G^{\Sigma\Sigma} & G^{\Sigma s} \\ 0 & 0 & G^{s\Sigma} & G^{ss} \end{array}\right] \left[\begin{array}{c} \boldsymbol{V}^f \\ \boldsymbol{V}^{\Sigma} \\ \hdashline \boldsymbol{U}^{\Sigma} \\ \boldsymbol{D}^s \end{array}\right] = \left[\begin{array}{c} \boldsymbol{b}^f \\ \boldsymbol{0} \\ \hdashline \boldsymbol{b}^{\Sigma} \\ \boldsymbol{b}^s \end{array}\right], \tag{3.63}$$

where the superscript $f$ refers to internal fluid variables, $s$ to internal variables for the vessel wall, $\Sigma$ to the FS interface variables; $C$ (with superscripts) refers to fluid matrices, $G$ to vessel wall matrices, $M^{\Sigma}$ is the FS interface mass matrix; $\boldsymbol{V}$ includes the fluid and pressure variables, $\boldsymbol{D}^s$ the vessel wall displacement internal variables, and $\boldsymbol{U}^{\Sigma}$ the vessel wall velocity interface variables; the vectors $\boldsymbol{b}$ denote the right-hand sides. The first row corresponds to the momentum and mass conservation for the fluid, the second and third rows to the interface kinematic and dynamic conditions, and the last row to the vessel wall problem. By eliminating $\boldsymbol{V}^f$, $\boldsymbol{V}^{\Sigma}$ and $\boldsymbol{D}^s$ from (3.63), we obtain the interface equation

$$(\widetilde{C}^{\Sigma} + \widetilde{G}^{\Sigma})\boldsymbol{U}^{\Sigma} = \widetilde{\mathbf{b}}^{\Sigma}, \tag{3.64}$$

where

$$\widetilde{C}^{\Sigma} = C^{\Sigma\Sigma} - C^{\Sigma f}(C^{ff})^{-1}C^{f\Sigma} \quad \text{and} \quad \widetilde{G}^{\Sigma} = G^{\Sigma\Sigma} - G^{\Sigma s}(G^{ss})^{-1}G^{s\Sigma}$$

are the fluid and vessel wall Schur complement matrices and

$$\widetilde{\mathbf{b}}^{\Sigma} = \mathbf{b}^{\Sigma} - C^{\Sigma f}(C^{ff})^{-1}\mathbf{b}^f - G^{\Sigma s}(G^{ss})^{-1}\mathbf{b}^s$$

is the corresponding right-hand side.

The Robin–Robin method (3.55, 3.56) could be obtained by applying the Richardson method to the interface equation (3.64) preconditioned by the matrix

$$P = \frac{1}{\sigma_f + \sigma_s}(\widetilde{C}^{\Sigma} + \sigma_f M^{\Sigma})(M^{\Sigma})^{-1}(\widetilde{G}^{\Sigma} + \sigma_s M^{\Sigma}). \tag{3.65}$$

This leads to a new family of partitioned schemes obtained by applying other Krylov methods to (3.64) with the same preconditioner. For example, GMRES preconditioned by the Dirichlet–Neumann preconditioner $P = \widetilde{G}^{\Sigma}$ is considered in Badia, Quaini and Quarteroni (2008*b*), whereas GMRES preconditioned with the RR preconditioner (3.65) is introduced in Badia, Nobile and Vergara (2009). The first of these two schemes highlighted better convergence properties with respect to the classical Dirichlet–Neumann method, whereas the second is more robust with respect to the choice of the interface parameters $\sigma_f$, $\sigma_s$ than the classical Robin–Robin method.

In some works, a non-linear interface equation is written directly for the non-linear problem (3.44) and a Newton method is then applied to this equation (Fernández and Moubachir 2005, Degroote and Vierendeels 2011).

**Remark 3.2** In the partitioned schemes introduced above, the vessel wall subproblem appearing at each iteration is still non-linear, that is, we have not discussed how to tackle point (iii) in the list of issues reported at the beginning of the subsection. The simplest way to treat vessel wall non-linearity – very appropriate when a non-linear structural solver is available – is to introduce inner Newton sub-iterations at each Robin–Robin iteration. Alternatively, Kuttler *et al.* (2010) have proposed a scheme based on integrating the management of the five sources of non-linearities/coupling (geometric coupling and adherence, fluid and structure constitutive non-linearities, physical coupling) in a single inexact-Newton loop. Other possible combinations will be discussed later on as specific monolithic procedures. For a detailed overview with numerical comparisons we refer to Nobile *et al.* (2014).

*Monolithic solvers*

As an alternative to partitioned schemes, monolithic procedures have been successfully considered in haemodynamics for the solution of the FSI problem (3.45). These methods consist in applying an exact or inexact Newton method to the whole non-linear FSI problem. Referring to the notation introduced above, by considering a finite element space discretization and the inexact Newton method, we obtain from (3.45)

$$\widetilde{J}(\boldsymbol{x}_{(k-1)})\delta\boldsymbol{x}_{(k)} = \boldsymbol{G} - \boldsymbol{A}(\boldsymbol{x}_{(k-1)}) \tag{3.66}$$

(for simplicity we omit the temporal index $n$), where $\widetilde{J}$ is the Jacobian matrix or a suitable approximation of it, $\boldsymbol{x} = [\boldsymbol{V}^f\ \boldsymbol{V}^\Sigma\ \boldsymbol{U}^\Sigma\ \boldsymbol{D}^s]^{\mathrm{T}}$, and $\boldsymbol{A}(\boldsymbol{x}) = \boldsymbol{G}$ is the non-linear system related to (3.45). The exact Jacobian matrix is given by

$$J(\boldsymbol{x}_{(k-1)}) = \left[\begin{array}{cc:cc} C^{ff} & C^{f\Sigma} & 0 & 0 \\ 0 & M^\Sigma & -M^\Sigma & 0 \\ \hdashline C^{\Sigma f} & C^{\Sigma\Sigma} & J_G^{\Sigma\Sigma}(\boldsymbol{U}^\Sigma_{(k-1)}) & J_G^{\Sigma s}(\boldsymbol{D}^s_{(k-1)}) \\ 0 & 0 & J_G^{s\Sigma}(\boldsymbol{U}^\Sigma_{(k-1)}) & J_G^{ss}(\boldsymbol{D}^s_{(k-1)}) \end{array}\right], \tag{3.67}$$

where the submatrices $J_G$ are the exact Jacobians of $\boldsymbol{A}$ related to the structure variables. For the solution of the linear systems (3.66) with the exact Jacobian, classical strategies used so far for haemodynamics include GMRES preconditioned by a one-level additive Schwarz method (Barker and Cai 2010*a*) and global algebraic multigrid (Gee, Kuttler and Wall 2011). Barker and Cai (2010*b*) use a two-level Newton method in combination with a two-level hybrid Schwarz preconditioner, where the solution on a coarse grid is used to provide a good initial guess to the Newton method. Alternatively, inexact Newton methods have been considered, for example by means of block approximations $\widetilde{J}$ of $J$ splitting the fluid velocity, pressure and vessel wall unknowns (Heil 2004, Crosetto, Deparis, Fourestey and Quarteroni 2011).

A particular class of inexact Newton methods is obtained by neglecting the term $-M_\Sigma$ appearing in the upper-right block of the exact Jacobian (3.67). This yields in fact a class of partitioned schemes of Dirichlet–Neumann type where issues (iii) and (v) (vessel wall non-linearity and physical coupling) are treated within the same iterations. An example is given by the preconditioner proposed in Crosetto *et al.* (2011), where the fluid and structure blocks in (3.67) are approximated by the corresponding algebraic additive Schwarz preconditioners. This method is strongly scalable for haemodynamic applications. Recently, Deparis, Forti, Grandperrin and Quarteroni (2016) have introduced a variant of the above preconditioner. This new preconditioner, named FaCSI, is based on operating a static condensation of the fluid interface variables and using a SIMPLE preconditioner for the fluid block.

For the sake of exposition, we have discussed numerical strategies for the FSI problem based on finite elements for the space discretization and finite differences for the time discretization. Other strategies considered so far in haemodynamics are space-time finite elements (see *e.g.* Tezduyar *et al.* 2007, Bazilevs, Takizawa and Tezduyar 2012) and the methods based on isogeometric analysis (see Bazilevs, Calo, Zhang and Hughes 2006, Bazilevs *et al.* 2009).

In Figure 3.7 we illustrate some examples of numerical results obtained in real geometries reconstructed from radiological images (see the caption for details).

### *3.6.4 Numerical methods for defective boundary problems*

For the numerical solution of the augmented formulation (3.27), one could rely either on a monolithic strategy, where the full augmented matrix is constructed and solved, or on splitting techniques. For the latter, Formaggia

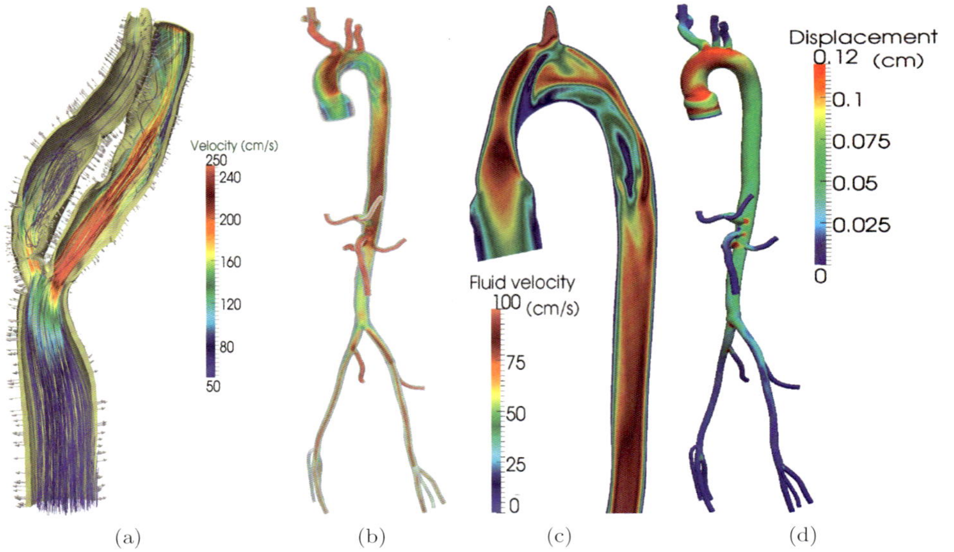


Figure 3.7 (a) Blood velocity streamlines and vessel wall displacement vectors in a stenotic carotid artery (data from MRI images provided by the Vascular Surgery and Radiology Divisions at Ospedale Maggiore Policlinico, Milan, Italy). (b–d) Results of a FSI simulation in the ascending and thoracic aorta (MRI images from www.vascularmodel.com/sandbox/doku.php?id=repository); courtesy of D. Forti (EPFL). Blood velocity magnitude in the whole domain (b) and on a selected longitudinal section (c), vessel wall displacements (d). All cases refer to the systolic peak. Numerical results were obtained using LifeV, P1-Bubble/P1 finite elements for the fluid problem and P1 finite elements for the vessel wall problem; the backward Euler scheme and the midpoint method was used for the time discretization of the fluid and vessel wall problems, respectively. The implicit Robin–Robin partitioned scheme was used in case (a) and the FaCSI preconditioner in cases (b–d).

*et al.* (2002) and Veneziani and Vergara (2005) propose writing the Schur complement equation with respect to the Lagrange multiplier of the linearized and discretized (in time and space) augmented formulation. This is a linear system whose dimension is equal to the number of flow rate conditions, say $m \geq 1$. By using the GMRES method to solve this system iteratively, the exact solution is reached after exactly $m$ iterations (in exact arithmetic). At each iteration, the solution of a standard fluid problem with Neumann conditions is needed (*exact splitting technique*). The solution of a further standard fluid problem is required to compute the initial residual in the GMRES algorithm. This approach is quite expensive, even for the case $m = 1$, which requires the solution of two fluid problems per time step. However, it preserves *modularity*; indeed, it can be implemented using available standard fluid solvers in a *black box* mode. This is an interesting property when applications to cases of real interest are addressed: see Viscardi *et al.* (2010), Vergara, Viscardi, Antiga and Luciani (2012), Piccinelli *et al.* (2013) and Guerciotti *et al.* (2015, 2017).

To reduce the computational time required by the exact splitting approach, Veneziani and Vergara (2007) propose a different (inexact) splitting procedure, requiring the solution of $m$ steady problems out of the temporal loop and of one unsteady null flow rate problem at each time step. This strategy introduces an error near the section which is smaller than the one based on conjecturing the velocity profile in the original (non-null) flow rate problem: see Section 3.4.1.

For the numerical solution of the control-based approach described in Section 3.4.3, Formaggia *et al.* (2008, 2009*b*) have considered classical iterative methods for the solution of the resulting KKT system.

Recently, a numerical approach based on the *Nitsche method* has been considered to prescribe a flow rate condition. In particular, the original idea of prescribing Dirichlet conditions with a consistent penalization approach (Nitsche 1970/71) has been extended by Zunino (2009) to the case of flow rate boundary conditions. This strategy does not introduce further variables other than those of the original problem, but it does require careful tuning of a penalization parameter. In addition, it deals with non-standard bilinear forms that need *ad hoc* implementation. However, it should be very effective if flow rate conditions are implemented in a DG code. Vergara (2011) has considered a similar approach to fulfilling the mean pressure condition (2.3) and the FSI case; see also Porpora, Zunino, Vergara and Piccinelli (2012).

For a more comprehensive overview of numerical strategies for defective boundary problems, we refer the reader to Formaggia and Vergara (2012).

### *3.6.5 Numerical methods for the geometric reduced models and multiscale approach*

For the numerical solution of the 1D reduced model (3.30), in principle any convenient approximation method for non-linear hyperbolic equations can be used. The peculiar feature of this model, however, is the lack of discontinuous solutions. A common approach relies on the finite element version of the Lax–Wendroff scheme, thanks to its excellent ability in containing numerical dispersion (Formaggia *et al.* 2001). As this scheme is explicit, a CFL-like condition is required to ensure absolute stability. In the presence of a viscoelastic term, the 1D model is usually discretized by means of a

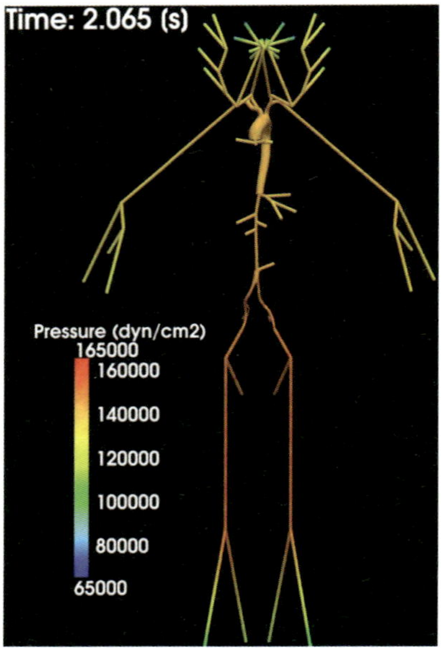


Figure 3.8 Pressure wave propagation in an ascending aorta (3D model) and in the 1D model of the systemic circulation. Numerical results were obtained using LifeV; the Newton method was used for the interface equation. Courtesy of C. Malossi.

splitting procedure where the solution is split into two components, one satisfying the pure elastic problem and the other satisfying the viscoelastic correction (Formaggia *et al.* 2003, Malossi, Blanco and Deparis 2012). High-order methods are suitable for capturing the (physical) reflections at bifurcations induced by the vessel tapering: see *e.g.* Sherwin, Franke, Peiró and Parker (2003*b*) and Sherwin, Formaggia, Peiró and Franke (2003*a*) for a discontinuous Galerkin discretization and Muller and Toro (2014) for a finite-volume scheme.

Regarding 0D models, they are in general described by systems of differential and algebraic equations, possibly non-linear due to the presence of diodes to represent the valves (Formaggia *et al.* 2009*a*). Usually, for haemodynamic applications, these systems can be reduced to classical Cauchy problems and solved by classical Runge–Kutta methods.

As in the case of the 3D/1D coupled problems described in Section 3.5.2, we can in principle identify three different strategies, namely *partitioned schemes*, *monolithic approaches*, and methods based on the solution of an *interface equation*. In partitioned schemes, the 3D and 1D problems are solved separately in an iterative framework. The coupling interface conditions can be enforced in many different ways. For example, we can prescribe the flow rate condition (3.39a) to the 3D problem and the pressure condition (3.42) to the 1D problem. Different algorithms are obtained by switching the role of the interface conditions in the iterative algorithm or by considering other interface conditions (*e.g.* (3.39b)). This is also the case when one of the two interface conditions is replaced by a condition expressing the continuity of the characteristic variable $W_1$ entering the 1D domain (Formaggia *et al.* 2001, Papadakis 2009), that is, according to (3.33),

$$W_1(t)|_{z=0} = \zeta_1\left(|\Gamma_f^t|, \int_{\Gamma_f^t} \boldsymbol{v} \cdot \boldsymbol{n} \, \mathrm{d}\gamma\right).$$

In any case, each of these approaches yields a 3D problem with a defective boundary condition, which could be tackled by one of the strategies described in Section 3.4. Formaggia *et al.* (2007) and Papadakis (2009) have successfully considered explicit algorithms based on the solution of the 3D and 1D problems only once per time step. These algorithms enforce a limitation on $\Delta t$, which, however, is milder with respect to that imposed by the numerical scheme adopted for the 1D model. As an alternative, Blanco, Feijóo and Urquiza (2007) and Blanco, Pivello, Urquiza and Feijóo (2009) have introduced iterative methods applied directly to the monolithic linearized system. A different approach to solving the 3D/1D coupled problem relies on writing an interface equation involving only the 3D/1D interface unknowns. We can interpret this equation as the geometric heterogeneous counterpart of the Schur complement equation. For its numerical solution, Leiva, Blanco and Buscaglia (2011), Malossi *et al.* (2013) and Blanco, Deparis and Malossi (2013) have used either the Broyden or the Newton method, in combination with GMRES. Methods relying on the numerical solution of the interface equation are simple to implement in the case of multiple interfaces, such as those arising in complex arterial networks.

In Figure 3.8 we provide a numerical result obtained by coupling the 3D model of an ascending aorta with a 1D model of the systemic circulation. This result highlights the suitability of the 1D model as provider of suitable absorbing conditions wfor the 3D model and in propagating the pressure wave along the whole network (Malossi 2012).

# PART TWO

# HEART FUNCTION

# 4

# Basic facts on quantitative cardiac physiology

In this chapter we present basic facts about the anatomy and functioning of the human heart. We discuss the propagation of the electric signal, the mechanics of heart contraction and cardiac fluid dynamics; finally we provide a brief summary of heart diseases.

## 4.1 Basic anatomy

The human heart is a hollow organ that pumps the blood into the arteries of the *systemic* and *pulmonary circulations* and collects it after its return through the veins; see *e.g.* (Klabunde 2012). Specifically, the heart supplies oxygenated blood and nutrients to the body through arteries and pumps instead de-oxygenated blood to the lungs for re-oxygenation. In a healthy heart, every second, blood is pumped to almost all the 75 trillion cells of the body, which amounts to 1.5 million barrels in an average lifetime. This endeavour is made possible by the *cardiac rhythm* – triggered by an electric signal initiating at the sinoatrial node – and the exceptional strength and resistance of our heart.

The human heart is made up of the *left* and *right heart*, each consisting of two chambers, an *atrium* and a *ventricle*. The left and right hearts are separated by the *interatrial* and *interventricular septa*, which do not allow the transfer of blood, whereas the atria and the ventricles are connected by the *atrioventricular valves* (*tricuspid valve* in the right heart, *mitral valve* in the left heart) that either allow or prevent the blood transfer from the atria to the ventricles depending on their configuration (open or closed, respectively): see Figure 4.1. In particular, these valves open when the atrial pressure is higher than the ventricular pressure and close as soon as the blood flow rate becomes negative, that is, when blood flow, which normally goes from the atrium to the ventricle, comes back into the atrium. In the

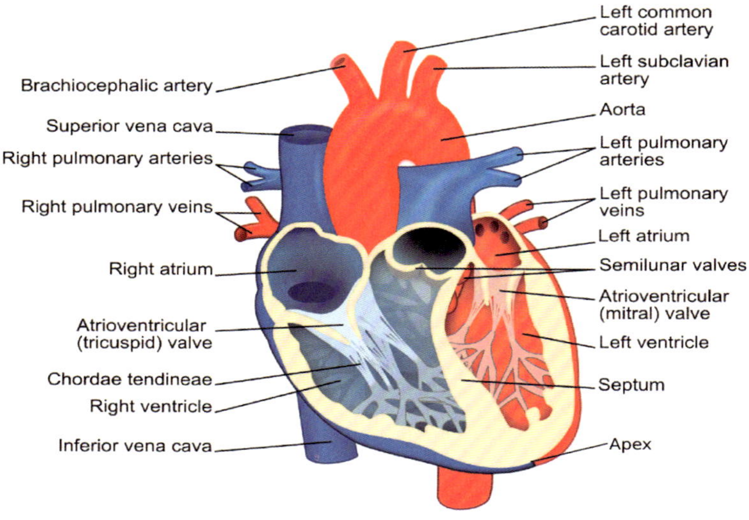


Figure 4.1 Schematic representation of the heart.

latter configuration, the blood flow rate starts to become negative; that is, the blood flow, which normally goes from the atrium to the ventricle, comes back into the atrium; however, this backflow is not significant in physiological conditions as the valves rapidly close. The *papillary muscles*, located in the ventricles, attach to the cusps of these atrioventricular valves via the *chordae tendineae*, preventing their inversion (prolapse) during closure.

All four chambers are connected to the circulatory system: the left ventricle through the aorta, the right ventricle through the pulmonary artery, the left atrium through the *pulmonary veins*, and the right atrium through the *superior* and *inferior venae cavae*. The ventricles are separated from the circulatory system by two further valves, the *aortic valve* on the left side and the *pulmonary valve* on the right side, whose opening/closure mechanism is similar to that of the atrioventricular valves; that is, they open when the pressure is higher in the ventricle with respect to the corresponding connected artery, whereas they close when the pressure jump across the valve reverses, thus preventing the blood flow rate from becoming negative (*i.e.* going from the artery to the ventricle). No valves are located between the atria and the corresponding terminal veins.

The heart wall is made up of three layers: the internal thin *endocardium*, the relatively thick muscular *myocardium* and the external thin *epicardium*. The myocardium of the left ventricle is almost twice as thick as that of the right ventricle. However, the walls of the atria are (much) less "muscular" and significantly thinner than those of the ventricles. The epicardium is surrounded by the *pericardium*, a serous membrane that isolates the heart from the closest organs, facilitating its movements.

## 4.2 The cardiac cycle

The main purpose of the heart is to pump blood in the circulatory system through the aorta and the pulmonary artery. To achieve this goal, the heart needs to exceed the resistance in the arteries where blood has pressure values of about 70 mmHg in the aorta and 10 mmHg in the pulmonary artery; these values are dependent, among other factors, on the reaction of the elastic vessel wall to the deformation induced by blood inside. Moreover, the heart supplies blood with the energy needed to reach the microvasculature in the peripheral areas of the body and the lungs. The total work done by the heart per heartbeat can be quantified as

$$W = Q\,\Delta P + \frac{1}{2}\,m\,v^2,$$

where $Q$ and $m$ are the blood flow rate and the blood mass ejected, $v$ is the blood velocity in the aorta or the pulmonary artery and $\Delta P = P - P_0$, with $P$ being the arterial blood pressure in either the aorta or the pulmonary artery and $P_0$ the reference pressure in the corresponding heart chamber. The above quantification of the cardiac work can be referred to either the left or right hearts. The kinetic component $\frac{1}{2}\,m\,v^2$ of the work $W$ is quite negligible with respect to the potential component $Q\,\Delta P$ (about 2% for the left heart and about 5% for the right heart), although it could become more relevant (up to 25%) under physical effort. The flow rate $Q$ in normal conditions is about $5 \times 10^3$ cm$^3$ min$^{-1}$, so that, assuming 60–90 heartbeats per minute, we have about 55.5–83.3 cm$^3$ of blood expelled at each heartbeat. The energetic requirements for pumping blood are obtained, as in all organs, by the consumption of oxygen that is provided to the heart by blood in the coronary arteries. The efficiency of the heart – that is, the ratio between the energy $W$ and the total energy consumption – is in physiological cases about 25%.

The *cardiac cycle* is the result of the concerted actions of several heart components. The *Wiggers diagram*, named for its developer (Wiggers 1915), is a standard representation used for understanding such cardiac cycles and, more generally, cardiac physiology (Mitchell and Wang 2014). In a Wiggers diagram, which is referred to the left heart as represented in Figure 4.2, the coordinated evolution along the heartbeat of the following quantities is highlighted: blood pressure in the left ventricle, left atrium and aorta;

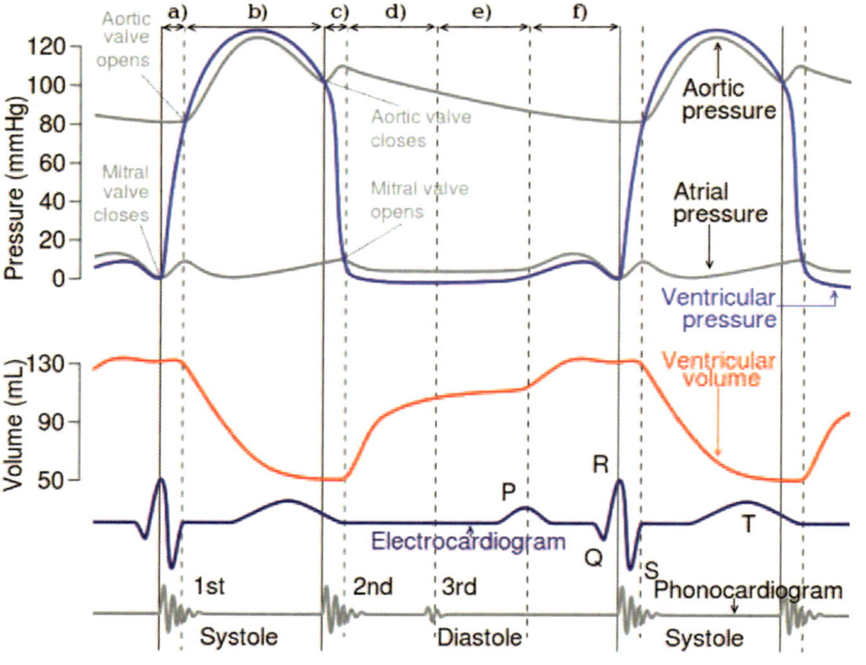


Figure 4.2 Wiggers diagram. The following quantities are displayed vs. time from top to bottom: blood pressure in the left ventricle (blue), atrium and aorta; left ventricular volume (red); electrocardiogram (dark blue); phonocardiogram. The left ventricle phases, systole and diastole, are highlighted: isovolumic contraction (a); ventricular ejection (b); isovolumic relaxation (c); ventricular filling (d–f), comprised of rapid blood inflow (d), diastasis (e) and atrial systole (f).

left ventricular volume; output of the electrocardiogram (ECG); output of the phonocardiogram; arterial flow (optional). Another representation of the cardiac function is provided by the *Pressure–Volume loop*, also known as PV diagram or loop, which illustrates the changes in volume and pressure in an heart chamber along the heartbeat; see Figure 4.3. Specifically, when referred to the left ventricle, the PV loop is the phase diagram of the pressure and volume variations represented in the Wiggers diagram. The PV loop is a useful tool for synthetically assessing the efficiency and functionality of the heart as a blood pump.

The cardiac cycle comprises different phases. For its description (see Figures 4.2 and 4.3), we consider the left heart and start from the situation where the left ventricle is filled with oxygenated blood coming from the left atrium, both the mitral and aortic valves are closed, and the left ventricle has reached its maximum volume.

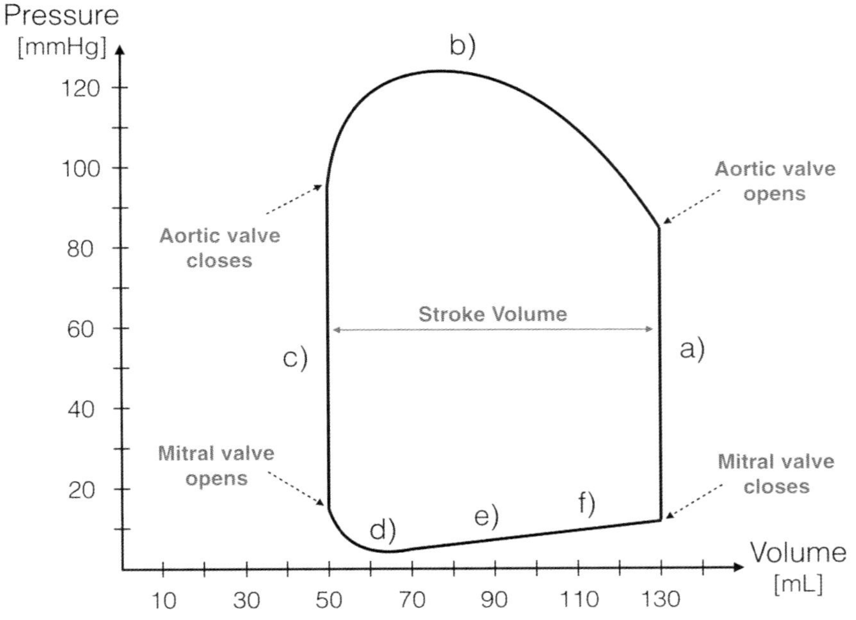


Figure 4.3 Pressure–Volume (PV) loop. The left ventricle phases, systole and diastole, are highlighted: isovolumic contraction (a); ventricular ejection (b); isovolumic relaxation (c); ventricular filling (d–f), comprised of rapid blood inflow (d), diastasis (e) and atrial systole (f). Opening and closing of mitral and aortic valves are indicated.

(a) *Isovolumic contraction.* After the atrial systole, the ventricular active contraction starts. This produces a rapid increase in the ventricular pressure in the chamber, whose valves are both closed. However, the ventricular pressure is still lower than the aortic pressure, so the aortic valve remains closed. Thus, during this phase ($\sim$ 0.05 s), there is a continuous and fast increase of ventricular pressure without appreciable change of blood volume in virtue of blood incompressibility.

(b) *Ventricular ejection.* As soon as the ventricular pressure overcomes the aortic pressure (about 70 mmHg), the aortic valve rapidly opens and blood is ejected into the systemic circulation. Since the ventricular contraction carries on after the valve opens, the ventricular pressure continues to increase. Accordingly, the aortic pressure also increases, in part due to the elastic adaptation of the vessel wall. In the first part of ejection ($\sim$ 0.15–0.20 s), the ventricular volume rapidly decreases until the peak pressure value is reached (about 120 mmHg); at this stage, the blood flow rate and velocity are maximum. Then ($\sim$ 0.15 s), the ventricle volume keeps decreasing, although at a smaller rate; this causes a gradual decrease of ventricular and aortic pressures. In particular, the pressure jump across the aortic valve decreases in magnitude, thus inducing a deceleration of the blood that however continues to flow into the aorta. At this stage, the active contraction of the ventricle stops, minor inertial effects allow some residual blood ejection, and the elastic energy accumulated starts to be released.

(c) *Isovolumic relaxation.* When the ventricular and aortic pressures become closer and hence the pressure jump across the aortic valve is nearly zero, the aortic valve closes. The release of energy of the ventricle continues with both the aortic and mitral valve closed; moreover, relaxation of the muscle starts. In this phase ($\sim 0.05\,\mathrm{s}$), changes in ventricular volume are negligible and the ventricular pressure rapidly drops. After valve closure, the aortic pressure may still increase (albeit slightly), due to the elastic recoil of the closing valve (*dicrotic wave*).

(d–f) *Ventricular filling.* While relaxing, the ventricular pressure becomes smaller that the left atrial pressure and soon reaches its minimum value (about 10 mmHg). The mitral valve opens and blood is allowed to flow into the ventricle from the atrium. This initial stage, (d), of (active) relaxation ($\sim 0.15\,\mathrm{s}$) is quite vigorous, ventricular volume changes rapidly, and suction determines the peak blood flow rate in the chamber ($E$–wave). The second stage, (e), of ventricular relaxation ($\sim 0.15\,\mathrm{s}$) is weaker, volume still increases at a smaller rate, and a limited amount of blood enters the chamber from the atrium; ventricular pressure gradually increases, while the mitral valve typically remains open (even if partial closing may occur). In the last stage, (f), of ventricular filling ($\sim 0.15\,\mathrm{s}$), the left atrium actively contracts and forces oxygenated blood to enter in the chamber. Ventricular volume increases, pressure slightly increases, and the blood flow rate reaches a second, albeit smaller, peak value ($A$–wave); atrial contraction is responsible of about the 20% change in ventricular volume during filling. When pressure values in the left atrium and ventricle become nearly equal, the mitral valve closes.

As anticipated, a meaningful characterization of the heart function can be inferred from the PV loop of Figure 4.3, which is referred to the left ventricle. For example, the *Stroke Volume* (SV) can be calculated from the End Diastolic Volume (EDV) and End Systolic Volume (ESV) as $\mathrm{SV} = \mathrm{EDV} - \mathrm{ESV}$; a typical value of SV is 95 mL. The *Ejection Fraction* (EF) of the left heart, computed as $\mathrm{EF} = 100\,\frac{\mathrm{SV}}{\mathrm{EDV}}$, measures the efficiency of pumping blood into the circulatory system; in a normal heart, EF is typically equal to 67%. Instead, the *Stroke Work* (SW) is the work done by the left ventricle to eject a given volume of blood (SV); specifically, $SW$ is estimated as the product of SV and the mean systolic pressure, and corresponds to the area enclosed in the pressure–volume diagram. The *Cardiac Output* (CO) is the volume of blood pumped by the left ventricle per unit time; specifically, $\text{CO} = \text{SV} \times \text{HR}$, where HR is the *Heart Rate*. As typically $\text{HR} = 60 - -100$ bpm (beats per minute), the cardiac output is in the range $\text{CO} = 4.0$–$8.0\,\text{L/min}$; therefore, in an average lifetime, this amounts to the previously mentioned 1.5 million barrels of blood pumped. Finally, the *Cardiac Work* (CW) – also known as cardiac minute work – represents the power of the ventricle, $\text{CW} = \text{SW} \times \text{HR}$.

Several other information can be extracted from the PV loop. For example, during ventricular ejection, the maximum pressure that can be developed by the left ventricle at any given volume basically follows the End Systolic Pressure–Volume Relationship (ESPVR), which represents the *inotropic* state of the ventricle; that is, roughly speaking, a measure of the contractility of the whole ventricle. A raise of inotropy increases the velocity of muscle fibre shortening, thus enabling an increment in the rate of pressure development and ejection velocity; in turn, this increases the SV and decreases ESV. Instead, ventricular filling basically occurs along the End Diastolic Pressure–Volume Relationship (EDPVR) – also known as the passive filling curve – which measures the ventricle "stiffness" (that is, the reciprocal of its *compliance*).

The right heart undergoes a cycle similar to the one of the left heart and experiences the same phases. The main difference is related to the peak pressure value reached in the right ventricle, which is significantly smaller than in the left ventricle (about 35 mmHg); as a consequence, the stroke work of the right heart is smaller than that of the left. This justifies the thicker myocardium of the left ventricle as higher values of resistances need to be exceeded; as a matter of fact, the right heart is responsible for pumping the de-oxygenated blood to the lungs and acts as "reservoir" of the circulatory system.

## 4.3 Electrical propagation

As seen in the previous section, the main driver of blood ejection in the circulatory system is active ventricular contraction. The heart itself is able to produce the electrical impulse that determines this contraction, triggered by an electric signal – in the form of an electric potential – that propagates

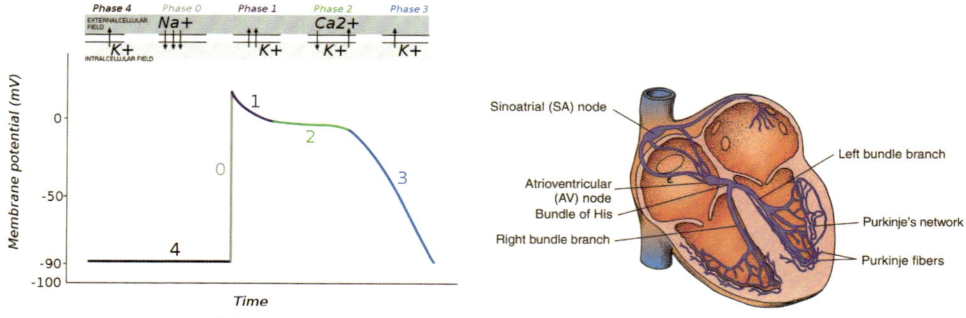


(a) (b)

Figure 4.4 (a) Characteristic action potential of cardiomyocytes and (b) anatomy of the cardiac conduction system (http://medical-dictionary.thefreedictionary.com).

along all the myocardium. This is possible owing to the excitability of the heart cells, the *cardiomyocytes*, which, when suitably stimulated, are able to produce a variation of the voltage – the potential – across the cellular membrane, which is called *transmembrane potential*. At rest, the transmembrane potential is negative ($\sim -90\,\mathrm{mV}$), whereas it reaches a positive value ($\sim 20\,\mathrm{mV}$) in a very short period (about $2\,\mathrm{ms}$) when the cell is stimulated. After this depolarization, a plateau around $0\,\mathrm{mV}$ is observed that corresponds to the refractory period (see Figure 4.4). Then, the repolarization phase starts, which brings the potential back to the rest value allowing for a new excitation (see Figure 4.4(a)). This action potential – the evolution of the transmembrane potential of the cell vs. time as depicted in Figure 4.4(a) – is generated by several ion channels that open and close, and by the resulting currents passing through the membrane. The most important channels are those of calcium, sodium and potassium. In particular, a fast inward sodium current is the main driver of rapid depolarization, a slow inward flux of extra-cellular calcium ions is the main agent behind the characteristic plateau appearing after the depolarization, whereas the outward potassium currents are responsible for the repolarization.

Unlike other cells in the human body, the cardiomyocytes obey the 'all-or-none' law, meaning that if the stimulus is above a suitable threshold, a complete action potential with peak value independent of the stimulus is generated, otherwise no response is provided by the cell. Another characteristic of the heart cells is the presence of a *refractory* period after the generation of an action potential, which inhibits any further stimulus independently of its intensity. Thus, during this period the cell is not excitable at all (*absolute refractory period*, infinite threshold). Afterwards, the cardiomyocytes recover their excitability with a value of the threshold needed to generate the action potential which decreases in time (*relative refractory period*). Finally, once the threshold value reaches its minimum, the cell returns to its excitable state and the threshold remains constant.

The cardiomyocytes act as a syncytium; that is, the stimulation of an individual cell produces the action potential and the corresponding current that results in the excitation of the neighbour cells, and thus of the whole myocardium. This is due to the *gap junctions*, intercellular channels characterized by low resistance and located between cardiomyocytes that permit the electric transmembrane potential to literally travel (propagate) from cell to cell through the whole tissue.

In normal conditions, the electric signal spontaneously originates at the *sinoatrial node*, located in the right atrium at the junction with the superior vena cava. It is made of self-oscillatory cells and is the natural pacemaker of the heart; the sinoatrial node imposes its rhythm on the entire myocardium (*sinusal rhythm*, $\sim$ 60–90 heartbeats per minute). The electric impulse generated by the sinoatrial node propagates through all the cardiomyocytes of the right atrium and then of the left atrium through the interatrial connections. This enables the activation of the atria tissues and drives their contraction. The electric wave propagation is faster along the fibres; that is mainly towards the ventricles ($\sim 200\,\mathrm{cm\ s^{-1}}$), allowing the electric signal to reach the *atrioventricular node*, which is located between the right atrium and the ventricles. When the signal arrives at this node, it is subjected to a delay ($\sim 0.12\,\mathrm{s}$) that allows the complete contraction of the atria before the electric propagation in the ventricles starts. Moreover, the atrioventricular node acts as a filter, which limits (damp) possible high frequencies of the electric signal coming from the atria – as induced, for example by atrial fibrillation – thus "protecting" the normal function of the ventricles. This node, when the sinoatrial node loses automatic function, becomes the leading pacemaker and is able to take on the role of giving the pace to ventricle stimulation. The electrical signal then enters the *bundle of His*, propagating in the ventricles through the two (left and right) *bundle branches* and then through the *Purkinje fibres* (see Figure 4.4(b)). The bundle of His, bundle branches and Purkinje fibres form the *cardiac conduction system* (CCS), a subendocardial specialized network responsible for the fast and coordinated propagation of electrical impulses in the ventricle. The propagation in the CCS is very fast ($\sim 350\,\mathrm{cm\ s^{-1}}$), and its role is to reach the whole endocardium via the dense network of Purkinje fibres, activating it almost simultaneously. Note that the cells of the CCS are dedicated to electrical propagation, so they are not involved in the muscular contraction. The electrical signal then enters the myocardium through the *Purkinje muscle junctions* which are the terminal points of the Purkinje network. At the Purkinje muscle junctions, the signal is subjected to a delay ($\sim 0.01\,\mathrm{s}$) and then propagates into the ventricular muscle towards the epicardium with reduced velocity ($\sim 80\,\mathrm{cm\ s^{-1}}$).

To better understand how the propagation of the electrical potential spreads into the ventricles, we observe that cardiomyocytes are of cylindrical type. This allows us to define the *fibre direction* of the cell, resulting in a macroscopic fibre direction intended as the average cell orientation in a sufficiently small control volume. A transmural variation of the fibre direction is measured between the epicardium and the endocardium ($\sim -70^\circ$ and $\sim 80^\circ$ with respect to the normal direction to the surface, respectively). The fibres are in turn organized into *sheets* of collagen. The velocity of propagation of the electrical potential is about twice as fast along the fibre direction compared to the directions tangential to the fibres.

## 4.4 Mechanisms of contraction and cardiac blood fluid dynamics

The propagation of the electrical signal through the cardiomyocytes is responsible for their contraction (*electromechanical coupling*), resulting in the atrial and, more importantly, ventricular contractions. The characteristic connections between the cardiomyocytes resulting in a syncytium allows coordinated contraction of the heart.

At the cellular level, as discussed in the previous section, there is an inward flux of extra-cellular calcium ions just after the depolarization of the cell. Once in the intracellular space, calcium ions bind to *troponin*, which allows *myosin* heads to bind to *actin* filaments and generate the upstroke, which in turn leads to the cell contraction.

At the macroscopic level, ventricle contraction results in a longitudinal shortening (from apex to base) of about 15% from the diastolic configuration, in a ventricular wall thickening of about 30%, and torsion around the longitudinal axis of about 15°. This is due to the particular fibre orientation of the cardiomyocytes, which also highly influences the mechanical response of the heart.

The overall heart behaviour can be partially explained by the so-called *Frank–Starling law*, stating that an increase (for any reason) of the end diastolic volume (*i.e.* the maximum ventricular expansion) results in an increase in the *stroke volume*; that is, the volume of blood pumped by the left ventricle per heartbeat. This is due to an increase in the load experienced by the cardiomyocytes as a result of the increased volume of blood filling the ventricle (*preload*). This extra stretching of the cells produces a larger number of actin–myosin bridges, resulting in augmented muscle contraction power. It should be noticed, however, that the Frank–Starling law holds true only up to a certain level of increased stretch: for higher values, the contractility power of the heart, and thus the stroke volume, decreases.

As well as the influence of electrical processes on mechanical behaviour, cardiomyocytes also experience mechano-electrical feedback. This is due to the formation of *stretch-activated* ion channels and to changes in cell conductivity by means of stretching the cell, which changes the membrane shape and the distance between gap junctions. This mechanism seems to be of utmost importance in describing the evolution of spiral waves and thus arrhythmias and fibrillation (Trayanova, Li, Eason and Kohl 2004, Keldermann, Nash and Panfilov 2009).

Blood flow in the cardiac chambers exhibits different characteristics with respect to the vascular flow. Peculiar factors are the large and complex deformations of the myocardium and the heart chambers, the complex interaction with valves leading to specific flow patterns, and the higher Reynolds number (about 5000 at peak). These combined effects determine a quite sophisticated blood flow regime whose characterization has not been fully understood yet. As a matter of fact, recent studies indicate that the blood flow regime is neither laminar not fully turbulent, but rather it can be referred as transitional, (Chnafa, Mendez and Nicoud 2014, Mittal *et al.* 2016, Menghini, Dede' and Quarteroni 2018, Tagliabue, Dede' and Quarteroni 2017*a*). While fully developed turbulence may appear and be characteristic of some pathological conditions, this is generally not the case in normal conditions. A typical aspect of blood flow in the left ventricle is the formation of the so-called vortex ring in the long axis plane corresponding to the E-wave; that is, at the diastolic peak of the flow. Moreover, the asymmetry of the mitral valve leaflets forces the blood flow jet to impinge on the posterior wall (Charonko *et al.* 2013, Seo *et al.* 2014); as a result, the interaction of this vortex ring with the ventricular wall gives rise to a complex flow pattern and to the generation of smaller vortex structures. These latter allow mixing the blood in the ventricular cavity and, in normal conditions, take on the role of preventing the formation of blood clots.

Complex vortex structures can also be observed in the left atrium due to the blood flow coming from the pulmonary veins and the geometrical features of this chamber (Mittal *et al.* 2016, Menghini, Dede', Forti and Quarteroni 2017).

## 4.5 A brief summary of heart diseases

The principal heart diseases (cardiopathies) are *ischaemic cardiopathy*, the *cardiomyopathies*, *hypertensive cardiopathy* and *valvular pathologies*.

Ischaemic cardiopathy is the most important in terms of frequency and clinical impact. It is caused by a reduced coronary flow rate (due to atherosclerosis of coronary arteries) with consequent malnutrition of the myocardium. When, due to coronary occlusion, a decrease in oxygen supply is abrupt, long-lasting and total, an *infarct of the myocardium* occurs. This is the most classical event of ischaemic cardiopathy, resulting in necrosis of cardiomyocytes and leading, at the end of the process, to the formation of a *scar*.

In *dilated cardiomyopathy* the ventricle wall becomes thinner due to the partial replacement of cardiomyocytes with fibrosis and small scars, leading to dilatation of the ventricle. In this respect, the increment of the ventricular volume also has the effect of perturbing the normal blood flow patterns and, eventually, of increasing the residence time of red blood cells in the chamber. In turn, the increment of volume increases the risk of generating blood cloths in the ventricle, near the apex. In *hypertrophic cardiomyopathy* the ventricular wall thickens, with a consequent increase in ventricular blood pressure resulting in decreased filling of the ventricle. As in all cases of ventricular hypertrophy, this produces malnutrition of the myocardium, since the amount of blood supplied by the coronary arteries remains unchanged. Moreover, in this specific hypertrophic cardiomyopathy, the orientation of the fibres is not coordinated as in normal conditions (this is called *electrical disarray*).

In hypertensive cardiopathy there is an increase in blood pressure, resulting in increased work needed by the heart to pump blood, leading again to thickening of the myocardial wall and to malnutrition of the myocardium.

The main valvular pathologies are *stenosis* and *insufficiency*. In aortic valve stenosis, narrowing of the maximum opening of the aortic valve causes the heart to require increased work to pump blood into the aorta properly, again resulting in thickening of the myocardial wall and malnutrition. In mitral valve stenosis, there is an increase in the pressure of the left atrium and in the pulmonary circulation, with consequences for the right heart. Aortic and mitral valve insufficiency is due to the partial reversal of flow (going from the aorta to the left ventricle in aortic insufficiency, and from the left ventricle to the left atrium in mitral insufficiency), which occurs as a consequence of inadequate closure of the valve. In this case the heart dilates in order to supply this retrograde flow, resulting in an increase in its contraction power according to the Frank–Starling law. However, sooner or later the diastolic cell stretching overcomes the threshold of validity of the Frank–Starling law, resulting in decreased contractile power.

The two main events, possibly fatal, that the heart may encounter as a consequence of these cardiopathies are *cardiac arrest*, due to *ventricular fibrillation*, and *heart failure*.

In ventricular fibrillation, the cardiomyocytes are not excited in a coordinated way and thus do not contract homogeneously; instead, groups of cells contract continuously whereas other groups relax. This chaotic excitation, if the fibrillation continues, inhibits the normal functioning of the heart pump, which is no longer able to pump the blood around the circulatory system regularly, leading finally to death. All the cardiopathies described above could yield altered electrical properties (*i.e.* velocity of conduction and refractoriness), which could lead to ventricular fibrillation. For example, in a myocardial infarct, the arrhythmogenic substrate is formed by a matrix of healthy cardiomyocytes, necrotic cardiomyocytes and scars, whereas in hypertrophic cardiomyopathy it is provided by the electrical disarray.

When the blood pumped by the heart at each heartbeat is less than the amount required by the body (but not absent, as in ventricular fibrillation), on the one hand the heart increases its frequency so as to guarantee that the blood ejected per minute (*cardiac output*) is almost normal, and on the other hand it increases its diastolic filling to increase the stroke volume. However, the increase in frequency (*tachycardia*) is energetically disadvantageous for the heart, and possible excessive diastolic cell stretching leads to the loss of validity of the Frank–Starling law. When these two compensating mechanisms are no longer effective, cardiac output dramatically decreases, leading to heart failure. In the absence of other causes of death (cardiac arrest or death for non-cardiac reasons), all the cardiopathies described above will sooner or later lead to heart failure.

# 5

# An insight into cardiac data

As discussed in Chapter 2, the use of patient-specific data is needed for mathematical and numerical modelling if we are aiming for personalized understanding of biophysical processes and to support clinicians in medical decisions. This also holds true for heart modelling. The latter accounts for several processes that are intimately coupled: electrical propagation, mechanical activation at the cellular level, mechanical contraction and relaxation (macroscopic at the tissue level), blood fluid dynamics, and valves dynamics. The first three processes occur in the cardiac tissue (here called the muscle region), blood fluid dynamics occurs in the four hollow regions (chambers) delimited by the endocardium, whereas valves dynamics concerns the valves leaflets. As done in Chapter 2 for the circulatory system, in what follows we briefly discuss how to obtain geometric, boundary and biological cardiac data.

## 5.1 Cardiac geometric data

Let us set aside for the moment the problem of valve dynamics. Referring to Figure 5.1, we need to build two computational domains: the muscle region $\Omega_{\mathrm{mus}}$, delimited by the external surface of the epicardium $\Sigma_{\mathrm{epi}}$ and by the internal surface of the endocardium $\Sigma_{\mathrm{endo}}$, and the cavities $\Omega_{\mathrm{cav}}$, referred to below as heart cavities or chambers, delimited by the endocardium. The cavities are easily obtained once the endocardium has been reconstructed, so that in fact the cardiac image reconstruction process relies on identifying the endocardium and epicardium surfaces.

This problem presents several challenges. In the vascular case, the external wall surface is usually obtained by extruding the internal surface under the assumption of constant (or in any case known) wall thickness (see Section 2.1.3). This procedure is unsuitable for the reconstruction of

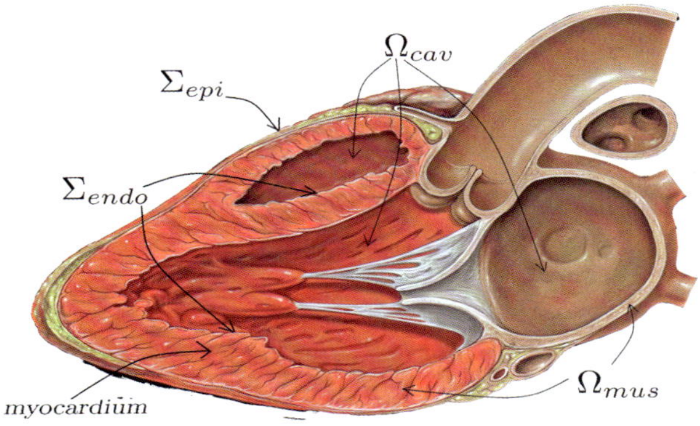


Figure 5.1 Longitudinal section of a complete heart domain.

the myocardium. On the one hand, the thickness changes significantly while moving from apex to base. On the other hand, changes can be dramatic from subject to subject, or from patient to patient. Moreover, due to the large displacements induced by heart motion, a dynamic acquisition procedure (allowing for the acquisition of several frames per heartbeat) is required to obtain a reconstruction of the heart other than at the end-diastolic phase, ideally along the whole heartbeat. The presence of the papillary muscles and wall irregularities given by *trabeculations* (trabecular structures) makes the reconstruction of the endocardium very problematic. Finally, the regions in proximity of the valves – those at the base of the ventricles – are also difficult to acquire through images and then to reconstruct; this is due to the complex morphology of the valve region, the motion of the muscle, and the lack of resolution of the dynamics acquisition procedures.

Let us briefly review the most common radiological procedures for acquisition of cardiac images. As in the vascular case, MRI and CT play a major role. Often, due to heart motion, temporally resolved acquisitions are performed, allowing us to obtain 20–30 frames per heartbeat.

The main interest is in the left ventricle, due to its vital importance, whose pronounced thickness ranges between 6 and 16 mm. The shape of its cavity is often approximated by an ellipsoid. In contrast, the right ventricle and the atria are characterized by a thickness that usually does not reach the spatial resolution of the acquisition technologies, so their reconstruction is hard and, consequently, less studied.

The standard cardiac acquisition plane is orthogonal to the long axis. Blood appears brighter whereas the myocardium and the surrounding tissue are darker: see Figure 5.2. Not all of the slices share the same degree of

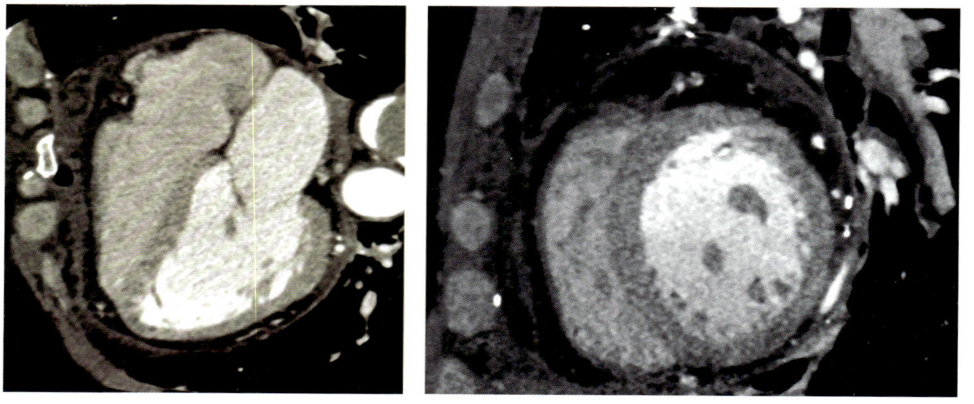

(a) (b)

Figure 5.2 (a) Longitudinal CT slice of the heart. Right atrium (top left), right ventricle (bottom left), left atrium (top right), left ventricle (bottom right). (b) CT slice in the plane orthogonal to the long axis. In both figures, on the right the thick left ventricle myocardium is detectable in darker grey. Data from radiological images provided by Ospedale Sacco, Milan, Italy; courtesy of E. Faggiano.

complexity in their reconstruction. In particular, apical and basal (upward) slice images are more difficult to segment than mid-ventricular slices.

Before the ventricle segmentation starts, a preliminary localization procedure is performed in order to identify a region of interest and reduce the computational effort. This step is usually performed automatically, taking advantage of the movement of the heart on a fixed background: see *e.g.* Cocosco *et al.* (2004). Another automatic heart location is based on extracting rectangular subwindows from the image and computing specific features for them. Then, based on *a priori* chosen class, the subwindows satisfying specific features are recognized as belonging to the heart.

An initial class of ventricle segmentation methods makes use of little (or even no) *a priori* information. Usually in these methods the endocardium is first segmented by means of thresholding (see Chapter 2 and Goshtasby and Turner 1995). Alternatively, *dynamic programming* methods have been considered, where the optimal path in a cost matrix is sought, assigning a low cost to boundaries. Taking advantage of the circular shape of the ventricle, polar coordinates are used and one-dimensional search is performed (Gupta *et al.* 1993). In order to exclude papillary muscles from the segmentation, possible strategies are the computation of the convex hull of the contour (van der Geest, Jansen, Buller and Reiber 1994) or a smoothing of the latter by fitting a parametric curve (Waiter *et al.* 1999). As in the vascular case, deformable models are used for cardiac segmentation (see Section 2). In particular, the functional to be minimized often includes a regularization term to control the smoothness of the reconstructed curves (Pham, Xu and Prince 2000).

Specific automatic methods that have been developed for cardiac image segmentation are based on strong *a priori* information concerning the shape of the ventricles, which is included in the segmentation algorithm by means of statistical models. These strategies are suited to cardiac segmentation because variability in heart shape among patients, as opposed to arteries, is very small in normal conditions. These statistical model-based segmentation strategies rely on identifying an average shape of available geometries forming a training set, and modelling the variability within the latter. This is usually done by means of *principal component analysis* of positions and, if needed, displacements, allowing computation of the eigenvalues and eigenvectors of the covariance matrix related to the training set. These strategies allow automatic segmentation without user intervention, at the expense of needing a training set. For example, deformable models have been extended to this framework by adding a term to the functional to be minimized that penalizes the distance to a reference model (*e.g.* the mean shape of the training set). Another very common statistical model-based strategy is *atlas-guided segmentation*. Given an atlas, that is, an integrated image from multiple segmentations, a registration procedure is performed based on mapping the coordinates of the image under investigation to those of the atlas (Lorenzo-Valdés *et al.* 2004). This transformation is then applied to the atlas obtaining the final segmentation. The registration process could be based on non-rigid transformations that account for elastic deformations. For a recent review of cardiac segmentation methods we refer to Petitjean and Dacher (2011).

Finally, we observe the importance of including the fibre orientation in the reconstructed geometries with respect to modelling electrical propagation and mechanical contraction in the muscle region. Indeed, as discussed in Chapter 4, the conduction velocity of the action potential propagation assumes different values along the fibres than in the tangential direction. Moreover, the stretching ability of the myocardium is facilitated along the fibre direction.

*Diffusion-tensor*-MRI is an MRI technology able to identify fibre orientation, but it is not yet used every day in clinical practice, and it is difficult to apply because of heart movement. See Nagler *et al.* (2015) for a preliminary study of the cardiac fibre estimation using synthetic diffusion-tensor-MRI

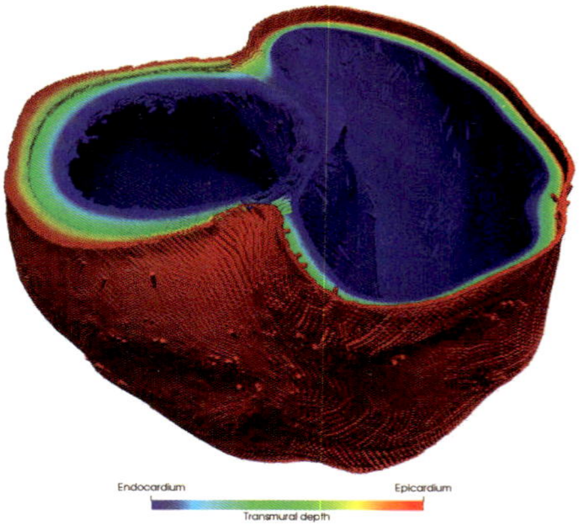


(a)

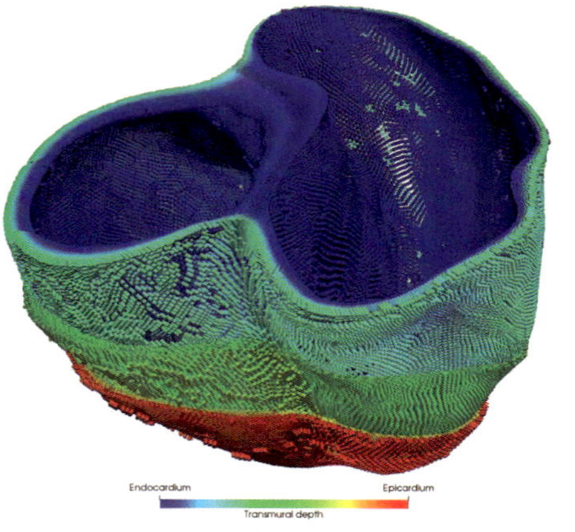


(b)

Figure 5.3 Rule-based construction of the fibres in a bi-ventricular geometry; blue colour represents fibres at the endocardium, while red colour fibres at epicardium. Different layers of fibres through the myocardium thickness are highlighted in (b). Images taken from Azzolin (2018).

datasets. Analytical representations of the fibres, suitably mapped onto the geometry under investigation, have been proposed to supply the lack of information provided by the imaging. For example, Peskin (1989) described fibres as geodesics, whereas Pravdin *et al.* (1989) represented them by means of spiral surfaces. Other strategies are based on computational generation of the fibre orientation to provide a plausible configuration, for example by means of rule-based approaches, that is, based on the solution of the Laplace equation (Bayer, Blake, Plank and Trayanova 2012, Patelli *et al.* 2017, Rossi *et al.* 2014, Wong and Kuhl 2014), or by using the unscented Kalman filter (Nagler, Bertoglio, Gee and Wall 2013). Examples of rule-based approaches for reconstructing fibre fields are reported in Figures 5.3 and 5.4.

Purkinje fibres are not detectable via classical radiological acquisition since their thickness falls below the spatial resolution. For this reason, Abboud, Berenfeld and Sadeh (1991), Sebastian, Zimmerman, Romero and Frangi (2011) and Ijiri *et al.* (2008) proposed exploiting the fractal nature of these fibres to generate a realistic Purkinje network, whereas Vergara *et al.* (2014), Palamara *et al.* (2014) and Palamara, Vergara, Faggiano and Nobile (2015) have personalized such fractal networks to the patient at hand by including patient-specific measurements of the activation times (see Section 5.2 for a description of the latter).

For muscle region mesh generation, the strategies described in Chapter 2

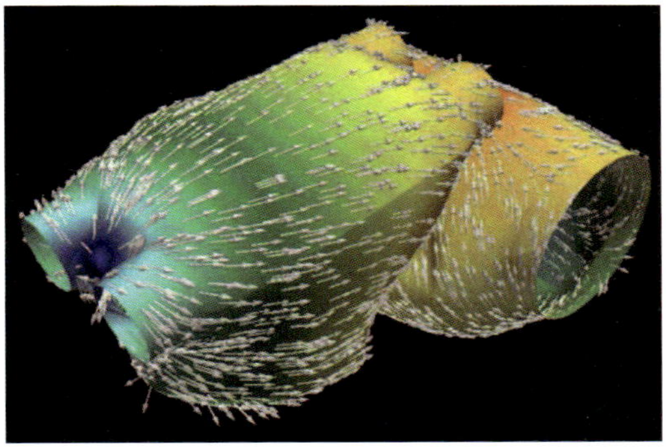

Figure 5.4 Rule-based construction of the fibres on the left and right atria modelled as surfaces; arrows represent the fibre fields, while colours indicate the solution of the Laplace equation used to generate the fibres. Result obtained by means of isogeometric analysis solver; see Pegolotti (2017). Courtesy of L. Pegolotti (EPFL).

can also be applied to cardiac geometries. For ideal ellipsoid geometries, usually considered in numerical experiments for testing the performance of the numerical algorithms, structured hexahedral meshes are often used, exploiting the symmetry of the ventricles around the long axis: see *e.g.* Pavarino, Scacchi and Zampini (2015). However, unstructured meshes composed of tetrahedra have also been considered (Goktepe and Kuhl 2010), in particular for real geometries reconstructed by MRI or CT (see *e.g.* Rossi *et al.* 2014, Wong, Goktepe and Kuhl 2013, Vergara *et al.* 2016), or for the atria (Virag *et al.* 2002). Hybrid unstructured meshes composed of tetrahedra and hexahedra have also been successfully considered (Gurev *et al.* 2015). We notice that for the solution of the mechanical problem in the muscle region, no particular requirements are needed for mesh generation, whereas for the electrical propagation problem, due to the very steep front (about 200 $\mu$m), the required mesh resolution should be at least of the order of 100 $\mu$m in order to spatially resolve this front (Clayton and Panfilov 2008). In view of the numerical solution of the fluid dynamics problem, for mesh generation of the heart chambers, unstructured tetrahedral elements are often considered: see *e.g.* Mittal *et al.* (2016). In this case the mesh resolution needs to be very fine, even smaller than that for CT or MRI technologies ($\simeq 0.5$ mm), in order to model the complex flow structures that arise, particularly in the left atrium and left ventricle.

## 5.2 Cardiac boundary data

The acquisition of boundary data on electrical activation in the muscle region is now possible thanks to specific therapeutic techniques. For example, the NavX system is able to locate accurately any electrode catheter inserted in the heart chambers, providing accurate, real-time recording of the local endocardial electrical activity at a point in contact with the catheter (Eitel *et al.* 2010, Vergara *et al.* 2014). In particular, this allows us to acquire endocardial maps of the activation times, defined as the time at which the action potential in a point reaches an intermediate value between the rest and the plateau potentials. However, this acquisition is performed only for specific therapeutic purposes, such as the ablation of anomalous electrical pathways.

For mechanical problems involving the muscle region, data that are commonly available include the stresses exerted by the blood on the endocardium of the left ventricle and the endocardial and/or epicardial vessel wall displacements. Stresses are indirectly recovered from measurements of aortic pressure (see Section 2.2). This is a good approximation; as a matter of fact the ventricular and circulatory pressures are not the same (thus allowing the acceleration and deceleration of blood) but they are very similar: see Figure 4.2. Heart wall displacements can be obtained from dynamic MRI or CT images, yielding 20–30 frames per heartbeat, providing the position of the endocardium and epicardium at multiple times; see Figure 5.5. After suitable postprocessing, these techniques can provide an estimate of the cardiac wall displacement (and thus velocity) by comparing two consecutive frames. The endocardial wall velocity, thanks to a continuity argument, could also be interpreted as the blood velocity at the interface with the endocardium (Khalafvand, Zhong and Ng 2014, Mittal *et al.* 2016).

Another useful measurement that can be provided quite easily by means of Doppler echocardiographic methods or PC-MRA (see Section 2.2) is the flow rate at the mitral and aortic valve orifices. With PC-MRA technology, measurement of blood velocity is possible in principle at any point of the ventricles and atria chambers.

In Chapter 6 we will see how these data can be used to provide boundary conditions for the different cardiac models we are about to introduce.

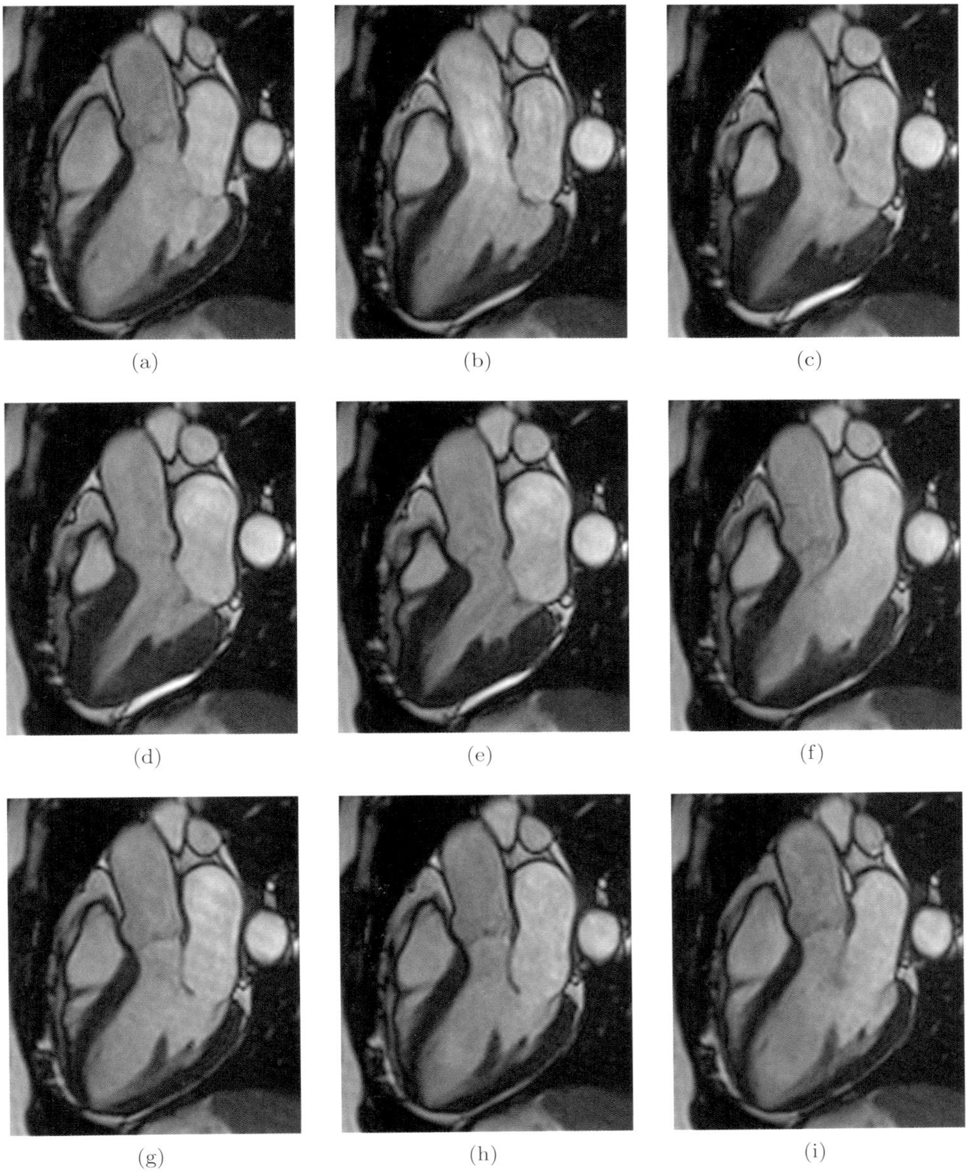


Figure 5.5 Dynamic MRI images: sequence of 9 longitudinal slices of the heart (out of 25); systole (a)–(e) and diastole (f)–(i) are highlighted. The left ventricle with the muscle wall (centre), left atrium (top-right), aortic root and aorta (top-centre), and right heart (mid-left) appear in the images; aortic (left) and mitral (right) valves' leaflets are visible too. Data from radiological images provided by CHUV, Centre Hospitalier Universitaire Vaudois, Lausanne, Switzerland.

### 5.3 Cardiac biological data

The classical *monodomain* and *bidomain* models, widely used to describe the electrical propagation in the muscle region and Purkinje network (see Section 6.1), require the following data: the membrane capacitance per unit area $C$, the membrane surface-to-volume ratio $\chi$, and the conductivities $\sigma$ (see the next section). Their subject-specific acquisition is generally out of reach. An acceptable range of values for the capacitance $C_m$ in the myocardium is 0.8–1.0 $\mu\mathrm{F\,cm^{-2}}$ (Roth 1991, Huiskamp 1998); the capacitance $C_p$ in the Purkinje network is higher ($\sim 1.3\ \mu\mathrm{F\,cm^{-2}}$: Legato 1973). The value of the membrane surface-to-volume ratio in the muscle region $\chi_m$ varies in the range 200–3000 $\mathrm{cm^{-1}}$ (Niederer *et al.* 2011, Potse *et al.* 2006), whereas for the Purkinje network, a measurement in a pig heart gives $\chi_p = 1467\ \mathrm{cm^{-1}}$ (Stankovičová *et al.* 2003). In the myocardium, we need to distinguish between conductivity along the fibre direction (index $f$) and conductivity in the direction of sheets (index $s$). Sometimes, a third direction (orthogonal to sheets) is also considered (if this is the case we will use the index $n$). Moreover, with the bidomain model in mind, we also distinguish between the intra-cellular (index $i$) and extra-cellular (index $e$) conductivities. Following Roth (1997), acceptable ranges used in the numerical experiments are $\sigma_f^i \in (0.17, 0.34)\ \mathrm{S\,m^{-1}}$, $\sigma_s^i \in (0.02, 0.06)\ \mathrm{S\,m^{-1}}$, $\sigma_f^e \in (0.12, 0.62)\ \mathrm{S\,m^{-1}}$, $\sigma_s^e \in (0.08, 0.24)\ \mathrm{S\,m^{-1}}$.

Another classical model used for describing the activation of Purkinje and muscle cells is provided by the *eikonal* equation (see Section 6.1). In this case, one needs to prescribe the conduction velocity $V$ explicitly, unlike the monodomain and bidomain models where this is determined by the conductivity and the membrane capacitance. Acceptable ranges of values of the conduction velocity are $V_f \in (0.6, 1.0)\,\mathrm{m\,s^{-1}}$ (Kerckoffs *et al.* 2003), $V_s \simeq V_f/2$ (Frazier *et al.* 1988), $V_n \simeq V_f/4$ (Clayton *et al.* 2011), and $V_p \in (3.0 - 4.0)\,\mathrm{m\,s^{-1}}$ (Iaizzo 2009), where again index $f$ refers to the direction along the fibres in the muscle region, $s$ to the direction along sheets, and $p$ to the Purkinje network.

These electrical data are barely measurable *in vivo*, so subject-specific measurements are not usually available. Nevertheless, the use of extra data, such as the activation time at the endocardium provided by the NavX system, could be used to estimate some of these parameters by solving a suitable inverse problem; see *e.g.* Sermesant *et al.* (2012) and Vergara *et al.* (2014) for the case of the Purkinje network.

The parameters involved in the cardiac mechanical model depend on the chosen constitutive law. In general, linearization of the stress–strain curves gives the following values for the corresponding time-varying Young's modulus $E$ (Rossi 2014): during a traction/compression test along the fibre direction, we have $E \simeq 20\,\text{kPa}$ during traction at small deformation and during compression, and $E \simeq 1500\,\text{kPa}$ during traction for deformation of about 15%; during traction the material behaves as transversally isotropic, so the stiffness in the two tangential directions (along sheets and orthogonal to fibres and sheets) is the same, whereas during compression the stiffness in the direction of the sheets is higher than that in the direction orthogonal to fibres and sheets. For the Poisson ratio, a value of 0.45 is usually considered.

Regarding the aortic valve leaflets, measurements in canine specimens exhibited low stiffness during systole ($\simeq 240\,\text{kPa}$) and increased stiffness during diastole ($\simeq 5000\,\text{kPa}$). For the mitral valve, different stiffness behaviour is observed for the two leaflets (anterior and posterior). In particular, Kunzelman *et al.* (1993) propose the following values for Young's modulus: for the anterior leaflet, $E = 6200\,\text{kPa}$ and $E = 2100\,\text{kPa}$ in the directions parallel and perpendicular to the annulus, respectively, and for the posterior leaflet, $E = 2300\,\text{kPa}$ and $E = 1900\,\text{kPa}$, respectively.

Physical characteristics of the blood in the heart are, in first instance, very similar to those in the circulatory systems, so its parameters (density and viscosity) are taken in the ranges reported in Section 2.3.

# 6

# Modelling the heart

In this chapter we discuss the main mathematical models introduced so far for describing heart function and the related numerical strategies developed for their solution. In particular, Section 6.1 is devoted to electrical propagation, Section 6.2 to cardiac mechanics and electromechanical coupling, Section 6.3 to ventricular fluid dynamics, Section 6.4 to valve modelling and its interaction with blood fluid dynamics, and finally Section 6.5 to the integration (coupling) of these models.

## 6.1 Cardiac electrical activity

We review in this section the most common mathematical and numerical models used for describing and simulating the physical processes at the basis of the cardiac electrical activity. Among the mathematical models, we consider the bidomain, monodomain and eikonal models for the cardiac tissue, together with the most common cardiac cell models.

### *6.1.1 The bidomain model*

As observed in Section 4.3, the electrical activation of the heart is the result of two processes: at the microscopic scales, the generation of ionic currents through the cellular membrane producing a local action potential, and at the macroscopic scales, the propagation of the action potential from cell to cell allowed by the presence of the gap junctions. The former is a discrete process, in the sense that there is a delay between the depolarization of a cardiomyocyte and its neighbours, whereas the latter can be assimilated to a smooth process (Durrer *et al.* 1970).

At the macroscopic level, the propagation of the electric signal, in the form of a *trans-membrane potential,* is described by means of partial differential

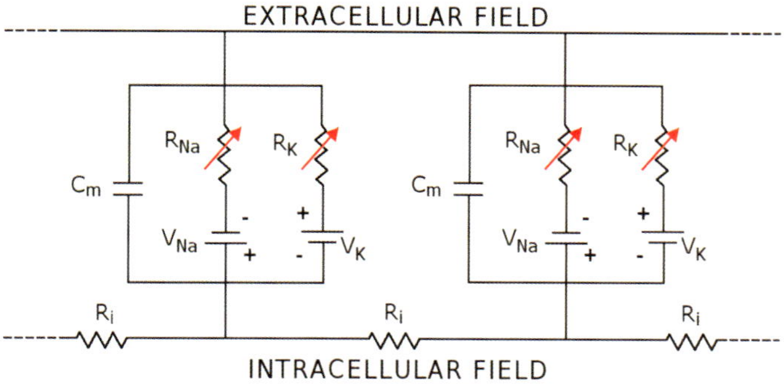


Figure 6.1 Electrical circuit for the sequence of two cardiac cells. Each consists of a capacitor and a series of resistances, one for each ionic current (here only sodium and potassium ionic channels are depicted). In the intracellular region, two adjacent cells are connected by a resistance representing a gap junction. However, the latter is not explicitly modelled at the macroscopic scales:instead its effect is hidden in the conductivity tensor (see the text).

equations, suitably coupled with ordinary differential equations modelling the ionic currents in the cells. In particular, the single membrane cell can be modelled as a capacitor separating charges that accumulate at its *intracellular* and *extracellular* surfaces. Moreover, as observed in Chapter 4, ionic currents cross the membrane through channels which open and close during excitation. A suitable model can therefore be expressed via a simple electric circuit as that depicted in Figure 6.1, for which

$$I_m = \chi_m \left( C_m \frac{\partial V_m}{\partial t} + I_{\text{ion}} \right),$$

where $I_m$ is the membrane current per unit volume, $C_m$ is the membrane capacitance, $\chi_m$ is the surface area-to-volume ratio (see Section 5.3 for a quantification of the latter two), $V_m(t, \boldsymbol{x})$ is the trans-membrane potential, and $I_{\text{ion}}(t, \boldsymbol{x})$ are the ionic currents. Due to the conservation of current and charge, this current should equal the divergence of both the intracellular and extracellular current fluxes $\boldsymbol{j}_i$ and $\boldsymbol{j}_e$:

$$\nabla \cdot \boldsymbol{j}_i = -I_m, \quad \nabla \cdot \boldsymbol{j}_e = I_m. \tag{6.1}$$

Ohm's law in the intracellular and extracellular regions gives

$$\boldsymbol{j}_i = -\boldsymbol{\Sigma}_i \nabla \phi_i, \quad \boldsymbol{j}_e = -\boldsymbol{\Sigma}_e \nabla \phi_e, \tag{6.2}$$

where $\boldsymbol{\Sigma}_i, \boldsymbol{\Sigma}_e$ are the conductivity tensors and $\phi_i(t, \boldsymbol{x}), \phi_e(t, \boldsymbol{x})$ are the intracellular and extracellular potentials, so that

$$V_m = \phi_i - \phi_e. \tag{6.3}$$

Note that, due to the anisotropy of the cardiac tissue induced by the presence of fibres and sheets, each conductivity tensor is in general expressed in terms of three scalar quantities representing the conductivities along the fibre direction $\boldsymbol{a}_f(\boldsymbol{x})$, the direction $\boldsymbol{a}_s(\boldsymbol{x})$ orthogonal to $\boldsymbol{a}_f$ and tangential to sheets, and the direction $\boldsymbol{a}_n(\boldsymbol{x})$ orthogonal to sheets; that is,

$$\boldsymbol{\Sigma}_\beta = \sigma_f^\beta \boldsymbol{a}_f \boldsymbol{a}_f^{\mathrm{T}} + \sigma_s^\beta \boldsymbol{a}_s \boldsymbol{a}_s^{\mathrm{T}} + \sigma_n^\beta \boldsymbol{a}_n \boldsymbol{a}_n^{\mathrm{T}}, \quad \beta = i, e. \tag{6.4}$$

Putting together all the above equations and using a homogenization procedure (see *e.g.* Colli Franzone *et al.* 2014 for a rigorous derivation), we obtain for each $t > 0$ the following system of two partial differential equations called the *parabolic–parabolic* (PP) *formulation of the bidomain* equations:

$$\chi_m C_m \frac{\partial V_m}{\partial t} - \nabla \cdot (\boldsymbol{\Sigma}_i \nabla \phi_i) + \chi_m I_{\mathrm{ion}} = I_i^{\mathrm{ext}} \quad \text{in } \Omega_{\mathrm{mus}}, \tag{6.5a}$$

$$-\chi_m C_m \frac{\partial V_m}{\partial t} - \nabla \cdot (\boldsymbol{\Sigma}_e \nabla \phi_e) - \chi_m I_{\mathrm{ion}} = -I_e^{\mathrm{ext}} \quad \text{in } \Omega_{\mathrm{mus}}, \tag{6.5b}$$

where $I_i^{\mathrm{ext}}(t, \boldsymbol{x})$, $I_e^{\mathrm{ext}}(t, \boldsymbol{x})$ are applied currents per unit volume.

Thanks to (6.1), $\nabla \cdot (\boldsymbol{j}_i + \boldsymbol{j}_e) = 0$; thus, using (6.2) and (6.3), we obtain the following *parabolic–elliptic* (PE) *formulation of the bidomain* equations:

$$\chi_m C_m \frac{\partial V_m}{\partial t} - \nabla \cdot (\boldsymbol{\Sigma}_i (\nabla \phi_e + \nabla V_m)) + \chi_m I_{\mathrm{ion}} = I_i^{\mathrm{ext}} \quad \text{in } \Omega_{\mathrm{mus}}, \tag{6.6a}$$

$$-\nabla \cdot (\boldsymbol{\Sigma}_i \nabla V_m) - \nabla \cdot ((\boldsymbol{\Sigma}_i + \boldsymbol{\Sigma}_e) \nabla \phi_e) = I_i^{\mathrm{ext}} - I_e^{\mathrm{ext}} \quad \text{in } \Omega_{\mathrm{mus}}. \tag{6.6b}$$

Due to the homogenization procedure, the effect of the gap junctions, which at the cellular level contributes to determining the current flux $\boldsymbol{j}_i$, is hidden in the conductivity tensor $\boldsymbol{\Sigma}_i$. We also notice that both bidomain problems (6.5) and (6.6) hold in the entire computational domain $\Omega_{\mathrm{mus}}$ given by the union of the myocardium with the endocardium and epicardium: see Figures 5.1 and 6.2. Indeed, again because of the homogenization procedure, no geometric distinction is made between the intracellular and extracellular regions, even if their different functionality is maintained in the bidomain models.

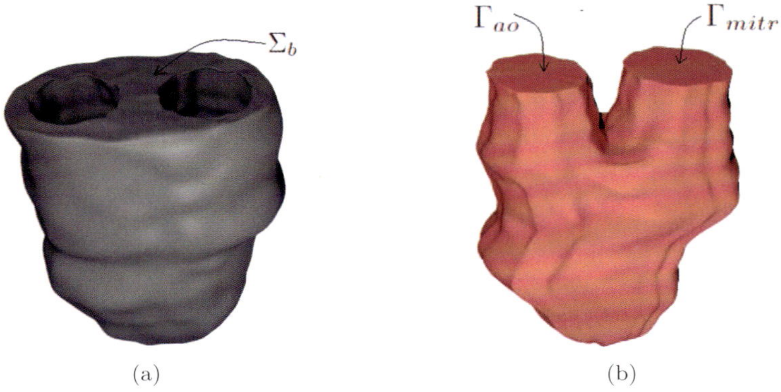


Figure 6.2 (a) Left ventricular myocardial domain obtained by the cut at the base (corresponding to $\Sigma_b$), and (b) corresponding fluid cavity domain.

### 6.1.2 Cardiac cell models

In order to close equations (6.5) and (6.6), we need to provide a model for the ionic current $I_{\text{ion}}$. In what follows we briefly describe three families of models, featuring different levels of complexity and accuracy.

The first family, the so-called *reduced* (phenomenological) *ionic models*, only provide a description of the action potential and disregard sub-cellular processes. Specifically, we have for each cell:

$$I_{\text{ion}} = f(V_m, \boldsymbol{w}), \tag{6.7a}$$

$$\frac{d\boldsymbol{w}}{dt} = \boldsymbol{g}_w(V_m, \boldsymbol{w}), \tag{6.7b}$$

where $f, \boldsymbol{g}_w$ are suitable functions, while $\boldsymbol{w} : [0, T] \to \mathbb{R}^M$ collects the so-called *gating variables* which represent the percentage of open channels per unit area of the membrane. If a cell is ideally attributed to each point $\mathbf{x} \in \Omega_{mus}$, then the function $\boldsymbol{w}$ reads $\boldsymbol{w} : [0, T] \times \Omega_{\text{mus}} \to \mathbb{R}^M$. The most celebrated reduced model for ventricular cells is the *FitzHugh–Nagumo* model (FitzHugh 1961), where

$$f(V_m, w) = -kV_m(V_m - a)(V_m - 1) - w, \qquad g_w(V_m, w) = \epsilon(V_m - \gamma w),$$

for suitable constant parameters $k$, $a$, $\gamma$. In this case the gating variable $w$ in fact plays the role of a *recovery* function, which allows us to model the refractoriness of cells. Other, more sophisticated ventricular cell models of this family include the *Rogers–McCulloch* model (Rogers and McCulloch 1994), the *Aliev–Panfilov* model (Aliev and Panfilov 1996), the *Fenton–Karma* model (Fenton and Karma 1998) and the *Bueno-Orovio* model (Bueno-

Orovio, Cherry and Fenton 2008). Like FitzHugh–Nagumo, the first two models are characterized by the dynamics of one gating variable and by a cubic non-linear expression of the ionic current. In contrast, the Fenton–Karma model and its Bueno-Orovio variant, specifically applied to human ventricular cells, include two and three gating variables, respectively, and a more complex non-linearity in the ionic current expression. These simple models are very appealing, especially because their parameters have a direct physical interpretation, such as the action potential duration, allowing easy setting of the model properties. For example, the Aliev–Panfilov model has been used successfully in the initial simulations of ventricular fibrillation in a real geometry (Panfilov 1999). However, they are not able to describe any process occurring at the level of the ionic channels or the cell, so they are recommended when one is only interested in electric activity of the heart.

The second family of ventricular cell models we consider is that of the so-called *first-generation* models. Unlike reduced models, which express the ionic current by means of the sole function $f$, they allow explicit description of the kinetics of different ionic currents by using several gating variables. They are given by

$$I_{\text{ion}} = \sum_{k=1}^{N} I_k(V_m, \boldsymbol{w}), \quad I_k = G_k \left( \prod_{j=1}^{M} w_j^{p_{j_k}} \right) (V_m - V_k), \quad \frac{d\boldsymbol{w}}{dt} = \boldsymbol{g}_w(V_m, \boldsymbol{w}),$$

where $N$ is the total number of ionic currents, $M$ is the total number of gating variables, $V_k$ is the Nernst potential of the $k$th ion (a constant value corresponding to the thermodynamic equilibrium of the ion at hand), $I_k$ is the current related to the $k$th ion, $p_{j_k}$ accounts for the influence of the $j$th gating variable on the $k$th ionic current (possibly vanishing) and $G_k$ is the maximal conductance of the $k$th ion. The $M$ components of $\boldsymbol{g}$ usually have the expression

$$g_{w,j} = (w_j^{\infty}(V_m) - w_j)/\tau_j(V_m),$$

where $w_j^{\infty}$ is the equilibrium state and $\tau_j$ the characteristic time constant. The most famous model of this family, the *Hodgkin–Huxley* (HH) model (Hodgkin and Huxley 1952), depends on three ionic currents, namely the sodium, potassium and leakage currents, and three gating variables:

$$I_{Na} = G_{Na} w_1^3 w_2 (V_m - V_{Na}), \quad I_K = G_K w_3^4 (V_m - V_K), \quad I_L = G_L(V_M - V_L).$$

Although introduced to describe the action potentials in nerves, the HH model inspired all the following models introduced specifically for the ventricle. Among these, we cite the *Beeler–Reuter* model (Beeler and Reuter 1977), the *Luo–Rudy I* model (Luo and Rudy 1991) and the *ten Tusscher–Panfilov* model (ten Tusscher and Panfilov 2006). These models have been widely used to study specific features of the ventricular electrical activation, such as re-entry and fibrillation (Xie *et al.* 2004).

Finally, we mention the family of *second-generation* ventricular cell models, such as the *Luo–Rudy dynamic* model (Luo and Rudy 1994*a*, 1994*b*), which, unlike first-generation models, provide a detailed description of ion concentration variables $\boldsymbol{c}$ and of many processes allowing for the study of channelopathies and drug action, for example. However, due to their increased complexity, the computational time required is huge for a complete heart model, and tuning of parameters is often very demanding. We refer to Clayton and Panfilov (2008) for a discussion of second-generation models and Rudy and Silva (2006) for a general review of cardiac cell models.

Although most research has focussed on ventricular cell models like those mentioned above, specific models have also been introduced for the atrial cells (*e.g.* Courtemanche, Ramirez and Nattel 1998 and Hilgemann and Noble 1987) and sinoatrial node cells (*e.g.* DiFrancesco 1993, Fabbri, Fantini, Wilders and Severi 2017 and Yanagihara, Noma and Irisawa 1980).

All the cardiac cell models belonging to the three families described above, used in combination with the bidomain problem (6.5) or (6.6), lead to a system of two PDEs coupled with two systems of ODEs; that is, the equations for the gating variables and ion concentrations at each point $\boldsymbol{x}$. The general form of this coupled problem is as follows (we only describe the PP case in detail). At each time $t > 0$, find the potentials $V_M$, $\phi_i$ and $\phi_e$, the gating variable $\boldsymbol{w}$ and the ion concentrations $\boldsymbol{c}$ such that, for each $t > 0$,

$$\chi_m C_m \frac{\partial V_m}{\partial t} - \nabla \cdot (\boldsymbol{\Sigma}_i \nabla \phi_i) + \chi_m I_{\text{ion}}(V_m, \boldsymbol{w}, \boldsymbol{c}) = I_i^{\text{ext}} \quad \text{in } \Omega_{\text{mus}}, \tag{6.9a}$$

$$-\chi_m C_m \frac{\partial V_m}{\partial t} - \nabla \cdot (\boldsymbol{\Sigma}_e \nabla \phi_e) - \chi_m I_{\text{ion}}(V_m, \boldsymbol{w}, \boldsymbol{c}) = -I_e^{\text{ext}} \quad \text{in } \Omega_{\text{mus}}, \tag{6.9b}$$

$$I_{\text{ion}} = \sum_{k=1}^{N} I_k(V_m, \boldsymbol{w}, \boldsymbol{c}) \quad \text{in } \Omega_{\text{mus}}, \tag{6.9c}$$

$$I_k = G_k \left( \prod_{j=1}^{M} w_j^{p_{j_k}} \right) (V_m - V_k(\boldsymbol{c})) \quad \text{in } \Omega_{\text{mus}}, \tag{6.9d}$$

$$\frac{\partial \boldsymbol{w}}{\partial t} = \boldsymbol{g}_w(V_m, \boldsymbol{w}) \quad \text{in } \Omega_{\text{mus}}, \tag{6.9e}$$

$$\frac{\partial \boldsymbol{c}}{\partial t} = \boldsymbol{g}_c(V_m, \boldsymbol{w}, \boldsymbol{c}) \quad \text{in } \Omega_{\text{mus}}, \tag{6.9f}$$

together with suitable initial and boundary conditions; by using the notation introduced above for the reduced and first-generation models, $\boldsymbol{c} : [0,T] \times \Omega_{\text{mus}} \to \mathbb{R}^S$ collects the $S$ ionic concentration variables and $\boldsymbol{g}_c$ is a suitable function: see *e.g.* Colli Franzone *et al.* (2014). We observe, in general, the dependence of the Nernst potential $V_k$ on the variable $\boldsymbol{c}$. Well-posedness results of the previous coupled problem are provided in Colli Franzone and Savaré (2002), where the existence and uniqueness of the solution of the PP formulation coupled with the FitzHugh–Nagumo model is proved, and in Bourgault, Coudière and Pierre (2006), where a Faedo–Galerkin technique is applied to the PE formulation coupled with a general first-generation cell model.

The ODE systems modelling the gating variables and the ionic concentration variables are in general stiff, since the Jacobians $\partial \boldsymbol{g}_w / \partial \boldsymbol{w}$ and $\partial \boldsymbol{g}_c / \partial \boldsymbol{c}$ associated with the cardiac cell models exhibit a wide range of eigenvalues and hence a large stiffness ratio.

For each $t > 0$, the weak formulation of the bidomain model (6.9) together with homogeneous Neumann conditions and initial conditions (see Section 6.1.4) reads as follows. Given $I_i^{\text{ext}}(t)$ and $I_e^{\text{ext}}(t) \in L^2(\Omega_{\text{mus}})$, find $V_m(t), \phi_e(t), \phi_i(t) \in H^1(\Omega_{\text{mus}})$, $\boldsymbol{w} \in [L^2(\Omega_{\text{mus}})]^M$ and $\boldsymbol{c} \in [L^2(\Omega_{\text{mus}})]^S$ such that

$$\begin{aligned} \chi_m C_m \int_{\Omega_{\text{mus}}} \frac{\partial V_m}{\partial t} z \,\mathrm{d}\omega &+ \int_{\Omega_{\text{mus}}} \boldsymbol{\Sigma}_i \nabla \phi_i \cdot \nabla z \,\mathrm{d}\omega \\ &+ \chi_m \int_{\Omega_{\text{mus}}} I_{\text{ion}}(V_m, \boldsymbol{w}, \boldsymbol{c}) z \,\mathrm{d}\omega = \int_{\Omega_{\text{mus}}} I_i^{\text{ext}} z \,\mathrm{d}\omega, \qquad (6.10\text{a}) \\ - \chi_m C_m \int_{\Omega_{\text{mus}}} \frac{\partial V_m}{\partial t} z \,\mathrm{d}\omega &+ \int_{\Omega_{\text{mus}}} \boldsymbol{\Sigma}_e \nabla \phi_e \cdot \nabla z \,\mathrm{d}\omega \\ &- \chi_m \int_{\Omega_{\text{mus}}} I_{\text{ion}}(V_m, \boldsymbol{w}, \boldsymbol{c}) z \,\mathrm{d}\omega = - \int_{\Omega_{\text{mus}}} I_e^{\text{ext}} z \,\mathrm{d}\omega, \qquad (6.10\text{b}) \\ \int_{\Omega_{\text{mus}}} \frac{\partial \boldsymbol{w}}{\partial t} \cdot \boldsymbol{y} \,\mathrm{d}\omega &= \int_{\Omega_{\text{mus}}} \boldsymbol{g}(V_m, \boldsymbol{w}) \cdot \boldsymbol{y} \,\mathrm{d}\omega, \qquad (6.10\text{c}) \\ \int_{\Omega_{\text{mus}}} \frac{\partial \boldsymbol{c}}{\partial t} \cdot \boldsymbol{\zeta} \,\mathrm{d}\omega &= \int_{\Omega_{\text{mus}}} \boldsymbol{g}_c(V_m, \boldsymbol{w}, \boldsymbol{c}) \cdot \boldsymbol{\zeta} \,\mathrm{d}\omega, \qquad (6.10\text{d}) \end{aligned}$$

for all $z \in H^1(\Omega_{\text{mus}})$, $\boldsymbol{y} \in [L^2(\Omega_{\text{mus}})]^M$ and $\boldsymbol{\zeta} \in [L^2(\Omega_{\text{mus}})]^S$, together with (6.9c, 6.9d).

### *6.1.3 Reduced continuous models: the monodomain and eikonal equations*

The bidomain models (6.5) and (6.6) are physically meaningful and rich enough to permit a very detailed description of a wide range of physiological and pathological scenarios; however, they are also very complex for which their analyses and simulations are quite involved.

The first step in reducing the complexity of the bidomain models is based on an assumption of proportionality between the intracellular and extracellular conductivities; that is, $\mathbf{\Sigma}_e = \xi \mathbf{\Sigma}_i$ for a suitable constant $\xi$. Substituting this relation in (6.6b), eliminating $\mathbf{\Sigma}_e$ and substituting the corresponding relation for $\mathbf{\Sigma}_i$ in (6.6a), we obtain the following *monodomain* equation. For each $t > 0$, find the trans-membrane potential $V_m$ such that

$$\chi_m C_m \frac{\partial V_m}{\partial t} - \nabla \cdot (\mathbf{\Sigma} \nabla V_m) + \chi_m I_{\text{ion}} = I^{\text{ext}} \quad \text{in } \Omega_{\text{mus}}, \tag{6.11}$$

where

$$\mathbf{\Sigma} = \frac{\xi}{1+\xi} \mathbf{\Sigma}_i \tag{6.12}$$

is the effective conductivity and

$$I^{\text{ext}} = \frac{\xi I_i^{\text{ext}} + I_e^{\text{ext}}}{1+\xi}.$$

Again, a ventricular cell model is needed to provide the ionic current $I_{\text{ion}}$. The same models discussed above for the coupling with the bidomain problem are used in combination with the monodomain problem too. Once the trans-membrane potential $V_m$ has been computed, the extracellular potential $\phi_e$ may be computed as a postprocessing by solving the elliptic problem (6.6b).

For each $t > 0$, the weak formulation of the monodomain problem (6.11) together with homogeneous Neumann conditions and initial conditions (see Section 6.1.4) reads as follows. Given $I^{\text{ext}}(t) \in L^2(\Omega_{\text{mus}})$, find $V_m(t) \in H^1(\Omega_{\text{mus}})$, $\boldsymbol{w} \in [L^2(\Omega_{\text{mus}})]^M$ and $\boldsymbol{c} \in [L^2(\Omega_{\text{mus}})]^S$ such that

$$\begin{aligned} \chi_m C_m \int_{\Omega_{\text{mus}}} \frac{\partial V_m}{\partial t} z \, \mathrm{d}\omega &+ \int_{\Omega_{\text{mus}}} \mathbf{\Sigma} \nabla V_m \cdot \nabla z \, \mathrm{d}\omega \\ &+ \chi_m \int_{\Omega_{\text{mus}}} I_{\text{ion}}(V_m, \boldsymbol{w}, \boldsymbol{c}) z \, \mathrm{d}\omega = \int_{\Omega_{\text{mus}}} I^{\text{ext}} z \, \mathrm{d}\omega, \end{aligned} \tag{6.13a}$$

$$\int_{\Omega_{\text{mus}}} \frac{\partial \boldsymbol{w}}{\partial t} \cdot \boldsymbol{y} \, \mathrm{d}\omega = \int_{\Omega_{\text{mus}}} \boldsymbol{g}(V_m, \boldsymbol{w}) \cdot \boldsymbol{y} \, \mathrm{d}\omega, \tag{6.13b}$$

$$\int_{\Omega_{\text{mus}}} \frac{\partial \boldsymbol{c}}{\partial t} \cdot \boldsymbol{\zeta} \, \mathrm{d}\omega = \int_{\Omega_{\text{mus}}} \boldsymbol{g}_c(V_m, \boldsymbol{w}, \boldsymbol{c}) \cdot \boldsymbol{\zeta} \, \mathrm{d}\omega, \tag{6.13c}$$

for all $z \in H^1(\Omega_{\text{mus}})$, $\boldsymbol{y} \in [L^2(\Omega_{\text{mus}})]^M$ and $\boldsymbol{\zeta} \in [L^2(\Omega_{\text{mus}})]^S$, together with (6.9c and 6.9d).

Although the hypothesis underlying the monodomain model – that is, the proportionality between the internal and external conductivities – is not physiological, as shown by experiments, in some cases this model provides a very accurate solution compared with the bidomain model. In particular, this is the case when there is no injection of current in the extracellular region (Colli Franzone, Pavarino and Taccardi 2005, Potse *et al.* 2006); the monodomain model is therefore fairly accurate and physically meaningful in physiological conditions. In contrast, when an external current is injected such as in defibrillation, the monodomain solution is no longer accurate, and the use of the more complex bidomain model is mandatory since the unequal anisotropy is fundamental to successful description of these scenarios (Trayanova 2006).

An alternative simplification is provided by the *eikonal* equation. Starting from the bidomain model coupled with a simplified representation of the ionic current that which does not consider any gating variable and allows for the description only of the depolarization phase, Colli Franzone, Guerri and Rovida (1990) derived the following *eikonal–diffusion* equation:

$$c_o\sqrt{\nabla\psi\cdot\boldsymbol{M}\nabla\psi}-\nabla\cdot(\boldsymbol{M}\nabla\psi)=1 \quad \text{in } \Omega_{\text{mus}}, \tag{6.14}$$

where $\psi(\boldsymbol{x})$ is the unknown *activation time* (see Section 5.2), $c_o$ denotes the velocity of the depolarization wave along the fibre direction for a planar wavefront, and $\boldsymbol{M}=\boldsymbol{\Sigma}/(\chi C_m)$. A different derivation was provided in Keener (1991), leading to the following *eikonal–curvature* equation:

$$c_o\sqrt{\nabla\psi\cdot\boldsymbol{M}\nabla\psi}-\sqrt{\nabla\psi\cdot\boldsymbol{M}\nabla\psi}\,\nabla\cdot\left(\frac{\boldsymbol{M}\nabla\psi}{\sqrt{\nabla\psi\cdot\boldsymbol{M}\nabla\psi}}\right)=1 \quad \text{in } \Omega_{\text{mus}}. \tag{6.15}$$

These are both steady equations providing information on the activation time of each cell in the tissue, *i.e.* of each point $\boldsymbol{x}\in\Omega_{mus}$. More specifically, the isocontours of $\psi(\boldsymbol{x})$ give the position of the action potential wavefront at time $t=\psi$. The eikonal–diffusive model (6.14) is an elliptic equation, where the propagation speed is influenced by the tissue surrounding the wavefront. Once the activation time $\psi$ has been computed, it is possible to obtain an approximate value of the extracellular potential $\phi_e$ by solving at each time step a suitable elliptic problem: see Colli Franzone and Guerri (1993).

In contrast, the eikonal–curvature model (6.15) is of parabolic type since the 'diffusive' term lacks the second derivative in the direction of propagation. This term is also proportional to an anisotropic generalization of the mean curvature (Tomlinson, Hunter and Pullan 2002). This implies that the propagation is faster when the wavefront is concave. This is in accordance with the diffusion of charge, which allows for faster depolarization in regions close to already depolarized tissues.

The eikonal equations are not suitable for recovering the action potential and the ionic currents. However, they provide accurate results about the activation of cells even in complex scenarios such as front-to-front collision: see *e.g.* Colli Franzone and Guerri (1993) for the eikonal–diffusive model.

The eikonal models are, however, very appealing from the computational point of view. First of all, they consist of a single steady PDE. Although non-linear, they do not require coupling with ODE systems. More importantly, the activation time, unlike the trans-membrane potential, does not feature any internal or boundary layer, so no special restriction on the mesh is needed in this case (see Section 5.1).

### *6.1.4 Boundary conditions and Purkinje network models*

We discuss here the initial and boundary conditions of the problems introduced above. The bidomain and monodomain equations and the ODE systems for the gating variables and ionic concentrations need to be equipped with suitable initial conditions; that is,

$$V_m|_{t=0} = V_{m,0}, \quad \boldsymbol{w}|_{t=0} = \boldsymbol{w}_0, \quad \boldsymbol{c}|_{t=0} = \boldsymbol{c}_0 \quad \text{in } \Omega_{\text{mus}},$$

for given functions $V_{m,0}(\boldsymbol{x}), \boldsymbol{w}_0(\boldsymbol{x}), \boldsymbol{c}_0(\boldsymbol{x})$.

For the boundary conditions for the bidomain, monodomain and eikonal-diffusion problems, a homogeneous Neumann condition is commonly prescribed at the external surface $\Sigma_{\text{epi}}$ of the epicardium and, for a ventricular domain only, at the base $\Sigma_b$ (see Figures 5.1 and 6.2(a)) to prescribe null outgoing current fluxes. In particular, the following conditions have to be prescribed on $\Sigma_{\text{epi}} \cup \Sigma_b$:

$$\begin{aligned}
&(\boldsymbol{\Sigma}_\beta \nabla \phi_\beta) \cdot \boldsymbol{n} = 0 \quad \beta = i, e && \text{for PP (6.5)},\\
&\left.\begin{aligned}&(\boldsymbol{\Sigma}_i \nabla (V_m + \phi_e)) \cdot \boldsymbol{n} = 0\\ &((\boldsymbol{\Sigma}_i + \boldsymbol{\Sigma}_e)\nabla \phi_e) \cdot \boldsymbol{n} + (\boldsymbol{\Sigma}_i \nabla V_m) \cdot \boldsymbol{n} = 0\end{aligned}\right\} && \text{for PE (6.6)},\\
&(\boldsymbol{\Sigma} \nabla V_m) \cdot \boldsymbol{n} = 0 && \text{for monodomain (6.11)},\\
&(\boldsymbol{M} \nabla \psi) \cdot \boldsymbol{n} = 0 && \text{for eikonal-diffusion (6.14)}.
\end{aligned}$$

As $\phi_e$ is defined up to a constant for the PE formulation (6.6) together with previous boundary conditions, the constraint

$$\int_{\Omega_{mus}} \phi_e \, d\omega = 0$$

is often employed and henceforth adopted in this section. Moreover, for the bidomain problems in both the formulations (6.5) and (6.6), the following compatibility conditions on the applied external currents must be enforced:

$$\int_{\Omega_{\text{mus}}} I_i^{\text{ext}} \, d\omega = \int_{\Omega_{\text{mus}}} I_e^{\text{ext}} \, d\omega.$$

On the internal surface $\Sigma_{\text{endo}}$ of the endocardium, Neumann boundary conditions are again prescribed. In this case, however, they could be non-homogeneous at specific stimulation points (*e.g.* the atrioventricular node and the points of the bundle of His). For the eikonal problem, Dirichlet data on the activation time could be prescribed at some specific locations if they are available, thanks to measurements provided by the NavX system, for example; see Section 5.2 (Sermesant *et al.* 2012). When redundant (*e.g.* when the electrical problem in the myocardium is coupled with the Purkinje fibres network: see below) these data have been used to solve inverse problems, for example to estimate the conduction velocity in the myocardium (Sermesant *et al.* 2012) or to obtain personalized Purkinje networks (Vergara *et al.* 2014, Palamara *et al.* 2014, Palamara *et al.* 2015).

If the mathematical model accounts for the presence of the Purkinje network, interface conditions on $\Sigma_{\text{endo}}$ describing the continuity of the current and of the potential at the Purkinje muscle junctions (PMJs) are implicitly provided for the bidomain and monodomain problems by the solution of the coupled muscle region/Purkinje network problem (Vigmond and Clements 2007, Vergara *et al.* 2016). For the sake of exposition, we will not provide details of the bidomain and monodomain models for the Purkinje network, instead referring interested readers to Vigmond and Clements (2007), Bordas *et al.* (2012) and Vergara *et al.* (2016). We will only note that, unlike the muscular case, in the network the gap junctions connecting two consecutive Purkinje cells are often explicitly modelled by means of resistances. Specific Purkinje cell models have also been developed, with the same structure as those developed for the muscular cells: see *e.g.* DiFrancesco and Noble (1985). However, we will describe the mechanisms of coupling; in particular, we will refer to the coupled problem obtained by considering the monodomain problem both in the muscle region and in the Purkinje network (Vergara *et al.* 2016). We consider $N$ Purkinje muscle junctions located at $\boldsymbol{x} = \boldsymbol{s}_j$ and we assume that each of them could be modelled by means of a resistance $R_{\text{PMJ}}$. Then, the *monodomain–monodomain coupled problem* is as follows. For each $t > 0$, find $V_p$, $V_m$, $\boldsymbol{w}_p$, $\boldsymbol{w}$ and $\gamma_j$, $j = 1, \ldots, N$, such that

$$P_m\left(V_m, \boldsymbol{w}, \sum_{j=1}^{N} \frac{1}{A_r} \mathcal{I}_{\mathcal{B}_r(\boldsymbol{s}_j)} \gamma_j + I^{\text{ext}}\right) = 0, \tag{6.16a}$$

$$P_p(V_p, \boldsymbol{w}_p, \boldsymbol{\gamma}) = 0, \tag{6.16b}$$

$$\gamma_j = \frac{V_p(\boldsymbol{s}_j) - \frac{1}{A_r}\int_{\mathcal{B}_r(\boldsymbol{s}_j)} V_m \, \mathrm{d}\boldsymbol{x}}{R_{\text{PMJ}}} \quad j = 1, \ldots, N, \tag{6.16c}$$

where $P_m(V_m, \boldsymbol{w}, F) = 0$ denotes the monodomain problem in the myocardium with source term $F$, $P_p(V_p, \boldsymbol{w}_p, \boldsymbol{\eta}) = 0$ is the monodomain problem in the Purkinje network with Neumann conditions with data $\eta_j$ at the Purkinje muscle junctions, $V_p$ and $\boldsymbol{w}_p$ are the trans-membrane potential and the gating variables in the Purkinje network, $\gamma_j$ are the PMJ currents which are determined by Ohm's laws (6.16c), $\mathcal{I}_Y$ is the characteristic function related to the region $Y \subset \Omega_{\text{mus}}$, $\mathcal{B}_r(\boldsymbol{s}_j)$ is the ball of radius $r$ centred at the point $\boldsymbol{s}_j$, and $A_r$ is the volume of this ball. We observe that the two monodomain problems are coupled by means of the PMJ currents $\gamma_j$: for the 3D problem the latter act as source terms distributed in balls of radius $r$, whereas for the network they act as Neumann conditions (Bordas *et al.* 2012). A similar approach could be considered for the bidomain problems as well.

The coupling between eikonal muscular and Purkinje network problems has been addressed by Vergara *et al.* (2014) for normal propagation and Palamara *et al.* (2014) for pathological propagations.

### 6.1.5 Computing the surface electrocardiogram signals

The computation of the potentials related to electrical propagation in the heart could be used to numerically compute the surface electrocardiogram (ECG) signals, that is, electrical potential on the surface of the body, thus simulating what happens in normal clinical practice. This could be obtained by coupling the bidomain or monodomain problem with the propagation in the torso (see *e.g.* Sundnes *et al.* (2007)), modelled by a simple diffusion problem for the extracellular potential at each $t > 0$:

$$-\nabla \cdot (\boldsymbol{\Sigma}_T \nabla \phi_T) = 0 \quad \text{in } \Omega_T,$$

where $\Omega_T$ is the torso domain that surrounds the heart domain $\Omega_{\text{mus}}$ (*i.e.* the heart boundary surface $\Sigma_{\text{epi}} \cup \Sigma_b$ denotes the interface with the torso), $\Omega_T \cap \Omega_{\text{mus}} = \emptyset$, with $\phi_T$ denoting the extracellular potential in the torso. Homogeneous Neumann conditions have to be applied on the external torso surface $\Sigma_T$, whereas the following interface conditions, which replace the boundary conditions for the heart problem, need to be prescribed at the torso/heart interface:

$$\begin{aligned} &\phi_e = \phi_T && \text{on } \Sigma_{\text{epi}} \cup \Sigma_b, \\ &(\boldsymbol{\Sigma}_e \nabla \phi_e) \cdot \boldsymbol{n} = (\boldsymbol{\Sigma}_T \nabla \phi_T) \cdot \boldsymbol{n} && \text{on } \Sigma_{\text{epi}} \cup \Sigma_b, \\ &(\boldsymbol{\Sigma}_i \nabla (V_m + \phi_e)) \cdot \boldsymbol{n} = 0 && \text{on } \Sigma_{\text{epi}} \cup \Sigma_b. \end{aligned}$$

### *6.1.6 Numerical discretization*

The numerical solution of the bidomain and monodomain problems is very demanding. Together with the strict constraint on the spatial mesh size due to the propagation of a very steep front (see Section 5.1), a time step of the order of tenths or even hundredths of milliseconds must be used in order to capture the fast dynamics characterizing the propagation, with time constants of the order of 0.1 ms. Moreover, as discussed below, the algebraic solution of the linear systems arising at each time step using the finite element method, for example, requires careful treatment – due to the coupled nature of the problem, the singularity of some of the matrices involved, and the presence of the non-linear term due to the ionic currents.

Several time-discretization strategies have been considered so far. We can group them into four main categories: *explicit; semi-implicit; implicit;* and *operator splitting-based* methods, which we now briefly present. We start by introducing the finite element matrices and vectors:

$$\begin{aligned} (M)_{jk} &= \int_{\Omega_{\text{mus}}} \psi_k \psi_j \, \mathrm{d}\omega, \\ (A_\beta)_{jk} &= \int_{\Omega_{\text{mus}}} \boldsymbol{\Sigma}_\beta \nabla \psi_k \cdot \nabla \psi_j \, \mathrm{d}\omega, \quad \beta = i, e \\ (\boldsymbol{I}_{\text{ion}}(\boldsymbol{V}_m^n, \boldsymbol{W}^r, \boldsymbol{C}^s))_j &= \int_{\Omega_{\text{mus}}} I_{\text{ion}}(V_m^n, \boldsymbol{w}^r, \boldsymbol{c}^s) \psi_j \, \mathrm{d}\omega, \\ (\boldsymbol{G}(\boldsymbol{V}_m^n, \boldsymbol{W}^r))_j &= \int_{\Omega_{\text{mus}}} \boldsymbol{g}(V_m^n, \boldsymbol{w}^r) \cdot \boldsymbol{y}_j \, \mathrm{d}\omega, \\ (\boldsymbol{S}(\boldsymbol{V}_m^n, \boldsymbol{W}^r, \boldsymbol{C}^s))_j &= \int_{\Omega_{\text{mus}}} \boldsymbol{g}_c(V_m^n, \boldsymbol{w}^r, \boldsymbol{c}^s) \cdot \boldsymbol{\zeta}_j \, \mathrm{d}\omega, \end{aligned}$$

where $\psi_i$, $\boldsymbol{y}_j$ and $\boldsymbol{\zeta}_j$ denote the basis functions of the finite element spaces, and $n, r, s$ are integers denoting discretized times. The vectors $\boldsymbol{V}_m$, $\boldsymbol{\Phi}_e$, $\boldsymbol{\Phi}_i$, $\boldsymbol{W}$ and $\boldsymbol{C}$ denote the unknown coefficients of the finite element solutions associated with the unknowns $V_m$, $\phi_e$, $\phi_i$, $\boldsymbol{w}$, $\boldsymbol{c}$. Note that the dimensions of $\boldsymbol{W}$ and $\boldsymbol{C}$ are $MK$ and $SK$, respectively, where $K$ is the number of degrees of freedom associated with the mesh and the choice of finite elements (*e.g.*

the number of vertices for linear finite elements). In all the cases, in order to simplify the notation, we will set $I_e^{\text{ext}} = I_i^{\text{ext}} = 0$, and we assume that the running temporal index $^{n+1}$ is understood.

*Explicit methods.* In explicit methods, all the problems in (6.10) are discretized by means of an explicit scheme, for example forward Euler for both the PDE and ODE systems (Puwal and Roth 2007, Ethier and Bourgault 2008). This choice allows us to decouple the four blocks of the bidomain system (the two PDEs and the two ODEs systems), involving only the mass matrix in the PP formulation, and thus in principle avoiding the need to solve any linear system provided that mass lumping is performed. In contrast, for the PE formulation, the absence of time derivatives in the second PDE implies that a linear system in the unknown $\mathbf{\Phi}_e$ needs to be solved at each discrete time instance $t^n$; we detail the discrete formulation for the forward Euler method:

$$\chi_m C_m M \frac{\boldsymbol{V}_m - \boldsymbol{V}_m^n}{\Delta t} = -A_i(\boldsymbol{V}_m^n + \mathbf{\Phi}_e^n) - \chi_m \boldsymbol{I}_{\text{ion}}(\boldsymbol{V}_m^n, \boldsymbol{W}^n, \boldsymbol{C}^n),$$
$$A_i \boldsymbol{V}_m + (A_i + A_e)\mathbf{\Phi}_e = \mathbf{0},$$
$$M\frac{\boldsymbol{W} - \boldsymbol{W}^n}{\Delta t} = \boldsymbol{G}(\boldsymbol{V}_m^n, \boldsymbol{W}^n), \quad M\frac{\boldsymbol{C} - \boldsymbol{C}^n}{\Delta t} = \boldsymbol{S}(\boldsymbol{V}_m^n, \boldsymbol{W}^n, \boldsymbol{C}^n).$$

Explicit methods generally involve a severe restriction on the time discretization of the type $\Delta t < h^2/\Sigma$, where $\Sigma$ is a representative value of the conductivity (Puwal and Roth 2007). Dos Santos, Plank, Bauer and Vigmond (2005) showed for a model problem that an explicit method is not absolutely stable even for a value of $\Delta t$ much smaller than that required to capture the front propagation. For this reason and due to the increased availability of computational resources (CPUs), explicit methods have nowadays lost popularity.

*Semi-implicit methods.* ODE systems are usually solved at each time step by means of explicit or semi-implicit methods (in the latter case the dependence on $V_m$ is treated explicitly). This suggests using semi-implicit methods (Keener and Bogar 1998, Pennacchio and Simoncini 2002, Colli Franzone and Pavarino 2004) for the whole coupled PDE/ODE problem. These methods are the most widely used together with operator splitting-based methods (see below). They are based on treating the diffusive term implicitly and the non-linear term explicitly. A possible semi-implicit (first-order) scheme for the PP formulation (6.10) is as follows:

$$M\frac{\boldsymbol{W} - \boldsymbol{W}^n}{\Delta t} - \boldsymbol{G}(\boldsymbol{V}_m^n, \boldsymbol{W}) = \mathbf{0}, \quad M\frac{\boldsymbol{C} - \boldsymbol{C}^n}{\Delta t} - \boldsymbol{S}(\boldsymbol{V}_m^n, \boldsymbol{W}, \boldsymbol{C}) = \mathbf{0},$$

$$
\begin{aligned}
\chi_m C_m M \frac{\boldsymbol{V}_m - \boldsymbol{V}_m^n}{\Delta t} + A_i \boldsymbol{\Phi}_i + \chi_m \boldsymbol{I}_{\text{ion}}(\boldsymbol{V}_m^n, \boldsymbol{W}, \boldsymbol{C}) = \mathbf{0}, \\
- \chi_m C_m M \frac{\boldsymbol{V}_m - \boldsymbol{V}_m^n}{\Delta t} + A_e \boldsymbol{\Phi}_e - \chi_m \boldsymbol{I}_{\text{ion}}(\boldsymbol{V}_m^n, \boldsymbol{W}, \boldsymbol{C}) = \mathbf{0}
\end{aligned}
$$

(see *e.g.* Colli Franzone and Pavarino 2004).

A semi-implicit method like the one reported here has two nice properties. First of all, the two PDEs are decoupled by the ODE systems, thus significantly simplifying the numerical solution of the entire problem. This decoupling strategy is justified by noticing that the Jacobian matrices of a fully implicit discretization feature dominant values on the diagonal, suggesting weak coupling between potentials and gating/ionic concentration variables (Munteanu, Pavarino and Scacchi 2009). Second, it allows for a linearization of the non-linear reaction term given by the ionic currents, thus requiring the solution of a 2×2 block linear system.

Special attention has been paid to evaluation of the ionic current in a finite element context. In particular, two strategies have mainly been considered, namely *ionic current interpolation* (ICI) and *state variable interpolation* (SVI). In the first case, only the nodal values are used to build an interpolation of the ionic current, whereas in the second, the trans-membrane potential and the gating/ionic concentration variables are interpolated within each element and the ionic current is then evaluated by using these interpolated variables; see Pathmanathan, Mirams, Southern and Whiteley (2011) and also Krishnamoorthi, Sarkar and Klug (2013). The ICI approach is of course more efficient from the computational point of view, and allows us to express the reaction term by means of a mass matrix. However, it has lower accuracy with respect to state variable interpolation; in particular, the computed conduction velocity is generally larger than the true velocity: see Pathmanathan *et al.* (2011).

From the algebraic point of view, the solution of a semi-implicit discretized problem is very demanding, since the matrix of the linear system associated with the PDEs written in terms of the unknowns $\boldsymbol{\Phi}_i$ and $\boldsymbol{\Phi}_e$ is given by

$$
B = \frac{\chi_m C_m}{\Delta t} \begin{bmatrix} M & -M \\ -M & M \end{bmatrix} + \begin{bmatrix} A_i & 0 \\ 0 & A_e \end{bmatrix}.
$$

Both the terms of this block matrix are singular, the first because of the degenerate parabolic nature of the PP bidomain formulation and the second since each block $A_\beta$ is related to a pure Neumann diffusive problem. However, the matrix $B$ is positive semidefinite, so the preconditioned conjugate gradient method is often used for its numerical solution (Pennacchio and Simoncini 2002, Colli Franzone and Pavarino 2004). Preconditioning is needed since $B$ is highly ill-conditioned, due to the block 2×2 mass matrix which, unlike the classical mass matrix, worsens the spectrum of the stiffness matrix. Efficient preconditioners include block Jacobi and Gauss–Seidel (Mardal, Nielsen, Cai and Tveito 2007), block SSOR (Pennacchio and Simoncini 2002), multilevel additive Schwarz (Pavarino and Scacchi 2008), multigrid (Plank *et al.* 2007, Vigmond *et al.* 2008), and a functional block preconditioner obtained by the monodomain solver (Gerardo-Giorda *et al.* 2009).

Semi-implicit methods have also been proposed for the PE formulation: see *e.g.* Fernández and Zemzemi (2010). For example, with respect to the unknowns $\boldsymbol{V}_m$ and $\boldsymbol{\Phi}_e$, we have

$$B = \frac{\chi_m C_m}{\Delta t}\begin{bmatrix} M & 0 \\ 0 & 0 \end{bmatrix} + \begin{bmatrix} A_i & A_i \\ A_i & A_i + A_e \end{bmatrix}.$$

Again the matrix is singular, ill-conditioned, and semidefinite positive. In this context, we cite Pierre (2012) for an incomplete block LU factorization preconditioner, and Vigmond, Aguel and Trayanova (2002), where the two PDEs are decoupled by treating $V_m$ explicitly in (6.6a) and $\phi_e$ in (6.6b).

In any case, semi-implicit methods are conditionally stable with a bound on $\Delta t$ which is, however, independent of the mesh size (Fernández and Zemzemi 2010, Colli Franzone *et al.* 2014).

A variant of the semi-implicit method reported above arises from treating the reaction term $I_{\text{ion}}$ implicitly. In this case, Newton–Krylov–Schwarz methods have been proved to be very efficient (Munteanu *et al.* 2009). Second-order semi-implicit schemes have been successfully considered as well: see *e.g.* Ethier and Bourgault (2008).

*Operator splitting-based methods.* These methods separate the reaction operator from the diffusive operator, in a similar way to what is done in fractional step methods for fluid problems. They were first introduced for the monodomain problem by Qu and Garfinkel (1998). Here we limit ourselves to present an operator splitting-based method for the PP formulation of the bidomain problem (Sundnes, Lines and Tveito 2005, Colli Franzone *et al.* 2014), but we refer the interested reader *e.g.* to (Spiteri and Torabi Ziaratgahi 2016) for a wider overview on the topic of operator-splitting methods for electrophysiology models.

(1) Given the quantities at time step $t^n$, solve the reaction problem and the

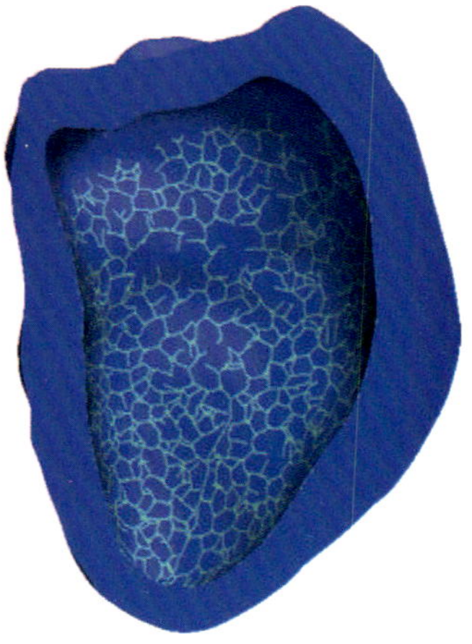

(a)

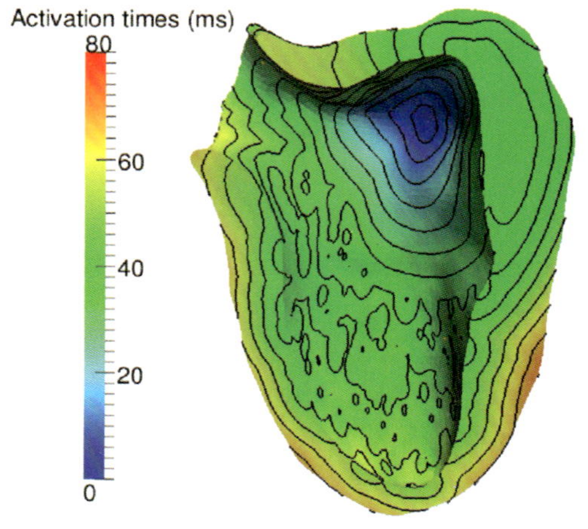


(b)

Figure 6.3 (a) Purkinje network generated by the algorithm proposed in Palamara *et al.* (2015) in the case of a real, subject-specific left ventricle. (b) Map of the activation times computed by means of the eikonal equation. The time marching scheme and P1 finite elements have been used. The source term (dark blue) is located within the myocardium, as typically happens in Wolff–Parkinson–White syndrome. Results were obtained by means of a code implemented in the VMTK environment (www.vmtk.org). Data from CT images provided by the Cardiology Division at Ospedale S. Maria del Carmine, Rovereto (TN), Italy, and from the Radiology Division of Borgo-Trento (TN), Italy.

ODE systems in $(t^n, t^n + \theta\Delta t]$:

$$
\begin{aligned}
\chi_m C_m M \frac{\widetilde{\boldsymbol{V}}_m^{n+\theta} - \boldsymbol{V}_m^n}{\Delta t} + \chi_m \boldsymbol{I}_{\text{ion}}(\boldsymbol{V}_m^*, \boldsymbol{W}^*, \boldsymbol{C}^*) &= \mathbf{0},\\
M \frac{\widetilde{\boldsymbol{W}}^{n+\theta} - \boldsymbol{W}^n}{\Delta t} - \boldsymbol{G}(\boldsymbol{V}_m^*, \boldsymbol{W}^*) &= \mathbf{0},\\
M \frac{\widetilde{\boldsymbol{C}}^{n+\theta} - \boldsymbol{C}^n}{\Delta t} - \boldsymbol{S}(\boldsymbol{V}_m^*, \boldsymbol{W}^*, \boldsymbol{C}^*) &= \mathbf{0}.
\end{aligned}
$$

(2) Given $\widetilde{\boldsymbol{V}}_m^{n+\theta}$, solve the diffusion problems in $(t^n, t^{n+1}]$:

$$
\begin{aligned}
\chi_m C_m M \frac{\widehat{\boldsymbol{V}}_m^{n+1} - \widetilde{\boldsymbol{V}}_m^{n+\theta}}{\Delta t} + A_i \boldsymbol{\Phi}_i^* &= \mathbf{0},\\
-\chi_m C_m M \frac{\widehat{\boldsymbol{V}}_m^{n+1} - \widetilde{\boldsymbol{V}}_m^{n+\theta}}{\Delta t} + A_e \boldsymbol{\Phi}_e^* &= \mathbf{0}.
\end{aligned}
$$

(3) Given $\widehat{\boldsymbol{V}}_m^{n+1}$, $\widetilde{\boldsymbol{W}}^{n+\theta}$, $\widetilde{\boldsymbol{C}}^{n+\theta}$, solve the reaction problem and the ODE

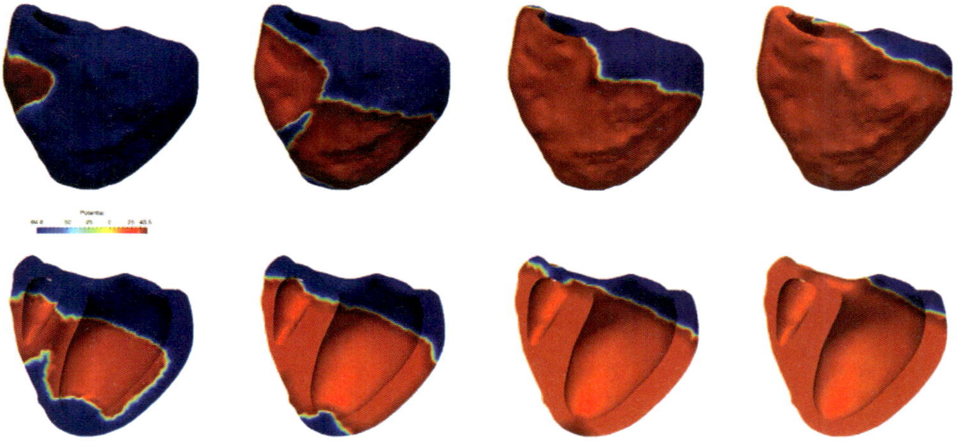

Figure 6.4 Propagation of the trans-membrane potential in the two ventricles at eight different instants during a heartbeat. Monodomain simulation, semi-implicit method, P1 finite elements. Results were obtained using LifeV; the computational mesh was obtained by an open source biventricular geometry segmented from CT images: see Rousseau (2010).

systems in $(t^n + \theta\Delta t, t^{n+1}]$:

$$\chi_m C_m M \frac{\boldsymbol{V}_m^{n+1} - \widehat{\boldsymbol{V}}_m^{n+1}}{\Delta t} + \chi_m \boldsymbol{I}_{\text{ion}}(\boldsymbol{V}_m^*, \boldsymbol{W}^*, \boldsymbol{C}^*) = \boldsymbol{0},$$
$$M \frac{\boldsymbol{W}^{n+1} - \widetilde{\boldsymbol{W}}^{n+\theta}}{\Delta t} - \boldsymbol{G}(\boldsymbol{V}_m^*, \boldsymbol{W}^*) = \boldsymbol{0},$$
$$M \frac{\boldsymbol{C}^{n+1} - \widetilde{\boldsymbol{C}}^{n+\theta}}{\Delta t} - \boldsymbol{S}(\boldsymbol{V}_m^*, \boldsymbol{W}^*, \boldsymbol{C}^*) = \boldsymbol{0}.$$

The superscript $^*$ means that the quantity at hand could be treated either explicitly or implicitly. The variable $\theta$ could assume value 1/2 or 1. In the latter case, step (3) is unnecessary and we simply set

$$\boldsymbol{V}_m^{n+1} = \widehat{\boldsymbol{V}}_m^{n+1}, \quad \boldsymbol{W}^{n+1} = \widetilde{\boldsymbol{W}}^{n+1}, \quad \boldsymbol{C}^{n+1} = \widetilde{\boldsymbol{C}}^{n+1};$$

this case corresponds to a first-order method (*Godunov splitting*). Instead, for $\theta = 1/2$, we have a second-order method provided that all the subproblems are solved with a second-order strategy (*Strang splitting*). Note that if step (2) is solved implicitly, then the same preconditioners introduced above for the semi-implicit schemes could be applied as well, since it applies to the same operator.

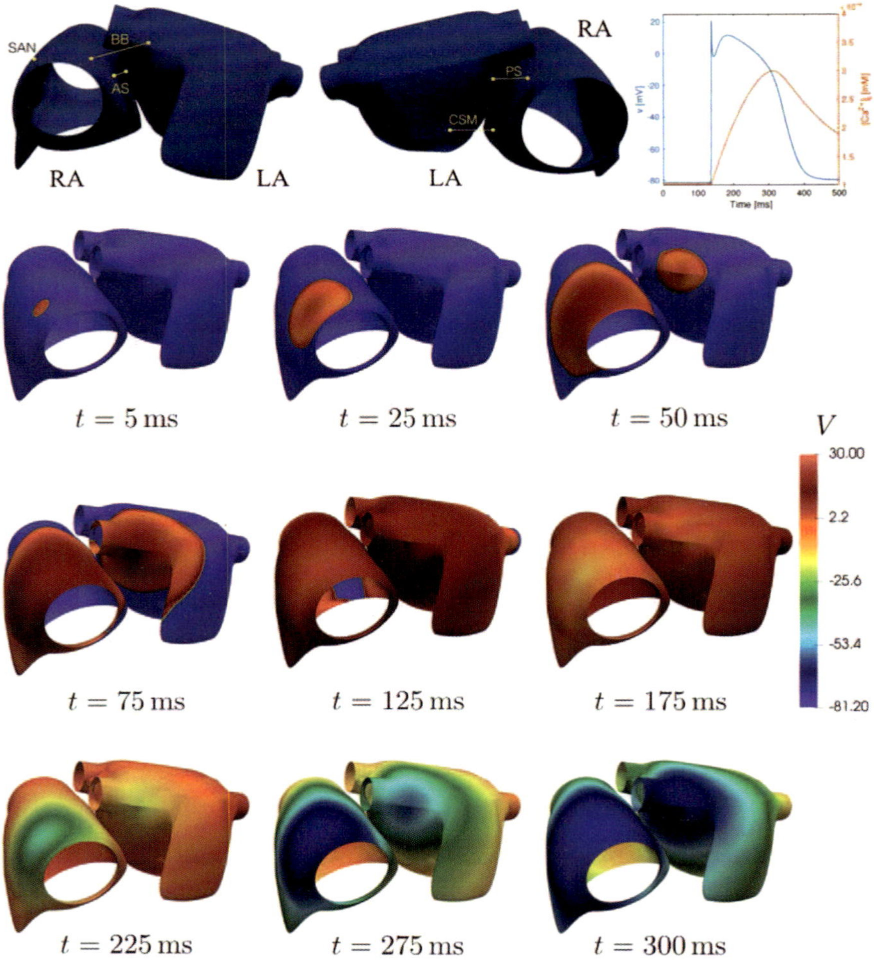


Figure 6.5 Numerical simulation of the electrophysiology problem on the left and right atrial surfaces according to the methods developed in Collin *et al.* (2013), Patelli *et al.* (2017), Pegolotti (2017), and Pegolotti *et al.* (2019); spatial discretization by Isogeometric Analysis (Cottrell *et al.* 2009). Idealized surface representations of the left (LA) and right (RA) atria generated by means of NURBS from different viewpoints; the sinoatrial node (SAN) and bundle interatrial connections are highlighted in yellow (top). Evolution of the trans-membrane potential on the atrial surfaces and propagated from the SAN node according to the bidomain equation together with the Courtemanche-Nattel-Ramirez cellular ionic model in Courtemanche *et al.* (1998) (bottom); fibres direction as highlighted in Figure 5.4. Results obtained by means of isogeometric analysis solver; courtesy of L. Pegolotti (EPFL).

*Implicit methods.* Some authors have considered a fully implicit discretization of the full bidomain problem (6.9): see *e.g.* Bourgault, Ethier and LeBlanc (2003) and Murillo and Cai (2004). In this case the whole Jacobian is built and the Newton method is applied. Due to the small time step required in bidomain simulations to capture the propagating front and because of the excellent stability properties of semi-implicit and operator splitting-based methods, fully implicit method are currently no longer popular.

We provide some examples of numerical results related to the solution of the electrophysiology problem in the myocardium and in the atria in Figures 6.3, 6.4 and 6.5.

## 6.2 Cardiac mechanics and electromechanical coupling

We review in this section the models used for the description of cardiac mechanics, both in its *active* and *passive* components. In particular, *active mechanics* refers to the model introducing the contraction and relaxation of the muscle independently of the action of external forces on the tissue. In this respect, we recall the two paradigms commonly used to model active mechanics: *active stress* and *active strain.* We consider then the coupling of electrophysiology and mechanical models into the integrated *electromechanics* (EM) model and we finally review the numerical strategies for the solution of such coupled problem.

### *6.2.1 The continuous mechanics problems*

We present the models commonly used for both active and passive cardiac mechanics.

*Active stress approach*

During a physiological contraction, the cardiac cells change in length by up to 20–30%, so finite elasticity models are needed to describe heart contraction and relaxation. In particular, the first Piola–Kirchhoff tensor is written as the sum of two terms (Nash and Panfilov 2004, Niederer and Smith 2008): a *passive component*, $\widehat{\boldsymbol{T}}_s^P$, describing the stress required to obtain a given deformation of the passive myocardium (similarly to arteries), and an *active component*, $\widehat{\boldsymbol{T}}_s^A$, denoting the tension generated by the depolarization of the propagating electrical signal that provides the internal active forces responsible for the contraction (see Section 4.4):

$$\widehat{\boldsymbol{T}}_s = \widehat{\boldsymbol{T}}_s^P + \widehat{\boldsymbol{T}}_s^A, \tag{6.23}$$

where, using the notation of Part 1, $\widehat{\ }$ refers to quantities computed in the reference domain.

The passive component of the stress is obtained as the derivative of a suitable strain energy function: see (3.8). The heart's mechanical response (just like the electrical propagation: see Section 6.1) is highly dependent on the presence of fibres and sheets. For this reason, the passive myocardium is modelled as an hyperelastic *orthotropic* material, characterized by two principal directions and with different material responses on three mutually orthogonal planes, identified by these directions. This is in accordance with the shear tests performed on pig hearts, which highlighted an elevated resistance to shear deformations producing an extension along the fibre direction, an intermediate resistance in the direction orthogonal to fibres and tangential to sheets, and the least resistance in the third orthogonal direction (Dokos, Smaill, Young and LeGrice 2002). Letting $\widehat{\boldsymbol{a}}_f$, $\widehat{\boldsymbol{a}}_s$, $\widehat{\boldsymbol{a}}_n$ denote the unit vectors along these directions (see Section 6.1) in the reference configuration, the following strain energy function has been proposed in Holzapfel and Ogden (2009):

$$\begin{aligned}\Theta(I_1, I_{4,f}, I_{4,s}, I_{8,fs}) \\ = \frac{a}{2b}\mathrm{e}^{b(I_1-3)} + \sum_{i=f,s}\frac{a_i}{2b_i}\left[\mathrm{e}^{b_i(I_{4,i}-1)^2}-1\right] + \frac{a_{fs}}{2b_{fs}}\left[\mathrm{e}^{b_{fs}I_{8,fs}^2}-1\right],\end{aligned} \tag{6.24}$$

where, referring to the notation introduced in Section 3.2, $I_1 = \operatorname{tr}\boldsymbol{C}$, $I_{4,i} = \widehat{\boldsymbol{a}}_i \cdot (\boldsymbol{C}\widehat{\boldsymbol{a}}_i)$, $i = f, s$, $I_{8,fs} = \widehat{\boldsymbol{a}}_f \cdot (\boldsymbol{C}\widehat{\boldsymbol{a}}_s)$ are invariants of $\boldsymbol{C}$, and $a$, $b$, $a_f$, $b_f$, $a_s$, $b_s$, $a_{fs}$, $b_{fs}$ are material parameters. The quantity $I_1$ is the first isotropic invariant and the related term in $\Theta$ accounts for the isotropic response of the myocardium at small deformations;$I_{4,f}$ and $I_{4,s}$ are the squares of the stretch of $\widehat{\boldsymbol{a}}_f$ and $\widehat{\boldsymbol{a}}_s$ in the deformed configuration, and the related terms in the energy are associated with the increased stiffness of the material along the two principal directions $\boldsymbol{a}_f$ and $\boldsymbol{a}_s$ for large deformations; finally, $I_{8,fs}$ denotes the angle spanned by the two principal directions in the deformed configuration, and the related term in the energy describes the coupling between the two principal directions. Convexity of the strain energy function $\Theta$ of Eq. (6.24) is guaranteed for positive parameter values (Holzapfel and Ogden 2009). Other orthotropic models have been proposed, for example by Hunter, Nash and Sands (1997) and Costa, Holmes and McCulloch (2001), whereas *transversally isotropic* models with only one principal direction (along the fibres) were introduced by Humphrey and Yin (1987) and Guccione, McCulloch and Waldman (1991), for example; however, the constitutive law of Eq. (6.24) is commonly accepted as the golden standard in cardiac passive mechanics.

Some authors (Holzapfel and Ogden 2009) model the myocardium as incompressible material in accordance with the experiments reported by Vossoughi, Vaishnav and Patel (1980). In this case the term $p_s(J-1)$ is added to the strain energy functions, as in (3.13), with $p_s$ playing the role of Lagrangian multiplier for the enforcement of the incompressibility constraint. Conversely, some other authors, *e.g.* (Cheng *et al.* 2005) and (Rossi *et al.* 2014), model the material as nearly-incompressible, for which moderate volumetric changes (2–15%) are allowed to account for blood perfusion (see (Yin, Chan and Judd 1996)). In this case a volumetric contribution $\Theta_{vol}(J)$ is added to the strain energy function $\Theta$ to penalize deformations which substantially depart from the fully incompressible case; a common choice is the following convex function endowed with global minimum in $J=1$ (see *e.g.* (Simo and Taylor 1991)):

$$\Theta_{vol}(J) = \frac{B}{2}(J-1)\log(J);$$

the larger is the bulk modulus $B>0$, the stronger is the penalization of volumetric changes. On the basis of experimental evidence, reported by Dokos *et al.* (2002), for example, highlighting hysteresis under shear deformations, viscoelastic orthotropic models have recently been proposed for the passive myocardium: see Gultekin, Sommer and Holzapfel (2016). The viscoelastic behaviour is probably due to the extracellular fluid that filtrates through the solid part.

The active contribution of the cardiac cells to the contraction is regulated by the opening of calcium channels as a response to the depolarization, with a consequent entry of calcium ions in the cells. As detailed in Section 4.4, this process is responsible for cardiac contraction. Since the latter occurs along the axial direction of the cardiac cells – that is, along the fibre direction – the active part of the stress tensor usually takes the form

$$\widehat{\boldsymbol{T}}_s^A = P^A \widehat{\boldsymbol{a}}_f \otimes \widehat{\boldsymbol{a}}_f \tag{6.25}$$

(Nash and Panfilov 2004), where the scalar function of time and space $P^A$ denotes the pointwise *active stress*, and should be properly modelled.

In the classical model for the active stress function proposed in Nash and Panfilov (2004), $P^A$ depends only on the trans-membrane potential $V_m$. In particular, for each spatial point $\boldsymbol{x} \in \Omega_{mus}$, the following ODE equation is introduced:

$$\frac{\mathrm{d}P^A(t)}{\mathrm{d}t} = \varepsilon(V_m(t))\big[k_P(V_m(t) - V_r) - P^A(t)\big], \tag{6.26}$$

where $V_r$ is the resting potential, $k_P$ is a suitable parameter controlling the amplitude of $P^A$, and $\varepsilon$ controls the delay of the contraction with respect to the action potential. For example, Goktepe and Kuhl (2010) proposed the expression

$$\varepsilon(V_m) = \varepsilon_0 + (\varepsilon_\infty - \varepsilon_0)\mathrm{e}^{-\mathrm{e}^{-\xi(V_m - \bar{V}_m)}},$$

where $\varepsilon_0$, $\varepsilon_\infty$, $\xi$, $\bar{V}_m$ are suitable parameters.

Since cardiac cell contraction is regulated by calcium ion concentration, the active stress function $P^A$ can be assumed to depend directly on this specific concentration, say $c_{\mathrm{ca}}$, rather than on the more general variable $V_m$. For example, Wong, Goktepe and Kuhl (2013) proposed a system of ODEs of the same structure as (6.26), but using $c_{\mathrm{ca}}$ instead of $V_m$ on the right-hand side.

In more sophisticated models, the active stress function also depends on the stretch in the fibre direction $\lambda = (\widehat{\boldsymbol{a}}_f^{\mathrm{T}} C \widehat{\boldsymbol{a}}_f)^{1/2}$ and on the fibre stretch rate $\mathrm{d}\lambda/\mathrm{d}t$ (Niederer, Hunter and Smith 2006, Land *et al.* 2012). In compact form, these models are written as

$$\begin{aligned} \frac{\mathrm{d}\boldsymbol{y}}{\mathrm{d}t} &= \boldsymbol{g}_y\left(P^A, \lambda, \frac{\mathrm{d}\lambda}{\mathrm{d}t}, \boldsymbol{c}, \boldsymbol{y}\right), \\ P^A &= g_{P^A}(\lambda, \boldsymbol{y}), \end{aligned} \tag{6.27}$$

for suitable functions $\boldsymbol{g}_y$ and $g_{P^A}$ and where $\boldsymbol{c}$, as in Section 6.1, is the ionic concentration variable (in particular the calcium one), whereas $\boldsymbol{y}$ collects other myofilament and electrophysiology state variables.

*Active strain approach*

As an alternative to the decomposition (6.23), where the stress tensor is split into a passive and an active component (the active stress approach), Cherubini, Filippi, Nardinocchi and Teresi (2008) and Ambrosi, Arioli, Nobile and Quarteroni (2011) have instead proposed a different strategy based on an *active strain* approach. In this case, the following factorization of the deformation tensor is used,

$$\boldsymbol{F} = \boldsymbol{F}^P \boldsymbol{F}^A,$$

where $\boldsymbol{F}^A$ is the active factor acting at the microscales, describing fibre distortion not preserving geometric compatibility, whereas $\boldsymbol{F}^P$ describes passive macroscale deformation and the deformation needed to restore compatibility. With this choice, quite common when analyzing plasticity, growth and remodelling of living tissues, the microscale information related to the fibre contraction is directly incorporated in the body kinematics, allowing for the inclusion of fibre contraction driven by the depolarization as a prescribed active deformation rather than a further contribution to stress. In this case, the first Piola–Kirchhoff stress tensor is generally written as

$$\widehat{\boldsymbol{T}}_s = J^A \frac{D\Theta}{D\boldsymbol{F}^P}(\boldsymbol{F}^A)^{-T},$$

where $J^A = \det(\boldsymbol{F}^A)$. In analogy with (6.25), a possible expression for $\boldsymbol{F}^A$ is

$$\boldsymbol{F}^A = \boldsymbol{I} - \beta V_m \widehat{\boldsymbol{a}}_f \otimes \widehat{\boldsymbol{a}}_f,$$

linking the trans-membrane potential to the active deformation tensor, where $\beta$ is a suitable parameter (Ambrosi *et al.* 2011). However, as the active deformation occurs mainly along the direction of the fibres, different active strain models have been proposed to account this aspect. In the transversely isotropic activation model of (Boyett, Frampton and Kirby 1991), the active deformation tensor assumes the expression

$$\boldsymbol{F}^A = \gamma_f \widehat{\boldsymbol{a}}_f \otimes \widehat{\boldsymbol{a}}_f + \frac{1}{\sqrt{\gamma_f}}(\boldsymbol{I} - \widehat{\boldsymbol{a}}_f \otimes \widehat{\boldsymbol{a}}_f) \tag{6.28}$$

in the variable $\gamma_f$, which represents the shortening of the fibres; here $\widehat{\boldsymbol{a}}_f$ stands for the fibre direction. Orthotropic activation models have instead been proposed in (Rossi *et al.* 2012) and (Rossi *et al.* 2014), which read

$$\boldsymbol{F}^A = \gamma_f \widehat{\boldsymbol{a}}_f \otimes \widehat{\boldsymbol{a}}_f + \gamma_s(\gamma_f) \widehat{\boldsymbol{a}}_s \otimes \widehat{\boldsymbol{a}}_s + \gamma_n(\gamma_f) \widehat{\boldsymbol{a}}_n \otimes \widehat{\boldsymbol{a}}_n, \tag{6.29}$$

where $\widehat{\boldsymbol{a}}_s$ stands for the normal to the sheets and $\widehat{\boldsymbol{a}}_n$ is orthogonal to both $\widehat{\boldsymbol{a}}_f$ and $\widehat{\boldsymbol{a}}_n$; the shortenings along $\widehat{\boldsymbol{a}}_n$ and $\widehat{\boldsymbol{a}}_s$ are determined by assuming isochoric active deformation, for which $\gamma_n = k'(1/\sqrt{1+\gamma_f} - 1)$ and $\gamma_s = 1/((1+\gamma_f)(1+\gamma_n(\gamma_f))) - 1$, where $k' > 0$ is a suitable parameter relating the microscale-to-macroscale shortening. More recently, a transmurally variable orthotropic model has been proposed in (Barbarotta 2014) and validated in (Barbarotta, Rossi, Dede' and Quarteroni 2018) to better reproduce the heterogeneous activation in the myocardium; in this case $k'$ becomes a function of a transmural coordinate, *i.e.* $k' = k'(\boldsymbol{x})$.

In order to link the fibres shortening $\gamma_f$ to cardiac electrophysiology, the use of a suitable mechanical activation model is in order within the active strain approach. Specifically, such model should describe the so-called crossbridge cycle occurring in the sarcomeres (Huxley and Kress 1985) and establish the dependence of $\gamma_f$ on the intracellular calcium concentration $\mathbf{c}$ (an output of the cell ionic model). Here we limit ourselves to recall the mechanical activation model proposed in (Ruiz-Baier *et al.* 2014), which assumes the compact form

$$\frac{d\gamma_f}{dt} = g_{\gamma_f}(\gamma_f, \mathbf{c}, \lambda) \tag{6.30}$$

for each $\boldsymbol{x} \in \Omega_{mus}$; here, $g_{\gamma_f}$ depends on the sarcomere force-length relationship, while $\lambda$ is the stretch in the fibre direction. We refer the interested reader to, *e.g.* (Regazzoni, Dede' and Quarteroni 2017) and the references therein for a more detailed sarcomere model and a review on the topic.

The active strain approach is probably more satisfactory from the modelling point of view, since, unlike active stress, it should provide (in principle) the expected fibre contraction without any tuning; moreover, it preserves the polyconvexity properties of the strain energy function along the mechanical activation. However, from the numerical point of view it is more involved, since standard finite element, finite elasticity solvers cannot be used directly and should be properly adapted; specifically, solvers based on the active strain approach should be properly integrated with the characteristic law of passive mechanics to achieve computational efficiency. As the active stress approach is more popular in literature, from now on we will mainly refer to it; however, we will also provide some indications on the use of the active strain approach. For a comparison between the two approaches we refer to Ambrosi *et al.* (2011) and Ambrosi and Pezzuto (2012), and for related computational results to Pezzuto (2013) and Rossi *et al.* (2014).

### *6.2.2 The coupled electromechanical problem*

The values of the trans-membrane potential $V_m$ or calcium ion concentration $c_{\text{ca}}$, to be used in (6.26) or (6.27) to compute the active stress function $P^A$, are sometimes prescribed as given data to the mechanics problem: see *e.g.* Eriksson, Prassl, Plank and Holzapfel (2013). However, in most cases these should be obtained from the bidomain or monodomain equations. This leads to a *coupled electromechanical* problem; see *e.g.* Dössel *et al.* (2007).

The electrical propagation problem needs to be solved in a domain that changes in time, because of the cardiac contraction and relaxation. Under suitable assumptions (Colli Franzone, Pavarino and Scacchi 2016), in an Eulerian framework, these problems assume the form (6.5), (6.6) or (6.11), provided that the conductivity tensors (6.4) or (6.12) are computed by using the deformed unit directions $\boldsymbol{a}_f$, $\boldsymbol{a}_s$, $\boldsymbol{a}_n$: see *e.g.* Keldermann *et al.* (2009).

However, for computational simplicity, the bidomain and monodomain equations are usually set in a Lagrangian framework and written in the reference undeformed configuration. Here we report the corresponding monodomain equation,

$$
\begin{aligned}
J\chi_m C_m\left(\frac{\partial \widehat{V}_m}{\partial t} - \boldsymbol{F}^{-T}\nabla\widehat{V}_m \cdot \frac{\partial \boldsymbol{\psi}}{\partial t}\right) - \nabla\cdot\left(J\boldsymbol{F}^{-1}\boldsymbol{\Sigma}\boldsymbol{F}^{-T}\nabla\widehat{V}_m\right)&\\
+ J\chi_m\widetilde{I}_{\text{ion}}\left(\widehat{V}_m, \widehat{\boldsymbol{w}}, \widehat{\boldsymbol{c}}, \lambda\right) = J\widehat{I}^{\text{ext}} \quad \text{in } \Omega_{\text{mus}}& \qquad (6.31)
\end{aligned}
$$

(using the notation of Part 1, we set $\Omega_{\text{mus}} = \Omega^0_{\text{mus}}$), coupled with the ODE systems (6.9e, 6.9f) (similar arguments hold true for the bidomain equations as well). The spatial derivatives have to be taken with respect to the undeformed domain, $\boldsymbol{\psi}$ is the deformation map between $\Omega^0_{\text{mus}}$ and $\Omega^t_{\text{mus}}$ and $\lambda$ is the stretch in the fibre direction introduced above.

From the above equation, we observe that there are three sources of *mechano-electrical feedback* – that is, three ways in which the mechanics problem influences the electrical problem:

(i) the effective conductivity tensor $\widehat{\boldsymbol{\Sigma}} = J\boldsymbol{F}^{-1}\boldsymbol{\Sigma}\boldsymbol{F}^{-T}$ depends on the deformation gradient $\boldsymbol{F}$;
(ii) the ionic current term $I_{\text{ion}}$ depends on the stretch in the fibre direction $\lambda$;
(iii) the relation between the spatial and material time derivatives introduces the advection term $-\boldsymbol{F}^{-T}\nabla\widehat{V}_m \cdot \partial\boldsymbol{\psi}/\partial t$, which depends on the solution of the mechanics problem (Colli Franzone *et al.* 2016).

Terms (i) and (iii) are due to the pull-back of the monodomain equation into the undeformed domain (geometric feedback). Term (ii) is due to a well-known physical process consisting of the opening of ion channels under the action of deformation (stretch-activated channels: see Section 4.4) (Kohl, Hunter and Noble 1999, Kohl and Sachs 2001). Accordingly, the ionic current term is written as the sum of two contributions:

$$
\widetilde{I}_{\text{ion}} = I_{\text{ion}}(\widehat{V}_m, \widehat{\boldsymbol{w}}, \widehat{\boldsymbol{c}}) + I^{\text{SAC}}(\widehat{V}_m, \lambda), \qquad (6.32)
$$

where $I_{\text{ion}}$ denotes one of the classical independent-stretch models described in Section 6.1.2, and $I^{\text{SAC}}$ is the current activated by the deformation. A fairly general expression for the latter term is given by

$$
I^{\text{SAC}} = \sum_i K_i(\widehat{V}_m)(\lambda - 1)(\widehat{V}_m - V_i)H(\lambda - 1), \qquad (6.33)
$$

where the $i$th term of the sum represents the stretch-activated currents related to the $i$th ion (usually sodium and potassium), $K_i$ is a suitable function, and $V_i$ is the Nernst potential introduced in Section 6.1.2. The Heaviside function $H(\cdot)$ guarantees that the stretch-activated ion channels open only under fibre tension ($\lambda > 1$) (Niederer and Smith 2007). Colli Franzone *et al.* (2016) showed (computationally) that these terms do not significantly alter the morphology of the action potential, but they strongly influence the action potential duration.

Stretch-activated ionic currents together with the active stress component of the stress tensor (or equivalently the active strain component of the deformation gradient) make the electromechanics problem a highly coupled system, which can be summarized as follows. Find the muscle displacement $\widehat{\boldsymbol{d}}$, the trans-membrane potential $\widehat{V}_m$, the gating variables $\widehat{\boldsymbol{w}}$, and the ionic concentration variables $\widehat{\boldsymbol{c}}$, such that, for all $t > 0$

$$-\nabla \cdot \left( \widehat{\boldsymbol{T}}_s^P(\widehat{\boldsymbol{d}}) + \widehat{\boldsymbol{T}}_s^A\left(\widehat{\boldsymbol{c}}, \widehat{\boldsymbol{d}}, \frac{\partial \widehat{\boldsymbol{d}}}{\partial t}\right)\right) = \mathbf{0} \quad \text{in } \Omega_{\text{mus}}, \tag{6.34a}$$

$$\widehat{\boldsymbol{T}}_s^A = P^A \widehat{\boldsymbol{a}}_f \otimes \widehat{\boldsymbol{a}}_f, \quad P^A = \mathcal{A}\left(\widehat{\boldsymbol{c}}, \widehat{\boldsymbol{d}}, \frac{\partial \widehat{\boldsymbol{d}}}{\partial t}\right) \quad \text{in } \Omega_{\text{mus}}, \tag{6.34b}$$

$$\widehat{V}_m = \mathcal{M}(\widehat{V}_m; \widehat{\boldsymbol{d}}, \widehat{\boldsymbol{w}}, \widehat{\boldsymbol{c}}) \quad \text{in } \Omega_{\text{mus}}, \tag{6.34c}$$

$$(\widehat{\boldsymbol{w}}, \widehat{\boldsymbol{c}}) = \mathcal{G}(\widehat{\boldsymbol{w}}, \widehat{\boldsymbol{c}}; \widehat{V}_m) \quad \text{in } \Omega_{\text{mus}}. \tag{6.34d}$$

Here, equation (6.34a) stands for the mechanical problem. Note that, unlike for the vessel case (see (3.7)), the time-dependent inertial term has been neglected, as is commonly done for cardiac mechanics. Moreover, $\widehat{\boldsymbol{T}}_s^P = \partial\Theta/\partial\boldsymbol{F}$, where $\Theta$ is given by the orthotropic law (6.24), for example, and $P^A$ is given by either (6.26) or (6.27). Equation (6.34c) represents the monodomain problem (6.31) in compact form, together with the ionic current expression given by (6.32, 6.9c, 6.9d, 6.33). Finally, (6.34d) is shorthand for the ODE systems (6.9e, 6.9f) for the gating and ionic concentration variables characterizing the cardiac cell model. The symbols $\mathcal{M}$ and $\mathcal{G}$ are abridged notations to identify the underlying PDE and ODEs, respectively. Note also that in writing system (6.34), we have exploited the fact that $\lambda$ and $\boldsymbol{F}$ could be written in terms of $\boldsymbol{d}$, allowing us to indicate the dependences of the monodomain problem on $\lambda$ and $\boldsymbol{F}$ and of $\widehat{\boldsymbol{T}}_s^A$ on $\lambda$ in compact form through $\boldsymbol{d}$.

If the active strain approach were instead to be used, the coupled electromechanics problem would read as follows. Find $\widehat{\boldsymbol{d}}$, $\widehat{\gamma}_f$, $\widehat{V}_m$, $\widehat{\boldsymbol{w}}$ and $\widehat{\boldsymbol{c}}$, such that, for all $t > 0$,

$$-\nabla \cdot \left( \widehat{\boldsymbol{T}}_s(\widehat{\boldsymbol{d}}) \right) = \mathbf{0} \qquad \text{in } \Omega_{\text{mus}}, \tag{6.35a}$$

$$\widehat{\boldsymbol{T}}_s = \widehat{J}^A \frac{D\Theta}{D\boldsymbol{F}^P} (\boldsymbol{F}^A)^{-T}, \quad \boldsymbol{F}^A = \boldsymbol{F}^A(\widehat{\gamma}_f) \qquad \text{in } \Omega_{\text{mus}}, \tag{6.35b}$$

$$\frac{\partial \widehat{\gamma}_f}{\partial t} = g_{\gamma_f}(\widehat{\gamma}_f, \widehat{\mathbf{c}}, \widehat{\boldsymbol{d}}) \qquad \text{in } \Omega_{\text{mus}}, \tag{6.35c}$$

$$\widehat{V}_m = \mathcal{M}(\widehat{V}_m; \widehat{\boldsymbol{d}}, \widehat{\boldsymbol{w}}, \widehat{\boldsymbol{c}}) \qquad \text{in } \Omega_{\text{mus}}, \tag{6.35d}$$

$$(\widehat{\boldsymbol{w}}, \widehat{\boldsymbol{c}}) = \mathcal{G}(\widehat{\boldsymbol{w}}, \widehat{\boldsymbol{c}}; \widehat{V}_m) \qquad \text{in } \Omega_{\text{mus}}. \tag{6.35e}$$

Here the active strain tensor in (6.35b) is expressed either by (6.28) or (6.29), while (6.35c) derives from (6.30).

Regarding the well-posedness of the electromechanical coupled problems (6.34) or (6.35), very few results have been obtained so far. We mention Pathmanathan, Chapman, Gavaghan and Whiteley (2010), who noticed that for the general active stress model (6.27), the equilibrium equation (6.34a) is not even elliptic when there is explicit dependence on the rate of stretch $\mathrm{d}\lambda/\mathrm{d}t$, and Andreianov, Bendahmane, Quarteroni and Ruiz-Baier (2015), who proved the existence of a weak solution for the case of a linearized elasticity equation in the active strain formulation coupled with the bidomain equations including the geometric feedback affecting the conductivity tensors.

### 6.2.3 The issue of boundary conditions for the mechanics problem

For the mechanical problem (6.34a) (or (6.35a)), proper boundary conditions should be prescribed at both the external epicardium and internal endocardium surfaces. For the former, the presence of both the pericardium and the surrounding tissue has to be accounted for, because of their effect on heart movement. Fritz *et al.* (2014) have proposed a sophisticated model of interaction with the pericardium accounting for a frictionless contact. More commonly, and similarly to the vascular case, a Robin condition such as (2.1) is prescribed at $\Sigma_{\text{epi}}$; see *e.g.* (Barbarotta *et al.* 2018) and (Gerbi 2018).

At the endocardium internal surface $\Sigma_{\text{endo}}$, in the presence of a fluid model in the atrial and ventricular cavities, the usual dynamic and kinematic conditions (3.19c, 3.19d), arising from the fluid–structure interaction model, implicitly provide both the endocardial displacement and normal stresses (see Section 6.5). When the fluid in the ventricular cavity is not modelled, suitable strategies for prescribing boundary conditions at $\Sigma_{\mathrm{endo}}$ are mandatory. A common strategy relies on prescribing a Neumann condition of the form

$$\widehat{\boldsymbol{T}}_s \widehat{\boldsymbol{n}} = P \widehat{\boldsymbol{n}}, \tag{6.36}$$

where $P$ is a suitable value of the blood pressure distribution at the endocardium.

During ventricular filling, condition (6.36) is prescribed both for atria and ventricles by means of selected values of blood pressures taken from the literature (see Figure 4.2).

During isovolumic contraction, the ventricular volume is kept constant often by means of fixed-point iterations, for example, where the value of the endocardial pressure to be prescribed in (6.36) at each time step is updated until satisfaction of the constraint given by the unchanged volume:

$$P_{(k+1)} = P_{(k)} + (V - V^n)/C_k,$$

(Usyk, LeGrice and McCulloch 2002, Eriksson *et al.* 2013), where $V$ is the current cavity volume, $k$ is the sub-iteration index and $C_k$ is a penalty parameter, and where the current temporal index $^{n+1}$ is as usual understood. Alternatively, a Lagrange multiplier approach can be employed (Gurev *et al.* 2015). During this phase the atrial pressure is kept constant to the values reached when the mitral and tricuspid valves close.

For ventricular ejection, a reduced 0D model (based on the analogy with electrical circuits: see Section 3.5.1) for the systemic (or pulmonary) circulation is usually coupled with the cardiac mechanics problem, assuming that the ventricular pressure equals the pressure in the aorta (or in the pulmonary artery) (Usyk *et al.* 2002, Eriksson *et al.* 2013). This is an approximation which is acceptable in first instance since, although the ventricular and circulatory pressures are different (thus allowing for the acceleration and deceleration of blood: see Figure 4.2), they are very similar. In this case one obtains a coupled problem between the cardiac mechanics and the lumped parameter model where the two subproblems exchange suitable interface conditions (*e.g.* in an iterative framework). For example, the 0D model could provide the pressure to be prescribed to the mechanics problem by means of (6.36), whereas the flow rate $Q = \rho_f(\mathrm{d}V/\mathrm{d}t)$ is prescribed to the 0D model. During the ejection phase the atrial pressure is determined by the venous pressure, which may be obtained with a 0D model or by values from the literature.

Finally, during isovolumic relaxation the endocardial pressure is decreased according to values from the literature until it reaches the pressure atrial value. Also during this phase the atrial pressure is determined by the venous pressure.

When only the ventricular mechanics is modelled (no atria), a truncated computational domain is considered, like the one depicted in Figure 6.2(a). In this case we have to provide suitable boundary conditions for the ventricular base $\Sigma_b$. Often, this surface is kept fixed by enforcing homogeneous Dirichlet conditions. In other cases, the tangential displacement is allowed by prescribing a homogeneous Neumann condition along the tangential directions.

### *6.2.4 Numerical approximation*

Let us consider the coupled electromechanical problem (6.34) in the active stress approach, which is commonly used in literature. Problem (6.34) is composed of four different blocks, namely the two PDEs (6.34a) and (6.34c) describing the heart mechanics and electrical propagation, respectively, the ODE system (6.34b) providing the active stress function, and the ODE systems (6.34d) modelling gating and ionic concentration variables. Moreover, the algebraic source of coupling (6.32, 6.33) needs to be accounted for to determine the stretch-activated ion currents. Their influence on the electrical problem has been included directly in the right-hand side of (6.34c).

A common numerical solution strategy for problem (6.34) addresses the two PDEs (6.34a) and (6.34c) separately by relying (when possible) on pre-existing mechanics and electrical codes: for instance, the mechanics subproblem is solved by Pavarino *et al.* (2015) using efficient Newton–Krylov iterations, while the electrical subproblem (monodomain equation together with a cell ODE model) is solved by means of one of the strategies described in Section 6.1.6 (see also Sundnes *et al.* 2014 for an operator splitting method).

In this context, at each time step the electrical subproblem is solved first and the mechanics problem later (Nash and Panfilov 2004, Gurev *et al.* 2015, Sundnes *et al.* 2014). In particular, after time discretization, the following scheme is employed (as usual the current temporal index $^{n+1}$ is understood and $^*$ means that the related term could be treated either implicitly or explicitly, depending on the temporal scheme used).

**Algorithm EM1.** At each time step:

(1) Solve the monodomain problem together with the cell model:

$$\widehat{V}_m = \mathcal{M}(\widehat{V}_m^*; \widehat{\boldsymbol{d}}^n, \widehat{\boldsymbol{w}}^*, \widehat{\boldsymbol{c}}^*) \quad \text{in } \Omega_{\text{mus}}, \tag{6.37a}$$

$$(\widehat{\boldsymbol{w}}, \widehat{\boldsymbol{c}}) = \mathcal{G}(\widehat{\boldsymbol{w}}^*, \widehat{\boldsymbol{c}}^*; \widehat{V}_m^*) \quad \text{in } \Omega_{\text{mus}}. \tag{6.37b}$$

(2) Then, solve the following mechanics problem:

(2a) Update the active stress contribution

$$\widehat{\boldsymbol{T}}_s^A = P^A \boldsymbol{a}_f \otimes \widehat{\boldsymbol{a}}_f, \quad P^A = \mathcal{A}\left(\widehat{\mathbf{c}}, \widehat{\boldsymbol{d}}^n, \frac{\widehat{\boldsymbol{d}}^n - \widehat{\boldsymbol{d}}^{n-1}}{\Delta t}\right) \quad \text{in } \Omega_{\text{mus}}.$$

(2b) Solve the equilibrium equation by means of the following Newton iterations. At each iteration $k$ solve

$$\begin{aligned}\nabla \cdot (D_F \widehat{\boldsymbol{T}}_s^P(\widehat{\boldsymbol{d}}_{(k-1)}))\delta\widehat{\boldsymbol{d}}_{(k)} \\ = -\nabla \cdot \left(\widehat{\boldsymbol{T}}_s^P(\widehat{\boldsymbol{d}}_{(k-1)}) + \widehat{\boldsymbol{T}}_s^A\left(\widehat{\mathbf{c}}, \widehat{\boldsymbol{d}}^n, \frac{\widehat{\boldsymbol{d}}^n - \widehat{\boldsymbol{d}}^{n-1}}{\Delta t}\right)\right) \quad \text{in } \Omega_{\text{mus}}.\end{aligned}$$

Using the notation introduced in Section 3.6.2, $D_F$ is the Gâteaux derivative with respect to $\boldsymbol{F}$, $\delta\widehat{\boldsymbol{d}}_{(k)} = \widehat{\boldsymbol{d}}_{(k)} - \widehat{\boldsymbol{d}}_{(k-1)}$, and, for simplicity, we have considered a Forward Euler approximation of $\mathrm{d}\lambda/\mathrm{d}t|_{t^n}$ (instead of $\mathrm{d}\lambda/\mathrm{d}t|_{t^{n+1}}$). The active stress contribution is treated explicitly, that is, it is updated once per time step. This choice may lead to numerical instabilities, as reported computationally in Niederer and Smith (2008). Pathmanathan *et al.* (2010) speculate that such instability could be ascribed to the (necessarily) explicit time discretization of the explicit stretch rate term $\mathrm{d}\lambda/\mathrm{d}t|_{t^n}$ (instead of $\mathrm{d}\lambda/\mathrm{d}t|_{t^{n+1}}$) in the active stress function solution.

To overcome these instabilities, Niederer and Smith (2008) proposed updating the active stress function at each Newton step, that is, to replace step (2) in Algorithm EM1 with the following:

**Algorithm EM1′.**

(2′). Solve the mechanics problem by means of the following Newton iterations. At each iteration $k$:

(2′a) Update the active stress contribution:

$$\widehat{\boldsymbol{T}}_s^A = P^A \boldsymbol{a}_f \otimes \widehat{\boldsymbol{a}}_f, \quad P^A = \mathcal{A}\left(\widehat{\mathbf{c}}, \widehat{\boldsymbol{d}}_{(k-1)}, \frac{\widehat{\boldsymbol{d}}_{(k-1)} - \widehat{\boldsymbol{d}}^n}{\Delta t}\right) \quad \text{in } \Omega_{\text{mus}}.$$

(2′b) Solve the equilibrium equation:

$$\begin{aligned}\nabla \cdot (D_F \widehat{\boldsymbol{T}}_s^P(\widehat{\boldsymbol{d}}_{k-1}))\delta\widehat{\boldsymbol{d}}_k \\ = -\nabla \cdot \left(\widehat{\boldsymbol{T}}_s^P(\widehat{\boldsymbol{d}}_{k-1}) + \widehat{\boldsymbol{T}}_s^A\left(\widehat{\mathbf{c}}, \widehat{\boldsymbol{d}}_{(k-1)}, \frac{\widehat{\boldsymbol{d}}_{(k-1)} - \widehat{\boldsymbol{d}}^n}{\Delta t}\right)\right) \quad \text{in } \Omega_{\text{mus}}.\end{aligned}$$

Note that step (2′) does not coincide with a Newton iteration for (6.34a, 6.34b). Although at the expense of a larger number of iterations, this scheme provides stable solutions and allows the use of a standard solver for the mechanics part.

A Newton method for the solution of the mechanics problem (6.34a, 6.34b), used in combination with a different explicit decoupled scheme, was successfully proposed by Pavarino *et al.* (2015), who split the electrical problem (6.34c, 6.34d) into the cellular and macroscopic parts (semi-implicit treatment), and solved the mechanics problem in between, as follows.

**Algorithm EM2**. At each time step:

(1) Solve the ODE system for the gating and ionic concentration variables

$$(\widehat{\boldsymbol{w}}, \widehat{\boldsymbol{c}}) = \mathcal{G}(\widehat{\boldsymbol{w}}^*, \widehat{\boldsymbol{c}}^*; \widehat{V}_m^*) \quad \text{in } \Omega_{\text{mus}}.$$

(2) Then, solve the mechanics problem by means of the following Newton method. At each iteration $k$ solve:

(2a) Update the active stress contribution:

$$\widehat{\boldsymbol{T}}_s^A = P^A \boldsymbol{a}_f \otimes \widehat{\boldsymbol{a}}_f, \quad P^A = \mathcal{A}\left(\widehat{\boldsymbol{c}}, \widehat{\boldsymbol{d}}_{(k-1)}, \frac{\widehat{\boldsymbol{d}}_{(k-1)} - \widehat{\boldsymbol{d}}^n}{\Delta t}\right) \quad \text{in } \Omega_{\text{mus}}.$$

(2b) Solve the equilibrium equation:

$$\begin{aligned} \nabla \cdot \left( D_F \widehat{\boldsymbol{T}}_s^P(\widehat{\boldsymbol{d}}_{(k-1)}) + D_F \widehat{\boldsymbol{T}}_s^A\left(\widehat{\boldsymbol{c}}, \widehat{\boldsymbol{d}}_{(k-1)}, \frac{\widehat{\boldsymbol{d}}_{(k-1)} - \widehat{\boldsymbol{d}}^n}{\Delta t}\right)\right) \delta\widehat{\boldsymbol{d}}_{(k)} \\ = -\nabla \cdot \left( \widehat{\boldsymbol{T}}_s^P(\widehat{\boldsymbol{d}}_{(k-1)}) + \widehat{\boldsymbol{T}}_s^A\left(\widehat{\boldsymbol{c}}, \widehat{\boldsymbol{d}}_{(k-1)}, \frac{\widehat{\boldsymbol{d}}_{(k-1)} - \widehat{\boldsymbol{d}}^n}{\Delta t}\right)\right) \quad \text{in } \Omega_{\text{mus}}. \end{aligned}$$

1 Solve the monodomain problem:

$$\widehat{V}_m = \mathcal{M}(\widehat{V}_m^*; \widehat{\boldsymbol{d}}, \widehat{\boldsymbol{w}}, \widehat{\boldsymbol{c}}) \quad \text{in } \Omega_{\text{mus}}.$$

Andreianov *et al.* (2015) have proposed a simplified variant of the above decoupled algorithms for the active strain formulation.[1] We provide the same variant below for the active stress formulation; in the second equation of (6.34b), however, the active stress function $P^A = \mathcal{A}(\widehat{\boldsymbol{c}})$ does not depend on the stretch and stretch rate.

[1] This is one of the very few papers that contain a convergence result for the finite element solution to the differential problem (6.34).

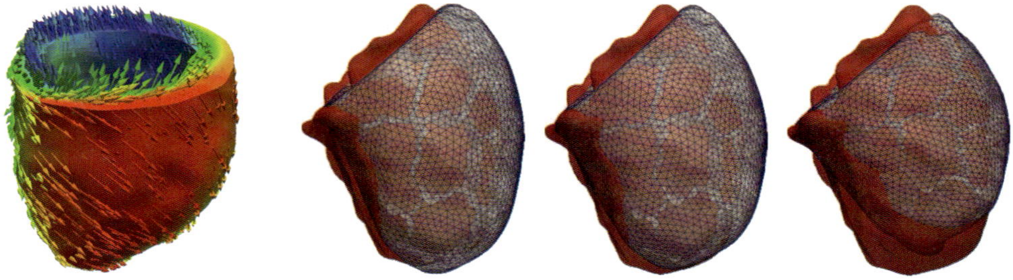

(a) (b)

Figure 6.6 (a) Fibre orientation in a real left ventricle obtained with the rule-based method proposed in Rossi *et al.* (2014). Data from CT images provided by the Cardiology Division of Ospedale S. Maria del Carmine, Rovereto (TN), Italy, and by the Radiology Division of Borgo-Trento (TN), Italy; courtesy of S. Palamara. (b) Displacement configuration of a real left ventricle during the contraction phase at three different times. Orthotropic model of activation: see Barbarotta (2014). Numerical results were obtained using LifeV and taken from Barbarotta (2014); data from CT images provided by the Cardio Surgery and Radiology Divisions at Ospedale Sacco, Milan, Italy.

**Algorithm EM3**. At each time step:

(1) Update the active stress contribution:

$$\widehat{\boldsymbol{T}}_s^A = P^A \boldsymbol{a}_f \otimes \widehat{\boldsymbol{a}}_f, \quad P^A = \mathcal{A}(\widehat{\boldsymbol{c}}^{n-1}) \quad \text{in } \Omega_{\text{mus}}.$$

(2) Solve the equilibrium mechanics problem by means of the following Newton method. At each iteration $k$ solve

$$\nabla \cdot \big(D_F \widehat{\boldsymbol{T}}_s^P (\widehat{\boldsymbol{d}}_{k-1})\big)\delta\widehat{\boldsymbol{d}}_k = -\nabla \cdot \big(\widehat{\boldsymbol{T}}_s^P (\widehat{\boldsymbol{d}}_{k-1}) + \widehat{\boldsymbol{T}}_s^A (\widehat{\boldsymbol{c}}^{n-1})\big) \quad \text{in } \Omega_{\text{mus}}.$$

(3) Then, solve the electrical problem:

$$\begin{aligned} \widehat{V}_m &= \mathcal{M}\big(\widehat{V}_m^*; \widehat{\boldsymbol{d}}^{n-1}, \widehat{\boldsymbol{w}}^*, \widehat{\boldsymbol{c}}^*\big) && \text{in } \Omega_{\text{mus}}, \\ (\widehat{\boldsymbol{w}}, \widehat{\boldsymbol{c}}) &= \mathcal{G}(\widehat{\boldsymbol{w}}^*, \widehat{\boldsymbol{c}}^*; \widehat{V}_m^*) && \text{in } \Omega_{\text{mus}}. \end{aligned}$$

Although segregated algorithms such as those reported above are the most widely used for numerical solution of the coupled electromechanics problem (6.34), a monolithic approach has been used by Goktepe and Kuhl (2010), who have successfully applied a Newton method to the whole coupled problem with a FitzHugh–Nagumo cardiac cell model (*i.e.* without the ODE systems (6.34d)); see also (Dal, Göktepe, Kaliske and Kuhl 2013) for the coupled electromechanics problem with the bidomain equations. More

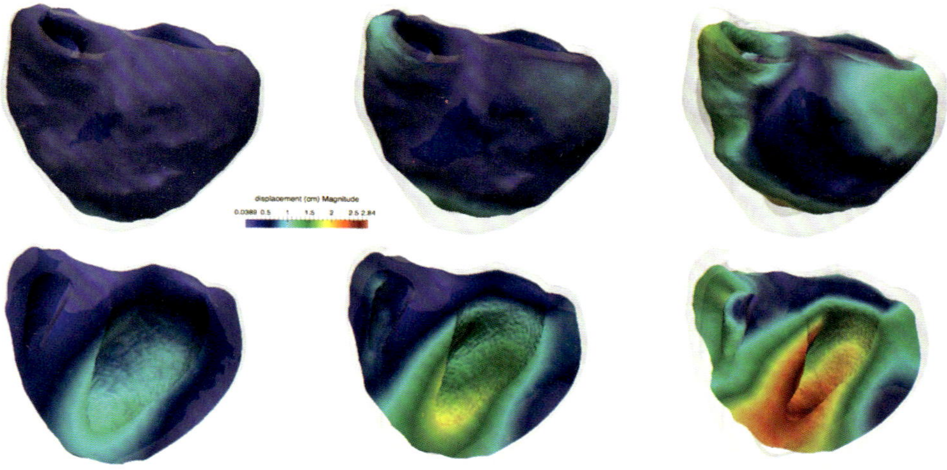


Figure 6.7 Displacements of the two ventricles at six different times during systolic contraction. Electromechanical coupled simulation, P1 finite elements. Numerical results were obtained using LifeV; the computational mesh was obtained from an open source biventricular geometry segmented from CT images: see Rousseau (2010).

recently, Hirschvogel *et al.* (2017) proposed a monolithic electromechanics solver including 0D models for the vascular system, atria and heart valves.

A monolithic algorithm for cardiac electromechanics within the active strain approach and based on the transmurally variable orthotropic activation model (6.29) was introduced and analyzed in Gerbi, Dede' and Quarteroni (2018); the same solver was used in Landajuela *et al.* (2018) for the electromechanical coupling in the left ventricle with the inclusion of the Purkinje network. Segregated and staggered algorithms for the same electromechanics model were alternatively proposed and analyzed in Gerbi (2018) and Gerbi, Dede' and Quarteroni (2018).

In Figure 6.6 we show an example of fibre configuration in the left ventricle, and in the same figure and Figure 6.7 we give the results of an electromechanical simulation.

## 6.3 The ventricular fluid dynamics

Blood flow in heart cavities $\Omega_{\text{cav}}$, shown in Figure 5.1, can be regarded as homogeneous, Newtonian and incompressible (Vierendeels, Riemslagh, Dick and Verdonck 2000, Watanabe *et al.* 2002). The displacements induced by the interaction with the myocardium can be larger than 30%, so it is mandatory to account for the geometric deformation of the fluid computational domain, either by prescribing its motion or through the solution of fluid–structure interaction (FSI) problems. Despite the large displacements, the ALE technique introduced in Section 3.6.3 is suitable for FSI in this context, as shown by several authors: see *e.g.* Cheng, Oertel and Schenkel (2005) and Nordsletten *et al.* (2011*a*). Alternatively, the immersed boundary method (Peskin 1972), which does not require remeshing or induced mesh deformation, has often been used since the celebrated paper by Peskin (Mittal *et al.* 2016, Choi *et al.* 2015, De Tullio *et al.* 2009, Meschini *et al.* 2018); see Section 6.4 for a mathematical description.

One of the main features of the intraventricular fluid dynamics is represented by the formation of a vortex ring (O-ring) during diastole (*i.e.* the filling phase) just downstream of the mitral valve; see *e.g.* Menghini *et al.* (2018) and Tagliabue *et al.* (2017*a*). This ring is generated during the peak flow due to a pressure gradient between left atrium and left ventricle, and it is distorted due to the asymmetry of the mitral valve leaflets (Seo *et al.* 2014). At the end of this phase, the vortex ring is broken up into small-scale structures that propagate towards the posterior wall and the apex. After the second mitral peak flow due to the atrium contraction, additional vortex rings pop up. However, due to the small duration of this phase, they are less intense and do not propagate far into the chamber (Le and Sotiropoulos 2013). Similar vortex rings are generated in the left atrium from the flow ejected by the pulmonary vein (Mittal *et al.* 2016, Menghini *et al.* 2017). This complex and disturbed fluid dynamics, in the presence of a fairly high Reynolds number ($\simeq 4000$), may lead to a nearly turbulent flow even in healthy cases; as a matter of fact, the ventricular blood flow can be characterized as transitional (Chnafa *et al.* 2014, Mittal *et al.* 2016, Querzoli, Fortini and Cenedese 2010). For this reason, it is common practice to include a suitable turbulence model in cardiac simulations; see *e.g.* Chnafa *et al.* (2014) for LES models, while Menghini *et al.* (2018) and Tagliabue, Dede' and Quarteroni (2017*b*) for the variational multiscale (VMS–LES) formulation. We refer the reader to Cimino *et al.* (2012) and Domenichini, Pedrizzetti and Baccani (2005) for a wider discussion of intraventricular blood flow in healthy and unhealthy conditions.

Regarding boundary conditions for the FSI problem, on the endocardium $\Sigma_{\text{endo}}$ (Figure 5.1) the kinematic and dynamic conditions are implicitly determined by the coupling with the structural problem holding in the myocardium, leading to a fluid–structure interaction problem (see Section 6.5). The solution of a coupled FSI problem can be avoided in those cases where the wall velocity can be derived from dynamic MRI or CT images as in

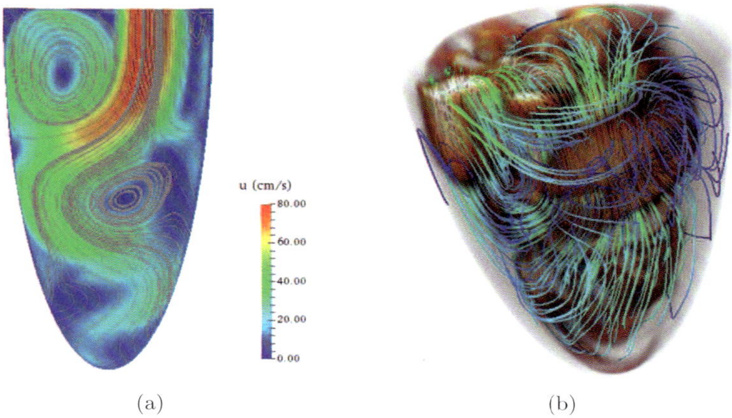


Figure 6.8 Blood flow modelling in idealized left ventricle geometries modelled as prolate ellipsoids (with prescribed deformation), 2D (a) and 3D (b): flow velocity and vortex structures at diastolic peak. Results obtained by means of isogeometric analysis solver; see Tagliabue *et al.* (2017*a*) and Tagliabue *et al.* (2017*b*). Courtesy of A. Tagliabue (EPFL).

(Chnafa *et al.* 2014) for the left ventricle and (Masci *et al.* 2017) for the left atrium. However, this requires us to have at our disposal several (20–30) wall displacement fields at different time instants during every heartbeat. The wall myocardium velocity (which provides the Dirichlet boundary condition for the fluid equations in the ventricle) can be generated by numerically differentiating the displacement field (Khalafvand *et al.* 2014, Mittal *et al.* 2016). Alternatively, the wall myocardium velocity could be provided by the solution of the electromechanics model if the latter were segregated from the fluid model (Choi *et al.* 2015). Finally, in reference or idealized geometries of the chambers, the deformation of the computational domain can be prescribed or inferred from the Wiggers diagram as done in Menghini *et al.* (2017), Menghini *et al.* (2018), Tagliabue *et al.* (2017*a*) and Tagliabue *et al.* (2017*b*). In these cases, the solution of FSI problems is not needed.

The heart also has four (virtual) sections that delimit it from the circulatory system, namely the aortic and pulmonary valve orifices (outlets) and the interfaces with the venae cavae and the pulmonary vein (inlets). In these cases, suitable conditions can be obtained by coupling the heart fluid dynamics with the aorta, the pulmonary artery, and the above-mentioned veins. These can be modelled by means of 3D, 1D or 0D models.

In the case of simulation in the left ventricle alone (see Figure 6.2(b)) we have to prescribe suitable boundary conditions at the mitral valve orifice

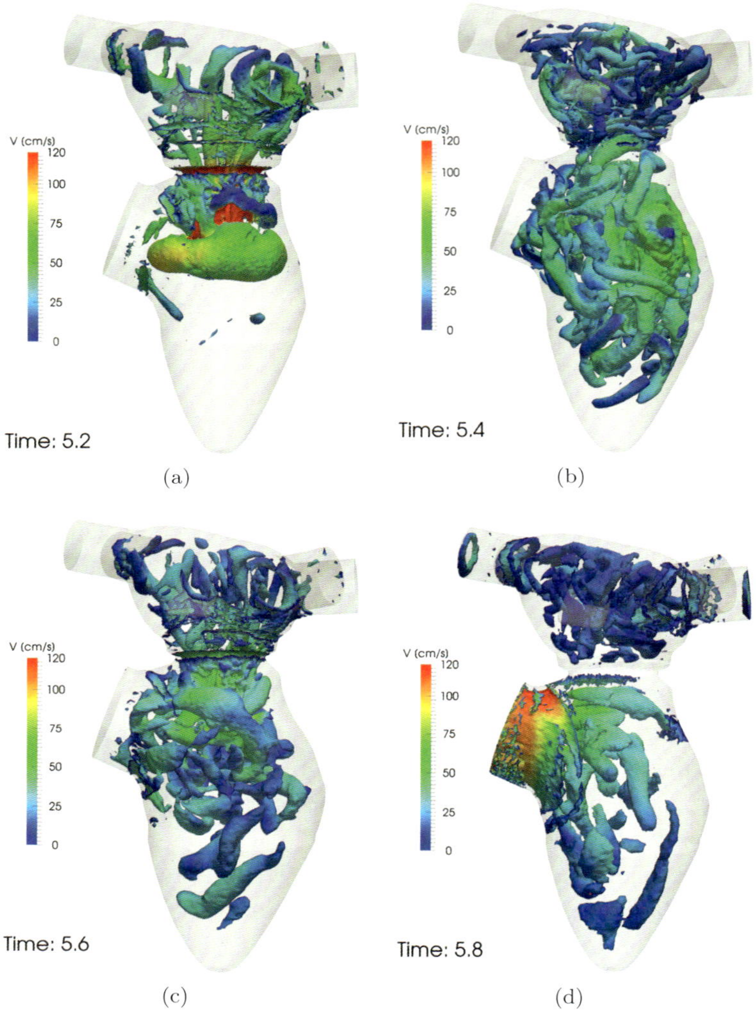


Figure 6.9 Numerical simulations of the blood flow in the left heart (left ventricle and left atrium) with prescribed deformation of the cavities: vortex structures by $Q$ criterion and velocity magnitude at different times of diastole. The vortex O-ring and smaller vortex structures in the left ventricle are highlighted. See Menghini *et al.* (2018); courtesy of F. Menghini (EPFL).

$\Gamma_{\text{mitr}}$ as well. For example, Khalafvand *et al.* (2014) propose prescribing the flow rates at $\Gamma_{\text{mitr}}$ and at the aortic valve outlet $\Gamma_{ao}$ obtained by MRI measurements of the volume changes of the left ventricle chamber, noticing that the two valves are never open simultaneously. Alternatively, flow rate curves

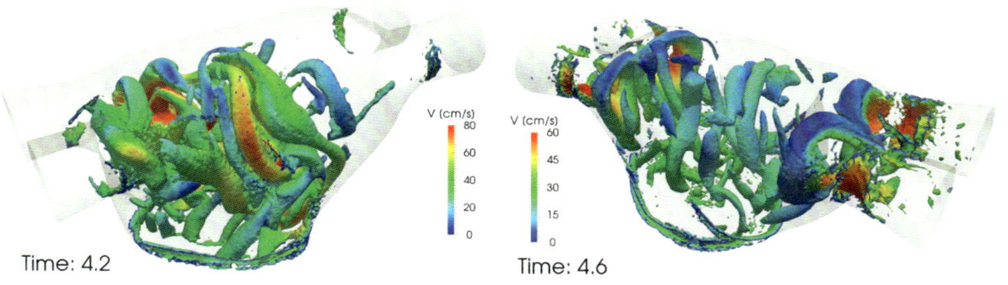


(a) (b)

Figure 6.10 Numerical simulations of the blood flow in the left atrium with prescribed deformation: vortex structures by $Q$ criterion and velocity magnitude at different times. The flow coming from the pulmonary veins is highlighted by O-ring vortexes in (b). See (Menghini *et al.* 2017); courtesy of F. Menghini (EPFL).

taken from the literature can be applied: see *e.g.* Nordsletten *et al.* (2011*a*). Special boundary conditions are instead proposed in Tagliabue *et al.* (2017*b*) as we will discuss in Section 6.4. In any case, fluid dynamical simulations of the blood flow in the heart chambers are strongly affected by the valve behaviour for which their action should be properly modelled.

We provide examples of numerical simulations related to the solution of the fluid dynamical problem in the left ventricle and in the left atria in Figures 6.8, 6.9 and 6.10.

## 6.4 Modelling the valves

Heart valves are made of thin leaflets. Aortic and pulmonary valves cause limited resistance to the blood during systole and sustain large pressure gradients during diastole. Moreover, unlike the vascular vessel wall, they are subjected to very large displacements. Because of these features, the mathematical and numerical modelling of the valve mechanics and their interaction with blood flow is very demanding, requiring *ad hoc* techniques for their description. This is further complicated by the fact that the opening and closing of the valves introduce topological changes to the computational domain of the fluid problem. Our main focus in this section will be on the aortic and mitral valves of the left ventricle, the most studied from the mathematical and clinical points of view. For recent reviews on valve modelling, see Marom (2015) and Votta *et al.* (2013), for example.

### *6.4.1 Mechanical models of the leaflets*

Due to fibre alignment, which occurs mostly in the circumferential direction $\boldsymbol{a}$, and to the presence of collagen, most of the valve mechanical models proposed so far are of the non-linear transversally isotropic type. In particular, they depend on the two invariants $I_1 = \operatorname{tr} \boldsymbol{C}$ and $I_4 = \widehat{\boldsymbol{a}} \cdot (\boldsymbol{C}\widehat{\boldsymbol{a}})$ of the left Cauchy tensor $\boldsymbol{C}$. For example, May-Newman, Lam and Yin (2009) and Prot, Skallerud and Holzapfel (2007) use the strain energy function

$$\Theta(I_1, I_4) = c\big[e^{b_1(I_1-3)^2+b_4(I_4-1)^2} - 1\big],$$

for suitable constants $c$, $b_1$, $b_4$. Variants of the above energy have been considered, for example by Humphrey and Yin (1987), May-Newman and Yin (1998) and Weinberg and Kaazempur-Mofrad (2006). For a comparison of numerical results obtained with these constitutive laws, see Auricchio, Ferrara and Morganti (2012). More sophisticated energy functions include the microstructure of the leaflet tissue: see *e.g.* Einstein *et al.* (2005).

Due to their thinness, heart valves are often modelled as membrane shells (see Ciarlet (2000)) by neglecting the shear bending forces, which are an order of magnitude smaller than the in-plane stresses (Hsu *et al.* 2015, Kim, Lu, Sacks and Chandran 2008, Merryman, Huang, Schoen and Sacks 2006, Morganti *et al.* 2015).

Some works on the mitral valve also consider the presence of the chordae tendinae (see Section 4.1). These comprise independent ring models, where the chordae are modelled as non-linear springs with zero elasticity during compression and exponential-like stiffness during traction (Kunzelman and Cochran 1990, Mansi *et al.* 2012), and one-dimensional models characterized by a non-linear energy function (Einstein *et al.* 2005, Votta *et al.* 2007, Padala *et al.* 2010).

Another difficulty arises when modelling the contact among the leaflets during closure. A common strategy to handle this process is a penalty method (Hsu *et al.* 2015, Marom 2015, Mansi *et al.* 2012). This is based on measuring the distance between each vertex of the finite element mesh discretizing the leaflet and the other closest leaflet, and on locating a spring between the vertex and the collision point when the distance becomes smaller than a critical value. Astorino, Gerbeau, Pantz and Traoré (2010) propose a more sophisticated algorithm, based on the introduction of sub-iterations that guarantee the satisfaction of the contact constraint via the introduction of Lagrange multipliers that act as a force of repulsion between the leaflets.

The numerical simulation of valve mechanics has usually been obtained by prescribing a pressure difference (jump) between the two sides of the leaflets, mimicking the effect of the fluid (Gnyaneshwar, Kumar and Balakrishnan 2002, Votta *et al.* 2013). However, more realistic models are obtained by considering the FSI problem arising between the blood flow and the leaflets. This is the topic of the next two subsections.

### 6.4.2 Reduced models for fluid–valve interaction

As already noted, the simulation of the fluid–structure interaction between blood and valve leaflets is computationally demanding. However, if one is interested only in the fluid dynamical quantities and not in the internal leaflet stresses, reduced models may be considered.

*Models for the valve orifice.* The first family does not explicitly represent the leaflets; rather, only the opening/closure mechanism of the valve is modelled through the description of the valve orifice. The simplest strategy consists in *a priori* operating the opening and closing of the valve on the basis of a flow rate or pressure profile obtained from the literature or from clinical data: see for instance Faggiano *et al.* (2013). For an example, see Bazilevs *et al.* (2009), Vergara *et al.* (2012) and Nestola *et al.* (2017) for the flow simulation in the aorta and Khalafvand *et al.* (2014) for that in the left ventricle. A more realistic situation is obtained by simulating the opening/closure mechanism of the aortic valve orifice by means of the following conditions prescribed to the fluid problem:

$$\begin{aligned} &\text{if } P_u > P_d \quad \text{then the valve opens,} \\ &\text{if } Q_d < 0 \quad \text{then the valve closes,} \end{aligned} \tag{6.38}$$

where $P_u$ is the upstream pressure and $P_d$ and $Q_d$ are the downstream pressure and flow rate (Formaggia *et al.* 1999). The quantities $P_u, P_d, Q_d$ could be prescribed as data or else be the results of the numerical computation of the flow field. For example, in a fluid dynamics simulation in the aorta, $P_u$ is the prescribed left ventricular pressure, and $P_d$ and $Q_d$ are the unknown aortic pressure and flow rate. For a left ventricular flow simulation, the situation is more involved as we have to distinguish between the mitral and the aortic valve: for the former, $P_u$ is the prescribed atrial pressure and $P_d$ and $Q_d$ are the unknown left ventricular pressure and flow rate; for the latter, $P_u$ is the unknown left ventricular pressure, and $P_d$ and $Q_d$ the prescribed aortic pressure and flow rate. Many works have considered a zero-dimensional model of the systemic circulation to provide the latter quantities (Wenk *et al.* 2013). In any case, the opening/closure mechanism is not prescribed *a priori*. This leads to a non-linear boundary condition for the fluid problem at the valve orifice which, in the electric circuit analogy of zero-dimensional models (see Section 3.5.1), is represented by an ideal diode. Similar models have been proposed by Korakianitis and Shi (2006*b*) and Blanco and Feijóo (2013), to account for diseased valves, by introducing a suitable non-ideal law for the diode. More refined reduced models consider the opening/closure mechanism not simply in an on–off mode: the open part of the orifice dynamically changes continuously by projecting the supposed leaflet position on the orifice plane. For example, in Sundaram, Balakrishnan and Kumar (2015) the dynamics of the valve orifice opening/closure is given by a prescribed law, whereas in Korakianitis and Shi (2006*a*) it is given by

$$A_V = \frac{(1-\cos\theta)^2}{(1-\cos\theta_{\max})^2},$$

where $A_V \in [0,1]$ is the fraction of open orifice area, $\theta$ is the (mean) opening leaflet angle ($\theta = 0$ means closed valve) and $\theta_{\max}$ is the maximum opening angle. The dynamics of the opening angle $\theta$ is determined by the ODE

$$\frac{\mathrm{d}^2\theta}{\mathrm{d}t^2} + k_1\frac{\mathrm{d}\theta}{\mathrm{d}t} + k_2(P_d - P_u)\cos\theta = 0, \tag{6.39}$$

for suitable parameters $k_1$ and $k_2$ and appropriate initial conditions on $\theta$ and $\mathrm{d}\theta/\mathrm{d}t$.

For all these models, which do not explicitly include the leaflets, there might be a need to switch between Dirichlet and Neumann (essential and natural) boundary conditions (and *vice versa*) along a single heartbeat in a fluid problem. Indeed, a Dirichlet condition is usually prescribed when the valve is closed (*e.g.* homogeneous in the physiological case), whereas a Neumann or a resistance condition might be preferred when the valve is open. This might be problematic at the numerical level, particularly in view of the definition of suitable algorithms and the implementation. Tagliabue, Dede' and Quarteroni (2017*b*) propose a new way to overcome this problem, based on a Robin-like condition called mixed time varying boundary condition, which implemented by means of the extended Nitsche's method proposed in Juntunen and Stenberg (2009); see (Tagliabue, Dede' and Quarteroni 2016) for the analysis of the method applied to parabolic PDEs. For simplicity we detail the case of a Neumann-like condition for the open valve, and we refer the reader to Tagliabue *et al.* (2017*b*) for the more physiological case of a resistance condition. Let $\Gamma$ be the valve orifice at hand, and suppose that one wants to prescribe at each time the following conditions:

$$\boldsymbol{v} = \boldsymbol{g} \qquad \text{if the valve is closed,} \tag{6.40a}$$

$$\boldsymbol{T}_f(\boldsymbol{v},p)\boldsymbol{n} = \boldsymbol{h} \qquad \text{if the valve is open.} \tag{6.40b}$$

For example, $\boldsymbol{g}$ might be obtained via a prescribed flow rate (null or equal to the fluid domain velocity in the physiological case) by assuming *a priori* the shape of the velocity profile (*e.g.* flat), whereas usually $\boldsymbol{h} = P\boldsymbol{n}$, where $P$ is a prescribed mean pressure. The boundary conditions (6.40) are replaced by the unique mixed time varying boundary condition

$$\boldsymbol{T}_f(\boldsymbol{v}, p)\boldsymbol{n} + \lambda \boldsymbol{v} = \boldsymbol{h} + \lambda \boldsymbol{g},$$

where $\lambda : \Gamma \times (0, T)$ is a suitable *switch* function dependent on space and time. If $\lambda \to 0^+$, then the natural (Neumann in this case) boundary condition is set on $\Gamma$ to mimic the open valve; conversely, if $\lambda \to +\infty$, the essential (Dirichlet) boundary condition is instead enforced to represent the closed valve. Such a mixed time-varying condition is set by means of the extended Nitsche method, for which the following terms are added to the weak formulation (3.6) of the fluid problem:

$$\begin{aligned}
&-\int_\Gamma \frac{\lambda h}{\xi + \lambda h} \boldsymbol{T}_f(\boldsymbol{v}, p)\boldsymbol{n} \cdot \boldsymbol{w} \,\mathrm{d}\gamma \\
&\quad - \int_\Gamma \frac{\lambda h}{\xi + \lambda h} (\boldsymbol{v} - \boldsymbol{g}) \cdot (\boldsymbol{T}_f(\boldsymbol{w}, q)\boldsymbol{n}) \,\mathrm{d}\gamma + \int_\Gamma \frac{\xi \lambda}{\xi + \lambda h} (\boldsymbol{v} - \boldsymbol{g}) \cdot \boldsymbol{w} \,\mathrm{d}\gamma \\
&\quad - \int_\Gamma \frac{h}{\xi + \lambda h} (\boldsymbol{T}_f(\boldsymbol{v}, p)\boldsymbol{n} - \boldsymbol{h}) \cdot (\boldsymbol{T}_f(\boldsymbol{w}, q)\boldsymbol{n}) \,\mathrm{d}\gamma + \int_\Gamma \frac{\xi}{\xi + \lambda h} \boldsymbol{h} \cdot \boldsymbol{w} \,\mathrm{d}\gamma,
\end{aligned}$$

where $\xi \in [0, +\infty)$ is a parameter and $h$ is the mesh size (possibly not constant); in particular, in order for the method to be effective, $\xi$ should be "large" when $\lambda \to +\infty$ and "small" for $\lambda \to 0^+$. This discrete problem preserves the usual finite element accuracy. Note that for $\lambda \to +\infty$ and $\xi$ "sufficiently large" we recover the classical Nitsche method for prescribing the Dirichlet condition (6.40a), whereas for $\lambda = 0$ and $\xi$ "small" the formulation is consistent with the Neumann condition (6.40b) with an additional stabilization term. Numerical results obtained with this method were presented in Figure 6.8. We remark that at this stage $\lambda$ and $\xi$ are assigned functions of the time; however, these could be used as unknowns of the fluid–valve problem.

Alternatively, the switch between a flow rate and mean pressure condition could be prescribed via the defective version of the extended Nitsche method proposed in Vergara (2011).

*Reduced models for valve leaflets.* A second family of reduced strategies includes a reduced model of the leaflets without solving the full 3D mechanical problem. These methods are very useful when one wants to determine to good accuracy the influence of the leaflets on the blood flow. A first simple model is based including the position of the open leaflets obtained by a preliminary mechanical simulation and considering an on–off opening/closure mode: see *e.g.* Bonomi *et al.* (2015). A similar model was proposed by Astorino, Hamers, Shadden and Gerbeau (2012), who considered an immersed *resistive method* to switch between the open and closed configuration. In particular, the following term is added to the variational formulation of the fluid problem:

$$\int_{\Gamma_o} R_o \boldsymbol{v} \cdot \boldsymbol{w} \, \mathrm{d}\gamma + \int_{\Gamma_c} R_c \boldsymbol{v} \cdot \boldsymbol{w} \, \mathrm{d}\gamma,$$

where $\Gamma_o$ and $\Gamma_c$ are the surfaces representing the open and closed leaflet configurations, respectively, and $R_o$ and $R_c$ are the corresponding resistance, which act as penalization terms to enforce the no-slip condition $\boldsymbol{v} = \boldsymbol{0}$ at the leaflet. Thus, when the value of the resistance is high, the corresponding surface configuration is physically included in the model, the velocity is zero at the leaflet and, accordingly, a pressure drop is generated across the leaflet; by contrast, when the value of the resistance is zero, the leaflet is invisible to the model, no constraint is prescribed on the velocity, and no pressure drop is generated. The switch between large and vanishing values of the resistances is determined by (6.38).

More sophisticated reduced fluid–valve models account not only for the open and closed configurations of the leaflets, but also provide a simplified dynamics of the entire valve opening/closure mechanism. For example, Laadhari and Quarteroni (2016) and Fedele, Faggiano, Dede' and Quarteroni (2017) represent a leaflet $\Gamma$ as a surface described by two embedded level-set functions which depend on a single scalar function of time; that is, the opening angle $\theta$. The latter is determined by a relation very similar to (6.39). At each time step, the term

$$\int_{\Gamma} R(\boldsymbol{v} - \boldsymbol{v}_{\mathrm{leaf}}) \cdot \boldsymbol{w} \, \mathrm{d}\gamma$$

is added to the weak formulation of the fluid problem, in order to guarantee a no-slip condition at the leaflet ($\boldsymbol{v} = \boldsymbol{v}_{\mathrm{leaf}}$, where $\boldsymbol{v}_{\mathrm{leaf}}$ is the leaflet velocity determined from $\theta$) by selecting a sufficiently large resistance $R$. We remark that in this case, the surface $\Gamma$ representing the valve leaflets through the level-set functions depends and varies over the time as determined by the opening angle $\theta$; the problem is therefore a reduced fluid–valve model in the unknowns $\boldsymbol{v}$, $p$ and $\theta$. A similar approach was adopted in Auricchio, Lefieux, Reali and Veneziani (2016), where however the leaflet was represented in a more simplified way by means of the opening angle alone (*i.e.* no level-set functions were involved). Suitable extensions of the SUPG and VMS–

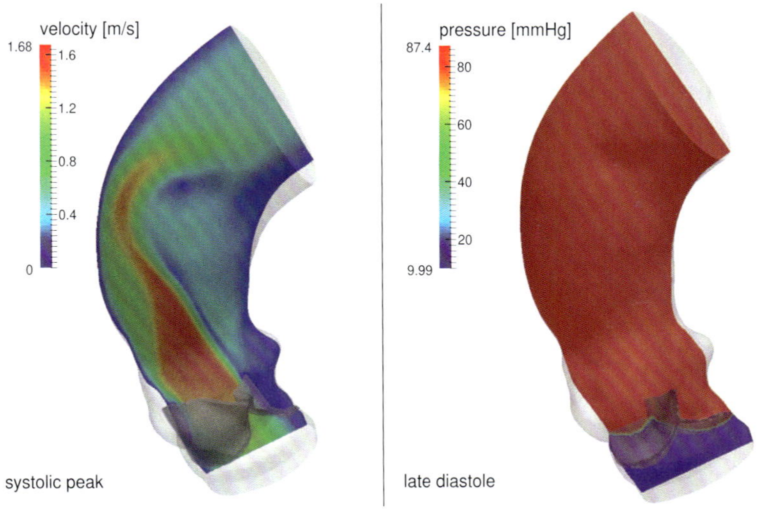


Figure 6.11 Fluid dynamics in the ascending aorta with a patient-specific aortic valve. Numerical results were obtained using LifeV. See Fedele *et al.* (2017) for a complete overview of the reduced fluid-valve interaction model and the results. Courtesy of M. Fedele (Politecnico di Milano).

LES stabilization techniques have been proposed in Fedele *et al.* (2017) and Menghini *et al.* (2018) to account for the resistive terms mimicking the presence of the valves.

In Figure 6.11 we give an example of the fluid dynamics across the aortic valve obtained by means of the method proposed in Fedele *et al.* (2017).

### *6.4.3 Interaction between blood and leaflets*

To accurately model the interaction between blood and valve leaflets, aimed, for example, at detailed computation of the internal leaflet stresses, the solution of a full FSI problem is required.

Unlike for the blood vessel and ventricular simulations, the arbitrary Lagrangian–Eulerian (ALE) formulation, described in Section 3.6, is not suited to handling the FSI problem arising between blood and heart valve leaflets. Indeed, due to the large displacements of the leaflets, the fluid mesh becomes highly distorted, producing severely stretched mesh elements and thus requiring a frequent remeshing of the grid. For this reason, specific FSI techniques have been developed specifically for the numerical solution of this problem. The most successful are the *immersed boundary* method, the *fictitious domain* approach and the *cut-FEM* method, together with their numerous variants; see *e.g.* (Hsu *et al.* 2015) and (Kamensky *et al.* 2015) for the recently proposed *immersogeometric* method. In general, all these methods are characterized by a fixed fluid mesh and enable us to treat non-conforming interface meshes.

*Immersed boundary method.* The celebrated immersed boundary method (IB) was specifically developed by Peskin (1972) for the fluid dynamics in the heart. The leaflets are represented by membranes in a Lagrangian framework regarded as part of the fluid, represented in an Eulerian framework, and exerting internal localized forces on the latter. This is achieved by introducing a Dirac *delta* distribution, $\delta$, on the membrane.

The IB method was originally developed for finite difference spatial discretization: see *e.g.* Peskin (1972), Mittal and Iaccarino (2005) and Peskin (2002). In this case, in order to avoid leaks, the Lagrangian grid should be sufficiently fine for the distance between two adjacent points to be less than the Eulerian mesh size. Then, the structural forces are interpolated into the fixed nodes of the fluid mesh. The major issue when finite differences are used is the approximation of $\delta$. This is usually obtained via a function $\delta_h$, which is non-singular for each $h$ and tends to $\delta$ for $h \to 0$ (Peskin 2002).

Here we describe the variational formulation of the IB method proposed in Boffi and Gastaldi (2003), which is useful for a finite element approximation and does not require any specific approximation of the delta distribution. Given a two-dimensional fluid domain $\Omega_f$, let $\Gamma_s$ be the immersed (one-dimensional) structure, whose material points are located at each $t$ in $\boldsymbol{X}(s,t)$, where $s \in [0, L]$ is the Lagrangian coordinate. We consider as an example the case of a massless linear elastic structure with elasticity constant $\kappa$. Thus, referring to the notation introduced in Section 3.1 and assuming homogeneous boundary conditions, the weak formulation of the IB method is as follows (Boffi, Gastaldi and Heltai 2007). For each $t > 0$, find $\boldsymbol{v} \in \boldsymbol{V}$, $\boldsymbol{v} = \boldsymbol{v}_0$ for $t = 0$, $p \in L^2(\Omega_f)$, and $\boldsymbol{X} = \boldsymbol{X}(t)$, $\boldsymbol{X} = \boldsymbol{X}_0$ for $t = 0$, such that

$$\rho_f \int_{\Omega_f} \frac{\partial \boldsymbol{v}}{\partial t} \cdot \boldsymbol{w}\, \mathrm{d}\omega + \mathcal{A}_f(\boldsymbol{v}, \boldsymbol{v}, \boldsymbol{w}) + \mathcal{B}(p, \boldsymbol{w}) = \int_0^L \kappa \frac{\partial^2 \boldsymbol{X}(s,t)}{\partial s^2} \boldsymbol{w}(\boldsymbol{X}(s,t))\, \mathrm{d}s, \tag{6.41a}$$

$$\mathcal{B}(q, \boldsymbol{v}) = 0, \tag{6.41b}$$

$$\frac{\partial \boldsymbol{X}}{\partial t}(s,t) = \boldsymbol{v}(\boldsymbol{X}(s,t), t), \tag{6.41c}$$

for all $\boldsymbol{w} \in \boldsymbol{V}$ and $q \in L^2(\Omega_f)$. In fact, the right-hand side of (6.41a) guarantees the satisfaction of the normal stress continuity at the membrane, whereas (6.41c) enforces the velocity continuity.

For the finite element approximation of the above problem, the forcing term is usually integrated by parts. For example, in the case of linear finite elements for the structure, for each $t > 0$ it becomes

$$\sum_{i=0}^{M-1} \kappa \left( \frac{\partial \boldsymbol{X}_h^{i+1}}{\partial s} - \frac{\partial \boldsymbol{X}_h^{i}}{\partial s} \right) \boldsymbol{w}(\boldsymbol{X}_h^i),$$

(Boffi *et al.* 2007), where $\boldsymbol{X}_h^i = \boldsymbol{X}_h(s_i)$, $i = 0, \ldots, M$, is the finite element approximation of $\boldsymbol{X}$ and $s_i$ are the nodes of the one-dimensional mesh.

Regarding the time discretization, a first approach is to consider a fully implicit scheme. For the backward Euler approximation, unconditional stability is guaranteed (Tu and Peskin 1992). However, this scheme requires the introduction of sub-iterations to handle the coupling between fluid and structure in (6.41). A more useful approach relies on treating the right-hand side of (6.41a) explicitly and the remaining part of the equation implicitly. The position occupied by the structure is then updated in a second step by means of a suitable implicit approximation of (6.41c). This scheme has been proved to be stable under a CFL-like condition (Boffi *et al.* 2007).

Several extensions and applications of the IB method have been provided. Among them, we mention the following: the variational formulation for the case of a thick immersed structure proposed in Boffi, Gastaldi, Heltai and Peskin (2008), for which the right-hand side of (6.41a) becomes

$$\int_{\Omega_s} \widehat{\boldsymbol{T}}_s(\widehat{\boldsymbol{d}}(\boldsymbol{s}, t)) : \nabla \boldsymbol{w}(\boldsymbol{X}(\boldsymbol{s}, t)) \, \mathrm{d}\boldsymbol{s},$$

where $\boldsymbol{s}$ in this case is a vectorial Lagrangian coordinate; a mesh-adaptive approach used in combination with a second-order scheme (see Griffith, Hornung, McQueen and Peskin 2007); the use of a curvilinear fixed fluid mesh to improve flexibility and efficiency (the CURVIB approach: see Borazjani, Ge and Sotiropoulos 2008); the application to realistic three-dimensional mitral and aortic valves successfully addressed in Griffith, Luo, McQueen and Peskin (2009) and Yin, Luo, Wang and Watton (2009).

*Fictitious domain approach.* The fictitious domain (FD) approach was first introduced by Glowinski, Pan and Periaux (1997) and Bertrand, Tanguy and Thibault (1997), and then used by de Hart, Peters, Schreurs and Baaijens (2000) and de Hart, Baaijens, Peters and Schreurs (2003) in the context of heart valves. The FD approach can be regarded as the dual of the IB method, in the sense that in the latter a weak enforcement of the normal stress continuity at the FS interface is added to the weak formulation of fluid problem, whereas in the FD approach the velocity continuity is weakly enforced at the FS interface. This is achieved by means of Lagrange multipliers, as detailed in what follows (we refer to Sections 3.1, 3.2 and 3.3 for the notation; in particular, variables with $\widehat{\ }$ are referred to the reference domain, and we assume homogeneous boundary conditions). Find

$$\boldsymbol{v}(t) \in \boldsymbol{V}^t, \quad \widehat{\boldsymbol{d}}(t) \in \boldsymbol{D}, \quad \boldsymbol{\lambda}(t) \in \boldsymbol{H}^{-1/2}(\Sigma^t) \quad \text{and} \quad p(t) \in L^2(\Omega^t),$$

such that

$$\begin{aligned}
&\rho_f \int_{\Omega^t} \frac{\partial \boldsymbol{v}}{\partial t} \cdot \boldsymbol{w} \, \mathrm{d}\omega + \mathcal{A}_f(\boldsymbol{v}, \boldsymbol{v}, \boldsymbol{w}) + \mathcal{B}(p, \boldsymbol{w}) \\
&\qquad + \rho_s \int_{\Omega_s} \frac{\partial^2 \widehat{\boldsymbol{d}}}{\partial t^2} \cdot \widehat{\boldsymbol{e}} \, \mathrm{d}\omega + \int_{\Omega_s} \widehat{\boldsymbol{T}}_s(\widehat{\boldsymbol{d}}) : \nabla \widehat{\boldsymbol{e}} \, \mathrm{d}\omega = \int_{\Sigma^t} \boldsymbol{\lambda} \cdot (\boldsymbol{w} - \boldsymbol{e}) \, \mathrm{d}\sigma, \\
&\mathcal{B}(q, \boldsymbol{v}) = 0, \\
&\int_{\Sigma^t} \boldsymbol{\mu} \cdot \left( \boldsymbol{v} - \frac{\partial \boldsymbol{d}}{\partial t} \right) \mathrm{d}\sigma = 0, \\
&\boldsymbol{d}_f = \boldsymbol{d} \quad \text{at } \Sigma^t,
\end{aligned} \tag{6.42}$$

for all $\boldsymbol{w} \in \boldsymbol{V}$, $\widehat{\boldsymbol{e}} \in \boldsymbol{D}$, $\boldsymbol{\mu} \in \boldsymbol{H}^{-1/2}(\Sigma^t)$ and $q \in L^2(\Omega^t)$, where $\Omega^t = \Omega_f^t \cup \Omega_s^t$ and $\boldsymbol{V}^t$ is defined over $\Omega^t$. For the well-posedness of the time-discretized version of problem (6.42) we refer to Formaggia *et al.* (2009*b*). We notice that the use of the same Lagrange multiplier $\boldsymbol{\lambda}$ from both the fluid and structure sides also guarantees the continuity of normal stresses (Formaggia *et al.* 2009*b*).

Stijnen, de Hart, Bovendeerd and van de Vosse (2004) have successfully reported a validation with experimental measurements, and Astorino *et al.* (2010) have reported an application of the FD approach to three-dimensional problems in combination with a contact model for the leaflets.

*Cut-FEM approach.* A natural strategy for handling an internal interface cutting the mesh in an arbitrary way is to write two weak formulations of the problem at hand, one for each of the two subdomains generated by the presence of the interface, and then sum them up. In this case, the meshes of the two subdomains are fixed (background meshes). Since some of the mesh elements are cut by the interface, their contribution to the matrices is split into two parts: see Figure 6.12(a). This method is known as cut-FEM (Hansbo and Hansbo 2002, Hansbo, Hansbo and Larson 2003). Here, the jump between the normal stresses at the interface is determined by the physical interaction with the interface, as happens for the blood/valve interaction.

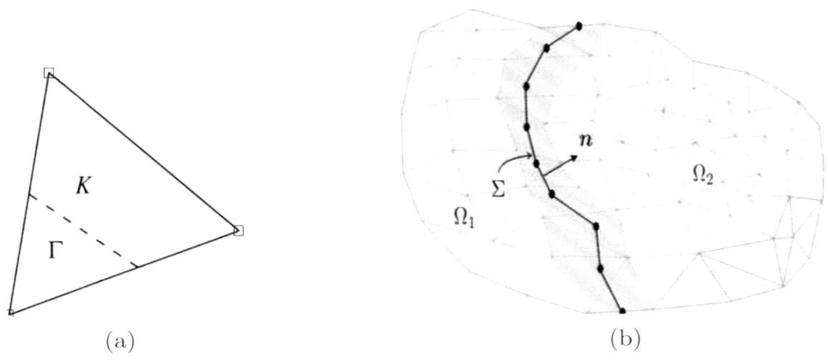


Figure 6.12 Element mesh $K$ cut by the interface $\Gamma$ (a) and FS domain (b). For the latter, we notice that $\Omega_f^1$ and $\Omega_f^2$ are two non-overlapping subdomains, whereas the related computational meshes have an overlap (in grey) in view of the X-FEM approach.

A common strategy used for guaranteeing the satisfaction of the interface continuity conditions is *discontinuous Galerkin* (DG) mortaring (often referred to as *Nitsche* mortaring). This is a very effective choice since the DG method prescribes interface conditions in a weak sense, thus allowing a great degree of flexibility of the solution at the interface (Hansbo and Hansbo 2002, Hansbo *et al.* 2003).

We notice however that the implementation of the cut-FEM method is not standard since in the cut elements we may have polygonal elements: see for example Figure 6.12(a), where the original triangle is split into a triangle and a trapezoid. A solution is offered by the *extended finite element* method (X-FEM), enriched in order to make the treatment of the cut elements easy. In particular, the basic idea is to duplicate the variables in the cut elements and to use the basis functions of the original triangle in both subdomains, to represent the finite element solution and to compute the integrals (Hansbo and Hansbo 2002).

To provide a concrete example of the cut-FEM method, we will give the weak formulation introduced and analyzed by Alauzet, Fabrèges, Fernández and Landajuela (2016), related to the case of a valve embedded in blood and represented by

$$\rho_s H_s \frac{\partial \boldsymbol{d}}{\partial t} + \boldsymbol{L}\boldsymbol{d} = -[\![\boldsymbol{T}_f \boldsymbol{n}]\!] \quad \text{in } \Sigma,$$

where $\Sigma$ is the embedded membrane, $\boldsymbol{L}$ is an elliptic operator, and $[\![\cdot]\!]$ denotes the jump across the membrane. In particular, referring to Figure 6.12(b), let

$\Omega_f^1$ and $\Omega_f^2$ be two non-overlapping subdomains separated by $\Sigma$, and $\Omega_{f,h}^1$ and $\Omega_{f,h}^2$ two meshes containing $\Omega_f^1$ and $\Omega_f^2$, respectively, with an overlap region (in grey in the figure) containing the membrane. Moreover, let $\boldsymbol{V}_h^i$ and $Q_h^i$ be velocity and pressure finite element spaces related to $\Omega_{f,h}^i$ and let $\mathcal{C}^i$ be one of the bilinear or trilinear forms $\mathcal{C}$ introduced in Chapter 3 restricted to $\Omega_{f,h}^i$. Thus we have

$$
\begin{aligned}
&\sum_{i=1}^{2}\left[\rho_f\int_{\Omega_f^i}\frac{\partial \boldsymbol{v}_h^i}{\partial t}\cdot\boldsymbol{w}\,\mathrm{d}\omega+\mathcal{A}_f^i(\boldsymbol{v}_h^i,\boldsymbol{v}_h^i,\boldsymbol{w})+\mathcal{B}^i(p_h^i,\boldsymbol{w})-\mathcal{B}^i(q,\boldsymbol{v}_h^i)\right]\\
&\qquad+s_h(\boldsymbol{v}_h,\boldsymbol{w})+\rho_s H_s\int_\Sigma\frac{\partial \boldsymbol{d}_h}{\partial t}\cdot\boldsymbol{e}\,\mathrm{d}\sigma+\int_\Sigma \boldsymbol{L}\boldsymbol{d}_h\cdot\boldsymbol{e}\,\mathrm{d}\sigma\\
&\quad+\sum_{i=1}^{2}\left[-\int_\Sigma \boldsymbol{T}_f(\boldsymbol{v}_h^i,p_h^i)\boldsymbol{n}^i\cdot(\boldsymbol{w}-\boldsymbol{e})\,\mathrm{d}\sigma-\int_\Sigma \boldsymbol{T}_f(\boldsymbol{w},q)\boldsymbol{n}^i\cdot\left(\boldsymbol{v}_h^i-\frac{\partial \boldsymbol{d}_h}{\partial t}\right)\mathrm{d}\sigma\right.\\
&\qquad\qquad\left.+\frac{\gamma}{h}\int_\Sigma\left(\boldsymbol{v}_h^i-\frac{\partial \boldsymbol{d}_h}{\partial t}\right)\cdot(\boldsymbol{w}-\boldsymbol{e})\,\mathrm{d}\sigma\right]=0.
\end{aligned}
$$

The terms in the third and fourth rows above are simply the usual DG terms guaranteeing consistency, symmetry and stability of the method, whereas $s_h(\cdot,\cdot)$ accounts for the *ghost node stabilization* (Burman *et al.* 2015), which guarantees an optimal convergence order. This formulation was introduced for infinitesimal displacements. However, the authors also treat the case of a moving interface: for details see Alauzet *et al.* (2016).

Finally, we notice that the cut-FEM approach has been also considered for the case of a thick structure: see Burman and Fernández (2014), (Zonca 2018) and Zonca, Formaggia and Vergara (2018). Alternatively to the X-FEM method, another strategy has been recently proposed in Antonietti *et al.* (2018) to manage the polygonal elements generated by the cut of the background mesh with the moving structure. This strategy is based on building the DG basis functions directly on the current polygon. This allows to easily consider high-order space discretizations.

## 6.5 Modelling the entire heart function

We conclude this chapter by providing some hints on the modelling of the complete heart function, a challenging and far-reaching endeavour. The latter is very complex and requires us to merge all the mathematical, numerical and computational issues highlighted previously in this chapter: see Chabiniok *et al.* (2016), Dössel and Loewe (2017), Lee *et al.* (2016), Nordsletten *et al.* (2011*b*) and Quarteroni *et al.* (2017).

Basically, an integrated model of the heart involves the coupling of the electromechanical problem (6.34), the blood fluid dynamics (see Section 6.3), and the valve functioning (see Section 6.4). The coupling between the first two subproblems occurs at the endocardium $\Sigma_{\text{endo}}$: see Figure 5.1. In particular, this is determined by the classical fluid–structure interaction coupling conditions, *i.e.*, the kinematic condition (3.19c) and the dynamic condition (3.19d). In particular, referring to the notation of Sections 3.1 and 6.2 and to Figure 5.1, we have the following problem in the framework of the active stress approach for electromechanics. Find the blood velocity $\boldsymbol{v}$ and pressure $p$, the muscle displacement $\boldsymbol{d}$, the trans-membrane potential $V_m$, the gating variables $\boldsymbol{w}$, and the ionic concentration variables $\boldsymbol{c}$, such that

$$\rho_f\left(\frac{\partial \boldsymbol{v}}{\partial t} + \rho_f(\boldsymbol{v}\cdot\nabla)\boldsymbol{v}\right) - \nabla\cdot\boldsymbol{T}_f(\boldsymbol{v},p) = \boldsymbol{0} \quad \text{in } \Omega^t_{\text{cav}}, \tag{6.43a}$$

$$\nabla\cdot\boldsymbol{v} = 0 \quad \text{in } \Omega^t_{\text{cav}}, \tag{6.43b}$$

$$\boldsymbol{v} = \frac{\partial \boldsymbol{d}}{\partial t} \quad \text{at } \Sigma^t_{\text{endo}}, \tag{6.43c}$$

$$\left(\boldsymbol{T}^P_s(\boldsymbol{d}) + \boldsymbol{T}^A_s\left(\boldsymbol{c},\boldsymbol{d},\frac{\partial \boldsymbol{d}}{\partial t}\right)\right)\boldsymbol{n} = \boldsymbol{T}_f(\boldsymbol{v},p)\,\boldsymbol{n} \quad \text{at } \Sigma^t_{\text{endo}}, \tag{6.43d}$$

$$-\nabla\cdot\left(\widehat{\boldsymbol{T}}^P_s(\widehat{\boldsymbol{d}}) + \widehat{\boldsymbol{T}}^A_s\left(\widehat{\boldsymbol{c}},\widehat{\boldsymbol{d}},\frac{\partial \widehat{\boldsymbol{d}}}{\partial t}\right)\right) = \boldsymbol{0} \quad \text{in } \Omega_{\text{mus}}, \tag{6.43e}$$

$$\widehat{\boldsymbol{T}}^A_s = P^A\widehat{\boldsymbol{a}}_f\otimes\widehat{\boldsymbol{a}}_f, \quad P^A = \mathcal{A}\left(\widehat{\boldsymbol{c}},\widehat{\boldsymbol{d}},\frac{\partial \widehat{\boldsymbol{d}}}{\partial t}\right) \quad \text{in } \Omega_{\text{mus}}, \tag{6.43f}$$

$$\widehat{V}_m = \mathcal{M}(\widehat{V}_m;\widehat{\boldsymbol{d}},\widehat{\boldsymbol{w}},\widehat{\boldsymbol{c}}) \quad \text{in } \Omega_{\text{mus}}, \tag{6.43g}$$

$$(\widehat{\boldsymbol{w}},\widehat{\boldsymbol{c}}) = \mathcal{G}(\widehat{\boldsymbol{w}},\widehat{\boldsymbol{c}};\widehat{V}_m) \quad \text{in } \Omega_{\text{mus}}. \tag{6.43h}$$

After numerical discretization in time and space, the corresponding nonlinear algebraic system is tremendously stiff and can have a very large numerical dimension. Devising computationally efficient numerical strategies for its solution is a very active research area.

An effective numerical strategy for solving the entire heart coupled problem is given by the iterative solution at each time step of the electromechanical and fluid subproblems and based on the exchange of the interface conditions (6.43c, 6.43d). In particular, one of the partitioned strategies described in Section 3.6.3 can be adapted and used for problem (6.43) as well. Of course, at each iteration of the partitioned algorithm, the electromechanical problem could be solved by means of one of the strategies reported in Section 6.2.

Another partitioned algorithm for the solution of problem (6.43) is obtained by considering the solution at each time step of the electrical problem first and the FSI problem later (Nordsletten *et al.* 2011*b*). This is simply an extension of EM1 and EM1′ algorithms described in Section 6.2, where steps (2b) and (2′b) are replaced by a Newton iteration over the FSI problem. Different segregated schemes were proposed in (Gerbi 2018) for the integrated problem in the framework of the active strain approach.

A different approach is based on the monolithic solution of the integrated heart problem (6.43) by means of a full Newton method. In particular, Quarteroni *et al.* (2017) describe fully implicit and semi-implicit methods. The latter is based on updating only a part of the Jacobian as a consequence of an operator splitting technique. By means of numerical experiments, the authors emphasized that particular choices of the splitting and of the temporal scheme could lead to numerical instabilities. Whatever strategy is adopted, the tangent problem at each Newton iteration is solved by means of a preconditioned iterative method, which in this case is particularly suitable due to the block structure of the Jacobian: see Quarteroni *et al.* (2017).

Stability and convergence analysis of the different numerical strategies and solvers is a field of current investigation.

As for today, the "UT heart simulator" developed by the research team of T. Hisada (Tokyo University) has provided the most comprehensive simulations of the entire cardiac function, including multiscale processes in the tissue, fluid dynamics in the heart chambers, and valves dynamics; see (Sugiura *et al.* 2012) and *e.g.* (Watanabe *et al.* 2002, Watanabe *et al.* 2004).

# PART THREE

# OPTIMIZATION, CONTROL, UNCERTAINTY AND COMPLEXITY REDUCTION

# 7
# Beyond direct simulation

In all the problems considered so far, for a given set of inputs (*e.g.* geometry, source terms, boundary and initial conditions) the goal has been to solve a forward (direct) PDE-based problem numerically, and, possibly, to evaluate some physical indices of clinical interest, such as the flow rate across a vessel section, the wall shear stress over a portion of the lumen boundary, or the oscillatory shear index. On the other hand, the efficient numerical algorithms and computational resources now available enable us to tackle several additional kinds of problem.

When simulating blood flows one has to deal with the variability of input data, such as geometric features of the vessel, boundary conditions and physical coefficients (*e.g.* the Reynolds number, the Womersley number, the structural model or material parameters related to the vessel wall). Very often, these data vary within a broad range and are almost impossible to characterize precisely. All these inputs affect the solution of the problem under investigation, as well as the outcomes of clinical interest. In the clinical context it is thus important to be able to characterize input/output relationships efficiently, in order to investigate both *intra-patient* and *inter-patient* variability. For the former case we include all those effects due to variations affecting a single patient, for example over time, or before/after clinical intervention. For the latter case, we mention for instance the morphological variability among vessel shapes due to age, size or pathological factors (see *e.g.* Xiong and Chong 2008 for the case of distal coronary anastomoses). It is thus of paramount importance to develop mathematical techniques capable of detecting the most relevant parameters, and then address the impact of their variation on the outputs of interest. This requires the solution of *many queries* to the *forward* problem. In this context, three classical situations we may face are (i) optimal control and optimal design, (ii) parameter identification and data assimilation, and (iii) uncertainty quantification.

(i) *Optimal control and optimal design problems.* When we pursue a suitable objective via an optimal strategy to be determined, we act on some *inputs* of the given partial differential equation, the *state* problem, such as boundary data, physical coefficients, or the shape of the domain itself, and the *control* variables, so that the solution of the corresponding state problem could meet the prescribed goal. This yields a PDE-constrained optimization problem; its numerical solution usually poses severe computational challenges, as the state problem needs to be solved several times while searching for the optimal control in an iterative way. Exploiting numerical optimization procedures for blood flow simulations is intended to (a) improve the design of prosthetic devices (such as stents, grafts, ventricular assist devices) with the aim of fulfilling a specific target, or (b) customize treatments or surgical procedures, provided that patient-specific information can be acquired. Examples include the optimal placement of electrodes in a defibrillation stage to damp the electrical activity in the myocardium in a desired way when dealing with the therapeutic treatment of cardiac arrhythmias (Nagaiah, Kunisch and Plank 2013*b*), the optimization of the shape of a cannula in order to maximize the flow rate through a ventricular assist device (Marsden 2014), and the improvement of the shape of a coronary bypass graft in order to possibly avoid vessel re-occlusion (Lei, Archie and Kleinstreuer 1997, Dur *et al.* 2011). The first example mentioned above is an optimal control problem, where the control variable is a current source for the monodomain (or bidomain) equation (see Section 6.1), that is, one of its data. The two other examples address a *shape optimization* or *optimal design* problem to be solved, the control variable being the *shape* of the domain where the state problem is set.

(ii) *Parameter identification and data assimilation.* In principle, cardiovascular models necessitate a huge amount of data, for example the patient's radiological images and measurements. In general, however, some of them may be missing; remember for instance the issue of missing or defective boundary conditions discussed in Section 3.4, or the lack of biological parameters characterizing the tissue properties. For example, it is very hard to estimate the electrical conductivity of the myocardium for electrophysiology models, whereas (pointwise) measurements of the electrical potential – whose mathematical modelling can be characterized by a PDE model requiring electrical conductivities as inputs – can be easier to acquire. By solving *inverse/identification problems* in cardiovascular modelling, we aim to identify those inputs which are unknown or affected by uncertainty. For that, we rely on suitable quantities which are (a) acquired from measurements, such as displacements, pressures or flow rates, and (b) obtained as the outcome of a numerical simulation, and match these two sets of values. In other words, to identify those input values yielding the acquired measurements, we need to drive the PDE outcome as near as possible to the measured quantity. In general, vastly different inputs may have produced the observed outcome: this is why, instead of finding the most likely input configuration resulting in the observation performed, we instead rely on statistical inversion theory, in order to incorporate all possible information about the unknown inputs we may have prior to the measurement. This requires us to reformulate inverse problems as problems of statistical inference, for example by means of Bayesian statistics. A second issue is *data assimilation*. This rather generic term encompasses a wide range of techniques exploited to merge measurements and images into the mathematical model in order to improve numerical simulations. Furthermore, a filtering effect induced by the numerical simulation can also be exploited in view of noise reduction in image and measurement acquisition.

(iii) *Uncertainty quantification and propagation.* Confidence in the outcome of a cardiovascular simulation depends directly on the level of accuracy and certainty at which inputs can be determined. In fact, although outcomes are computed from inputs via a deterministic process, input data are often contaminated by experimental noise, or cannot be fully ascertained. Common sources of uncertainty in cardiovascular simulations include (a) boundary conditions, (b) anatomical models, where each geometric model is contaminated by image noise, (c) flow split, since very often there is a lack of clinical data to determine flow distribution to multiple distal branches, and (d) material properties, related to vessel walls or blood (Sankaran and Marsden 2010). Because of uncertainty, computational simulations have to be performed for a set of different parameter configurations and then merged in order to determine how robust simulation outcomes are with respect to variations in uncertain inputs (Sankaran and Marsden 2011). This is indeed strictly related to the task of parametric studies and sensitivity analyses, and can be seen as a *forward uncertainty quantification* (UQ) *problem*. Investigating the propagation of input uncertainties via computed outputs means evaluating suitable statistics of the outputs (such as expected values, moments, confidence bands), which are functions of the parameters affected by uncertainty. On the other hand, the solution of optimal control and inverse identification problems also depends on the experimental noise affecting observations and measurements used during the identification process, or the set-up of a desired target. Evaluating uncertainties in this case, providing suitable *confidence* intervals for the estimated quantities (not simply point estimates) and characterizing the statistical distribution of the unknown parameters are all *inverse UQ problems*. In this second case, quantifying uncertainties is even more important because an inverse problem is intrinsically ill-posed.

In the following chapters we hone our understanding of these three classes of problems, showing relevant examples in cardiovascular modelling.

# 8

# Control and optimization

Solving a PDE-constrained optimization problem consists of reaching a target by acting on a system governed by PDEs. The goal is to act on a *state problem* $\mathcal{E}(y, u) = 0$ given by a PDE system modelling the behaviour of a state variable $y$, through a control variable $u$ in order to reach a desirable target. This is usually done by minimizing (or maximizing) a cost functional $J = J(y, u)$ expressing some physical index of interest encoding the desired objective – for instance, the squared distance from a target state. For a comprehensive presentation of the functional setting and well-posedness analysis of PDE-constrained optimization, see the monographs by Hinze, Pinnau, Ulbrich and Ulbrich (2009) and Gunzburger (2003). Other classes of problems of interest in cardiovascular applications, such as those related to *parameter estimation*, can also be cast in a PDE-constrained optimization framework; see *e.g.* Section 9.1 for further insights.

Generally speaking, a PDE-constrained optimization problem reads

$$\min_{y,u} J(y, u) \quad \text{subject to} \quad \mathcal{E}(y, u) = 0, \quad y \in V, \quad u \in \mathcal{U}_{\text{ad}} \subseteq \mathcal{U}. \tag{8.1}$$

Here $V$ and $\mathcal{U}$ denote the state and the control space, whereas $\mathcal{E} : V \times \mathcal{U} \to V^*$ and $J : V \times \mathcal{U} \to \mathbb{R}$ denote the state equation and the cost functional, respectively; $V^*$ is the dual space of $V$, and $\langle \cdot\, , \, \cdot \rangle_{V^*,V}$ denotes the duality between two elements in $V^*$ and $V$; similarly, $\langle \cdot\, , \, \cdot \rangle_{\mathcal{U}^*,\mathcal{U}}$ indicates the duality between two elements in $\mathcal{U}^*$ and $\mathcal{U}$. Additional constraints, depending on the problem at hand, can also be imposed, for example in the form of inequalities; we express this fact by saying that we seek the optimal control in a closed subset $\mathcal{U}_{\text{ad}} \subseteq \mathcal{U}$ of admissible controls.

We assume that the state equation $\mathcal{E}(y, u) = 0$ has a unique solution $y = y(u) \in V$, and that the Fréchet derivative (with respect to $y$) $\mathcal{E}_y(y(u), u)$ has a bounded inverse for each $u \in \mathcal{U}$. Under these assumptions, the solution operator of the state equation is continuously differentiable – we let $y'(u)$ denote its derivative – and the *reduced formulation*

$$\min_u \tilde{J}(u) = J(y(u), u), \quad u \in \mathcal{U}_{\text{ad}} \tag{8.2}$$

is equivalent to (8.1). Note that this is a convenient framework to embrace – upon defining suitable functional spaces and operators – both stationary and time-dependent state problems; in the following we will make it clear whether the proposed methods can be used to tackle both classes of problems.

## 8.1 Optimality conditions

The solution $(\hat{y}, \hat{u})$ of a PDE-constrained optimization problem such as (8.1) requires a system of optimality conditions to be fulfilled, including the state equation and an optimality condition which involves the gradient of the cost functional. Indeed, if $\hat{u} \in U_{\text{ad}}$ is a local minimum of $\tilde{J}$, then it satisfies the variational inequality (also referred to as the *optimality condition* or *minimum principle*)

$$\langle \tilde{J}'(\hat{u}), v - \hat{u} \rangle_{\mathcal{U}^*, \mathcal{U}} \geq 0 \quad \text{for all } v \in \mathcal{U}_{\text{ad}}. \tag{8.3}$$

The quantity appearing on the left-hand side is the so-called Gâteaux derivative of $\tilde{J}$, evaluated at $\hat{u}$, in the generic, admissible direction $v - \hat{u}$ (see *e.g.* Tröltzsch 2010); $\tilde{J}'(\hat{u})$ denotes the gradient of $\tilde{J}$ at $\hat{u}$. To express this latter quantity in terms of the state solution $y$, we can use either (i) the sensitivity approach or (ii) the adjoint approach. As we will see below, in both cases at least a second PDE problem has to be solved in order to evaluate $\tilde{J}'(u)$.

### *8.1.1 Sensitivity approach*

Computing *sensitivities* requires the evaluation of directional derivatives of both the cost functional and the state solution. For any $u, v \in \mathcal{U}$, we can write

$$\langle \tilde{J}'(u), v \rangle_{\mathcal{U}^*, \mathcal{U}} = \langle J_y(y(u), u), y'(u)v \rangle_{V^*, V} + \langle J_u(y(u), u), v \rangle_{\mathcal{U}^*, \mathcal{U}}. \tag{8.4}$$

The quantity $\delta_v y = y'(u)v$ denotes the sensitivity of the state with respect to the control, evaluated at $u$, for a given variation $v$, and can be obtained by solving a further PDE. Indeed, differentiating the state equation $\mathcal{E}(y(u), u) = 0$ along the direction $v$, we obtain

$$\mathcal{E}_y(y(u), u) y'(u) v + \mathcal{E}_u(y(u), u) v = 0, \tag{8.5}$$

where $\mathcal{E}_y(y,u), \mathcal{E}_u(y,u)$ are the Fréchet derivatives of the state operator with respect to $y$ and $u$, respectively; see *e.g.* Tröltzsch (2010). Then $\delta_v y = y'(u)v$ is given by the solution of the linearized state equation

$$\mathcal{E}_y(y(u),u)\delta_v y = -\mathcal{E}_u(y(u),u)v. \tag{8.6}$$

Note that $y'(u) : \mathcal{U} \to V$ is a linear operator so that, for any admissible $v \in \mathcal{U}$, a new problem has to be solved to evaluate $\delta_v y$. Numerically, this approach is very demanding if the whole gradient $\tilde{J}'(u)$ is required: in this case, the number of linearized state equations (8.6) to be solved is equal to the dimension of the control space $\mathcal{U}$, a task that becomes out of reach as soon as the control has dimension larger than $O(10)$.

### *8.1.2 Adjoint approach and Lagrange multipliers*

A convenient alternative is based on the so-called *adjoint approach*. By rewriting (8.4) as

$$\langle \tilde{J}'(u), v\rangle_{\mathcal{U}^*,\mathcal{U}} = \langle (y'(u))^* J_y(y(u),u) + J_u(y(u),u), v\rangle_{\mathcal{U}^*,\mathcal{U}} \tag{8.7}$$

and exploiting problem (8.5), we can express the first term on the right-hand side of (8.7) as

$$(y'(u))^* J_y(y(u),u) = -\mathcal{E}_u^*(y(u),u)((\mathcal{E}^*{}_y(y(u),u)))^{-1} J_y(y(u),u),$$

where $\mathcal{E}_u^*(y(u),u)$ is the adjoint operator[1] of $\mathcal{E}_u(y(u),u)$. Let us introduce an additional variable $\lambda = \lambda(u) \in V$, called the *adjoint state*, the solution of

$$\mathcal{E}_y(y(u),u))^* \lambda = -J_y(y(u),u). \tag{8.8}$$

Then $(y'(u))^* J_y(y(u),u) = \mathcal{E}_u^*(y(u),u)\lambda$; moreover, owing to (8.7), the evaluation of

$$\tilde{J}'(u) = \mathcal{E}_u^*(y(u),u)\lambda(u) + J_u(y(u),u) \tag{8.9}$$

simply requires us to solve the state problem and a further PDE problem, regardless of the dimension of the control space $\mathcal{U}$. Note that the adjoint problem is always a linear PDE.

The adjoint-based expression of the gradient of the cost functional (and more generally a system of first-order optimality conditions) can also be

[1] The adjoint operator of $\mathcal{E}$, denoted by $\mathcal{E}^*$, is given by the relation $(\mathcal{E}^*\varphi,\psi)_{L^2(\Omega)} = (\varphi,\mathcal{E}\psi)_{L^2(\Omega)}$ for any $\varphi,\psi \in C_0^\infty(\Omega)$; note that no boundary condition is involved in its definition. For this reason, $\mathcal{E}^*$ is also referred to as the *formal* adjoint operator.

obtained, in a more straightforward way, by relying on the Lagrange multiplier method (Hinze *et al.* 2009). Let us define the Lagrangian functional $\mathcal{L} : V \times \mathcal{U} \times V \to \mathbb{R}$,

$$\mathcal{L}(y, u, \lambda) = J(y, u) + \langle \lambda, \mathcal{E}(y, u) \rangle_{V,V^*},$$

where $\lambda \in V$ denotes a Lagrange multiplier enforcing the PDE constraint (playing the role of adjoint variable); note that in this case the three variables are independent.

By deriving $\mathcal{L}$ with respect to $\lambda$ and imposing that the derivative is equal to zero, we recover the state problem,

$$\langle \mathcal{L}_\lambda(y, u, p), \varphi \rangle_{V^*,V} = 0 \quad \text{for all } \varphi \in V \;\Leftrightarrow\; \mathcal{E}(y, u) = 0.$$

Similarly, by deriving $\mathcal{L}$ with respect to $y$, we obtain the expression of the adjoint problem (8.8),

$$\langle \mathcal{L}_y(y, u, p), \psi \rangle_{V^*,V} = 0 \quad \text{for all } \psi \in V \;\Leftrightarrow\; J_y(y, u) + \mathcal{E}_y^*(y, u) = 0. \quad (8.10)$$

Finally, at the optimum we impose

$$\begin{aligned} &\langle \mathcal{L}_u(y, u, \lambda), v - u \rangle_{\mathcal{U}^*,\mathcal{U}} = 0 \quad \text{for all } v \in \mathcal{U}_{\text{ad}} \\ &\quad\Leftrightarrow\; \langle J_u(y, u) + \mathcal{E}_u(y, u)^* \lambda, v - u \rangle_{\mathcal{U}^*,\mathcal{U}} \geq 0 \quad \text{for all } v \in \mathcal{U}_{\text{ad}}. \end{aligned}$$

In this way, a system of first-order necessary optimality conditions to be fulfilled by the optimal solution $(y, u)$ and the corresponding adjoint state $\lambda$ is given by the following Karush–Kuhn–Tucker (KKT) system:

$$\mathcal{E}(y, u) = 0, \quad (8.11a)$$

$$\mathcal{E}_y(y, u)^* \hat{\lambda} = -J_y(y, u), \quad (8.11b)$$

$$\langle J_u(y, u) + \mathcal{E}_u(y, u)^* \lambda, v - u \rangle_{\mathcal{U}^*,\mathcal{U}} \geq 0 \quad \text{for all } v \in \mathcal{U}_{\text{ad}}. \quad (8.11c)$$

In the unconstrained case $\mathcal{U}_{\text{ad}} \equiv \mathcal{U}$, the variational inequality reduces to the equation

$$\langle J_u(y, u) + \mathcal{E}_u(y, u)^* \lambda, v \rangle_{\mathcal{U}^*,\mathcal{U}} = 0 \quad \text{for all } v \in \mathcal{U},$$

so (8.11) can be viewed as the Euler–Lagrange system for the Lagrangian functional; that is, the solutions of (8.11) are the stationary points of $\mathcal{L}(\cdot, \cdot, \cdot)$:

$$\nabla \mathcal{L}(y, u, \lambda)[w, v, \eta] = 0 \quad \text{for all } (\phi, v, \psi) \in Y \times \mathcal{U} \times V.$$

The third inequality of system (8.11) allows us to recover the expression of the gradient $\tilde{J}'(u)$. Indeed, since $\mathcal{E}(y(u), u) = 0$, it holds that $\mathcal{L}(y(u), u, \lambda) =$

$\tilde{J}(u)$ for any arbitrary $\lambda \in V$, so that, by differentiating this latter equality with respect to $u$, we obtain

$$\begin{aligned}\langle \tilde{J}'(u), v\rangle_{\mathcal{U}^*,\mathcal{U}} &= \langle \mathcal{L}_y(y(u), u, \lambda), y'(u)v\rangle_{V^*,V} + \langle \mathcal{L}_u(y(u), u, \lambda), v\rangle_{\mathcal{U}^*,\mathcal{U}} \\ &= \langle \mathcal{L}_u(y(u), u, \lambda), v\rangle_{\mathcal{U}^*,\mathcal{U}}.\end{aligned}$$

Hence, $\tilde{J}'(u) = \mathcal{L}_u(y(u), u, \lambda(u))$, since $\langle \mathcal{L}_y(y(u), u, \lambda), \psi\rangle_{V^*,V} = 0$ for any $\psi \in V$, thanks to (8.10).

For illustration we discuss a specific example, by considering the problem of minimizing the energy

$$J(\boldsymbol{v}, \boldsymbol{u}) = \frac{1}{2}\int_{\Omega_{\text{obs}}} |\boldsymbol{v} - \boldsymbol{v}_d|^2 \, d\Omega + \frac{\alpha}{2}\int_{\Gamma_{\text{con}}} |\nabla \boldsymbol{u}|^2 \, d\Gamma,$$

of a fluid flow in a tract of blood vessel where a bypass is inserted. As a matter of fact, the bypass is not simulated. Its action is represented via a velocity control $\boldsymbol{u}$ acting on the boundary $\Gamma_{\text{con}} \subset \partial\Omega_f$, the interface where the bypass and the vessel meet: see Figure 8.1. The goal is to regularize the velocity pattern in a suitable observation region $\Omega_{\text{obs}} \subseteq \Omega_f$ by requiring $\boldsymbol{v}$ to be as close as possible to a desired distribution $\boldsymbol{v}_d$; see the related discussion in the next section. Referring to the notation of Chapter 3, for simplicity, we consider a steady version of the Navier–Stokes equations (3.1a, 3.1b), for which the velocity/pressure couple $y = (\boldsymbol{v}, p)$ solves the state problem

$$\begin{aligned}
& -\nabla \cdot \mathbf{T}_f(\boldsymbol{v}, p) + \rho_f(\boldsymbol{v}\cdot\nabla)\boldsymbol{v} = \mathbf{0} && \text{in } \Omega_f,\\
& \nabla \cdot \boldsymbol{v} = 0 && \text{in } \Omega_f,\\
& \boldsymbol{v} = \boldsymbol{v}_{\text{in}} && \text{on } \Gamma_{\text{in}},\\
& \boldsymbol{v} = \mathbf{0} && \text{on } \Gamma_w,\\
& \boldsymbol{v} = \boldsymbol{u} && \text{on } \Gamma_{\text{con}},\\
& \boldsymbol{T}_f(\boldsymbol{v}, p)\boldsymbol{n} = \mathbf{0} && \text{on } \Gamma_{\text{out}},
\end{aligned}$$

where the control variable is the velocity $\boldsymbol{u}$ imposed on the boundary $\Gamma_{\text{con}}$. Here $\alpha > 0$ is a parameter penalizing the control magnitude (or cost); this can also be seen as a regularization term, ensuring the convexity of the cost functional. The fluid Cauchy stress tensor $\mathbf{T}_f(\boldsymbol{v}, p)$ has been defined in (3.2).

Following the Lagrangian approach, we can derive a system of first-order optimality conditions, where the adjoint problem for the adjoint variables $\lambda = (\boldsymbol{z}, q)$ is given by

$$\begin{aligned}
& -\nabla \cdot \mathbf{T}_f(\boldsymbol{z}, q) + \rho_f(\nabla^{\mathrm{T}}\boldsymbol{v})\boldsymbol{z} - \rho_f(\boldsymbol{v}\cdot\nabla)\boldsymbol{z} \\
& \qquad\qquad = (\boldsymbol{v} - \boldsymbol{v}_d)\mathcal{I}_{\Omega_{\text{obs}}} && \text{in } \Omega_f,\\
& \nabla \cdot \boldsymbol{z} = 0 && \text{in } \Omega_f,
\end{aligned}$$

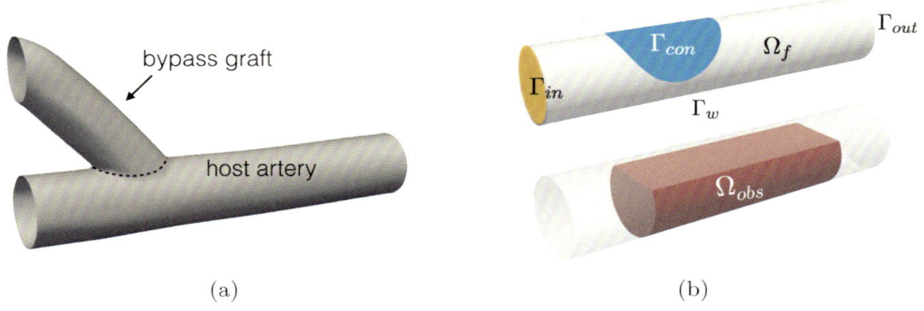


Figure 8.1 (a) Schematic representation of a bypass graft. (b) Domain, boundary portion and observation region for the bypass model problem.

$$
\begin{aligned}
&\boldsymbol{z} = \mathbf{0} && \text{on } \Gamma_{\text{in}} \cup \Gamma_w \cup \Gamma_{\text{con}}, \\
&\boldsymbol{T}_f(\boldsymbol{z}, q)\boldsymbol{n} = \mathbf{0} && \text{on } \Gamma_{\text{out}},
\end{aligned}
$$

where $\mathcal{I}_{\Omega_{\text{obs}}} = \mathcal{I}_{\Omega_{\text{obs}}}(\mathbf{x})$ is the characteristic function of the region $\Omega_{\text{obs}}$. Note that the adjoint problem is linear in $(\boldsymbol{z}, q)$, and comes from the linearization of the Navier–Stokes equations around the state solution; the optimality condition instead reads

$$\alpha \boldsymbol{u} + \boldsymbol{z} = \mathbf{0} \quad \text{on } \Gamma_{\text{con}}.$$

**Remark 8.1** In the case of time-dependent state problems, the adjoint problem is backward-in-time. Depending on the observation appearing in the cost functional – which can be either on the whole time interval $(0, T)$ or at the final time $T$ only – the dependence of the adjoint problem on the state is only at $t = T$ (thus, as initial condition) or on the whole interval $(0, T)$. The approach followed so far can still be employed to derive a system of optimality conditions: see *e.g.* Section 8.3.2 for further details of a case of interest.

## 8.2 Numerical approximation

Solving a PDE-constrained optimization problem entails a computational effort larger than that required for the solution of a forward (state) problem. The two formulations (8.1) and (8.2) yield two different paradigms for the approximation of such a problem. In the former case, both state and control variables are optimization variables and PDE constraints are explicitly specified; in the latter, only the control variable $u$ is an optimization variable, whereas the state variable $y$ is considered to be an implicit function of $u$ via the PDE constraint.[2] In this latter case, the solution of the state problem is *nested* in the evaluation of the gradient $\tilde{J}'(u)$ of the reduced cost functional.

Algorithms for solving PDE-constrained optimization problems can be sorted according to several criteria. An initial classification criterion is between *iterative methods*, rooted in iterative minimization algorithms for the reduced cost functional, and *all-at-once methods*, where the PDE constraint is kept explicitly and the three equations forming (8.11) are solved simultaneously. Another criterion is concerned with the highest order of derivatives exploited by the algorithm, yielding derivative-free methods, gradient-based methods and Hessian-based methods.

A different perspective is taken when addressing the interplay between *optimization* and *discretization*: numerical discretization can be performed before or after the derivation of a system of optimality conditions. More precisely, in the so-called *optimize-then-discretize* approach, optimization is carried out at the continuous level (*e.g.* to find system (8.11)) and then the discretization is operated on the resulting optimality system. Alternatively, using the *discretize-then-optimize* approach, we first approximate the state equation (and the cost functional) and then carry out the optimization at the discrete level. Here we address the former approach; further details are given at the end of this section. For brevity, we recall the main features of iterative and all-at-once methods in the case of *unconstrained* problems, that is, problems without further equality/inequality constraints or, equivalently, for which $\mathcal{U}_{\mathrm{ad}} \equiv \mathcal{U}$. In particular, $\boldsymbol{Y} \in \mathbb{R}^{n_y}$, $\boldsymbol{U} \in \mathbb{R}^{n_u}$ denote the discrete representation of the state and the control variable, respectively, whereas $\boldsymbol{\lambda} \in \mathbb{R}^{n_\lambda}$ is the discrete adjoint variable.

### 8.2.1 Iterative methods

Iterative (also referred to as *black-box*) methods treat the reduced problem

$$\min_{\boldsymbol{U}} \tilde{J}(\boldsymbol{U}) = J(\boldsymbol{Y}(\boldsymbol{U}), \boldsymbol{U}),$$

once $\boldsymbol{U}$ is known; $\boldsymbol{Y}(\boldsymbol{U})$ is obtained as the solution of the state equation. An existing algorithm for the solution of the state equation therefore has to be embedded into an optimization loop, and any available PDE and optimization routines can be freely combined. In particular, iterative methods are a popular choice when dealing with optimal control problems by extending an

[2] From the numerical standpoint, the former approach is often given the name of *simultaneous analysis and design* (SAND) and the latter is referred to as *nested analysis and design* (NAND).

existing code for the state problem. Within this class, a notable difference exists between gradient-based and non-gradient-based algorithms.

*Non-gradient-based* (or *derivative-free*) algorithms, such as the popular *Nelder–Mead algorithm*, exploit either comparisons between function evaluations in different directions at each step, or low-order local approximants of $\tilde{J}$, in order to assess its local behaviour and find the minimizer: see *e.g.* Marsden, Feinstein and Taylor (2008). Employing a finite-difference approximation of the gradient is an attractive alternative due to its ease of implementation, but it may suffer from limited accuracy and large costs in the presence of many design variables. Hence, these methods are feasible only in the case where the control space has very small dimension, for example if the control is expressed in terms of a vector of $n_u = O(10)$ design variables.

*Gradient-based* algorithms exploit the gradient $\tilde{J}'$ to iteratively update the control until a suitable convergence criterion is fulfilled. Notable instances are descent methods, such as the gradient, (non-linear) conjugate gradient, quasi-Newton or Newton methods. In the simplest case of a gradient method, starting from an initial guess $\boldsymbol{U}^{(0)}$ we iteratively generate a sequence

$$\boldsymbol{U}^{(k+1)} = \boldsymbol{U}^{(k)} - \tau_k \tilde{J}'(\boldsymbol{U}^{(k)}), \quad k = 0, 1, \dots,$$

where $\tau_k > 0$ is a step size, until *e.g.* $\|\tilde{J}'(\boldsymbol{U}^{(k)})\| < \varepsilon$, for a given tolerance $\varepsilon > 0$. Further details can be found in Nocedal (1992) and Kelley (1999), for example. The solver for the state equation has to be augmented with a routine which provides the gradient of the state with respect to the optimization variables, and hence the solution of the adjoint problem. Optimization algorithms with faster convergence rates are needed to speed up the execution of the whole algorithm. Although straightforward to implement, the gradient method suffers from a poor rate of convergence when dealing with the numerical solutions of PDE-constrained optimization problems. More efficient methods are more typically employed, such as quasi-Newton methods: see *e.g.* Borzì and Schulz (2011) for further details.

### 8.2.2 All-at-once methods

By treating both the control and the state variables as independent optimization variables, coupled via the PDE constraint, we deal with an equality constrained non-linear optimization problem, the state equation now playing the role of equality constraint. The goal of all-at-once (also referred to as *one-shot*) methods is to tackle the (possibly) non-linear optimality system (8.11) as a whole problem to be solved. After numerical discretization, in the unconstrained case we obtain the algebraic system

$$J_{\boldsymbol{Y}}(\boldsymbol{Y},\boldsymbol{U}) + \mathbf{e}_{\boldsymbol{Y}}^{\mathrm{T}}(\boldsymbol{Y},\boldsymbol{U})\boldsymbol{\lambda} = \mathbf{0}, \tag{8.12a}$$

$$J_{\boldsymbol{U}}(\boldsymbol{Y},\boldsymbol{U}) + \mathbf{e}_{\boldsymbol{U}}^{\mathrm{T}}(\boldsymbol{Y},\boldsymbol{U})\boldsymbol{\lambda} = \mathbf{0}, \tag{8.12b}$$

$$\mathbf{e}(\boldsymbol{Y},\boldsymbol{U}) = \mathbf{0}. \tag{8.12c}$$

Here $\mathbf{e}(\boldsymbol{Y},\boldsymbol{U})$ denotes the discrete state operator, $J_{\boldsymbol{Y}}$ and $J_{\boldsymbol{U}}$ are the gradients of $J$ with respect to state and control variables, respectively, whereas $\mathbf{e}_{\boldsymbol{Y}}$ and $\mathbf{e}_{\boldsymbol{U}}$ are the Jacobians of the state equations with respect to state and control variables, respectively. The three equations of system (8.12) can also be seen as the conditions obtained by requiring that the gradient of the discrete Lagrangian $\mathcal{L}(\boldsymbol{Y},\boldsymbol{U},\boldsymbol{\lambda}) = J(\boldsymbol{Y},\boldsymbol{U}) - \boldsymbol{\lambda}^{\mathrm{T}}\mathbf{e}(\boldsymbol{Y},\boldsymbol{U})$ vanishes.

The strategy above is well suited to PDE-constrained optimization problems involving stationary state systems, but it is more computationally involved in the time-dependent case. If $J(\boldsymbol{Y},\boldsymbol{U})$ is quadratic and $\mathbf{e}(\boldsymbol{Y},\boldsymbol{U})$ is linear in $\boldsymbol{Y}$ and $\boldsymbol{U}$, (8.12) is a linear system of equations in saddle-point form, such as those arising from quadratic programming. In this case, preconditioned iterative methods for linear systems could be employed, such as those based on Krylov subspaces. In this respect, several preconditioners have been proposed in the past decade, in which multigrid schemes are exploited as inner solvers (or preconditioners) for some blocks of the KKT matrix within an outer iterative solver; see *e.g.* Benzi *et al.* (2005) and Rees, Dollar and Wathen (2010). More recent extensions to constrained problems have been addressed, for example in Borzì and Schulz (2011) and the references therein.

If the state problem is non-linear, the optimality system has to be solved via appropriate linearization procedures (*e.g.* sequential quadratic programming methods) or modern penalty methods (*e.g.* augmented Lagrangian methods). Indeed, the equations of system (8.12) are still linear in $\boldsymbol{\lambda}$ but non-linear in $(\boldsymbol{Y},\boldsymbol{U})$. When a Newton-type method is applied to (8.12), each iteration on the KKT system entails the solution of the linear system

$$\begin{pmatrix} \mathcal{L}_{\boldsymbol{YY}} & \mathcal{L}_{\boldsymbol{YU}} & \mathbf{e}_{\boldsymbol{Y}}^{\mathrm{T}} \\ \mathcal{L}_{\boldsymbol{UY}} & \mathcal{L}_{\boldsymbol{UU}} & \mathbf{e}_{\boldsymbol{U}}^{\mathrm{T}} \\ \mathbf{e}_{\boldsymbol{Y}} & \mathbf{e}_{\boldsymbol{U}} & 0 \end{pmatrix} \begin{pmatrix} \delta\boldsymbol{Y} \\ \delta\boldsymbol{U} \\ \boldsymbol{\lambda}^{(k+1)} \end{pmatrix} = - \begin{pmatrix} J_{\boldsymbol{Y}} \\ J_{\boldsymbol{U}} \\ \mathbf{e} \end{pmatrix} \tag{8.13}$$

for the update $\delta\boldsymbol{X}^{\mathrm{T}} = (\delta\boldsymbol{Y},\delta\boldsymbol{U})^{\mathrm{T}}$ of the optimization variable and the new value $\boldsymbol{\lambda}^{(k+1)}$ of the adjoint variable. Then we set $(\boldsymbol{Y}^{(k+1)},\boldsymbol{U}^{(k+1)})^{\mathrm{T}} = (\boldsymbol{Y}^{(k)},\boldsymbol{U}^{(k)})^{\mathrm{T}} + (\delta\boldsymbol{Y},\delta\boldsymbol{U})^{\mathrm{T}}$. Here

$$\mathcal{H} = \begin{pmatrix} \mathcal{L}_{\boldsymbol{YY}} & \mathcal{L}_{\boldsymbol{YU}} \\ \mathcal{L}_{\boldsymbol{UY}} & \mathcal{L}_{\boldsymbol{UU}} \end{pmatrix}$$

denotes the Hessian of the Lagrangian functional, to be evaluated at $(\boldsymbol{Y}^{(k)}, \boldsymbol{U}^{(k)}, \boldsymbol{\lambda}^{(k)})^{\mathrm{T}}$. Note the saddle-point structure of system (8.13), where the adjoint variable indeed plays the role of multiplier for the constraint expressed by the (linearized) state equation. The system (8.13) can be equivalently obtained as the KKT system for the linear-quadratic optimization problem

$$\min_{\delta \boldsymbol{X}} \left[ \frac{1}{2} \delta \boldsymbol{X}^{\mathrm{T}} \mathcal{H} \delta \boldsymbol{X} + \begin{pmatrix} J_{\boldsymbol{Y}} \\ J_{\boldsymbol{U}} \end{pmatrix}^{\mathrm{T}} \delta \boldsymbol{X} \right] \quad \text{subject to} \quad \begin{pmatrix} \mathbf{e}_{\boldsymbol{Y}} \\ \mathbf{e}_{\boldsymbol{U}} \end{pmatrix} \delta \boldsymbol{X} + \mathbf{e} = 0$$

(*e.g.* Hinze *et al.* 2009, Borzì and Schulz 2011), whence the name *sequential quadratic programming* method, which is commonly used to refer to the Newton iterations on system (8.13). Indeed, a quadratic programming problem has to be solved at each step, for example by means of a preconditioned Krylov method such as MINRES, until a suitable convergence criterion is fulfilled. Suitable approximations of the Hessian, based for example on quasi-Newton methods, are required to make this algorithm more computationally attractive: see *e.g.* Borzì and Schulz (2011).

**Remark 8.2** Constraints on the control and/or state variables add nonlinearity to the optimization problem. A first option is to treat inequality constraints in an outer loop, via *penalty methods* which allow us to convert them into additional terms in the cost functional. For instance, if $u \leq b$ is a pointwise control constraint, the term $\frac{c}{2}\| \max\{0, u - b\}\|_{\mathcal{U}}^2$ can be added, where $c > 0$ is a penalty parameter to be properly selected, and then an iterative method can be used in the inner loop. Another option in iterative methods is to perform a projection over the space of admissible controls at each step. More efficient strategies to tackle constrained problems are usually obtained when dealing with constraints in the main optimization loop, such as in the case of *primal–dual active set* strategies: see *e.g.* the monographs by Borzì and Schulz (2011) and Hinze *et al.* (2009).

We finally point out that in this section we have opted for the optimize-then-discretize approach: that is, we have shown how to recover a system of optimality conditions and then proceed to its numerical discretization. The opposite strategy (discretize-then-optimize) would have led to substantially similar numerical methods, by choosing either an iterative or an all-at-once method for the system of optimality conditions derived once the original state system had been discretized. The two approaches do not generally yield identical solutions; see *e.g.* Hinze *et al.* (2009) for a discussion.

## 8.3 Applications to cardiovascular modelling

### 8.3.1 Optimal design of bypass grafts

PDE-constrained optimization problems are obtained when looking for the optimal design of prosthetic devices, such as ventricular assist devices or bypass grafts. For instance, coronary artery bypass grafting (CABG) is a standard surgical procedure to restore blood perfusion to the cardiac muscle by redirecting blood from the aorta through a graft vessel downstream of a coronary artery affected by stenosis or occlusion. The ability to design the graft–vessel connection (the so-called anastomosis, which we refer to as the domain $\Omega$) in an efficient way is a potentially critical factor in preventing post-operative recurrence of re-stenosis.

Today it is accepted that intimal wall thickening, caused by the accelerated growth of smooth muscle cells and the surrounding matrix, is one of the leading causes of long-term failure of end-to-side vascular grafts (Haruguchi and Teraoka 2003). Low and/or highly oscillatory patterns of wall shear stress (WSS), as well as strong vorticity and recirculations, cause intimal wall thickening (Ethier *et al.* 1998, Keynton *et al.* 2001) at sites where curvatures, bifurcations, tortuosity and branching occur, and, more generally, where flow departs from unidirectional patterns (Giordana *et al.* 2005, Loth, Fischer and Bassiouny 2008). In mathematical terms, an *optimal* graft is one that minimizes suitable cost functionals involving the area of low WSS, the spatial WSS gradient (Lei *et al.* 1997) or the vorticity (Quarteroni and Rozza 2003, Manzoni, Quarteroni and Rozza 2012*b*); see *e.g.* Kleinstreuer (2006) for a detailed review. Taking blood velocity $\mathbf{v}$ and pressure $p$ as state variables, and $u = \Omega$ (*i.e.* the shape of the domain itself) as the control variable, the goal is thus to find the optimal shape $\hat{\Omega}$ of the graft by minimizing the cost functional

$$J(\boldsymbol{v}, \Omega) = \int_0^{\mathrm{T}} \int_{\Omega_{\mathrm{obs}}} |\nabla \times \boldsymbol{v}|^2 \,\mathrm{d}\omega \,\mathrm{d}t,$$

where $\Omega_{\mathrm{obs}} \subset \Omega$ is a given observation region in the artery portion immediately after the anastomosis. Indeed, high downstream vorticity may lead to strong flow recirculation, yielding similar effects in terms of intimal thickening.

Other cost functionals that can be employed include the following.

- A tracking-type functional, in order to drive the blood velocity (and pressure, if $\delta > 0$) towards a specified velocity (and pressure) target state $\boldsymbol{v}_d$,

$p_d$, featuring a regular pattern:

$$J(\boldsymbol{v},\Omega)=\frac{1}{2}\int_0^{\mathrm{T}}\int_{\Omega_{\mathrm{obs}}}|\boldsymbol{v}-\boldsymbol{v}_d|^2\,\mathrm{d}\Omega\,\mathrm{d}t+\frac{\delta}{2}\int_0^{\mathrm{T}}\int_{\Omega_{\mathrm{obs}}}|p-p_d|^2\,\mathrm{d}\omega\,\mathrm{d}t.$$

A typical choice of $(\boldsymbol{v}_d, p_d)$ is provided by the Stokes (or a low-Reynolds Navier–Stokes) flow in the same domain.

- In two dimensions, a *Galilean invariant* vortex measure identifies a region as a vortex if $\nabla\boldsymbol{v}$ has complex eigenvalues; that is, if $\det(\nabla\boldsymbol{v})>0$. Following Hintermüller, Kunisch, Spasov and Volkwein (2004), Kunisch and Vexler (2007) and Lassila, Manzoni, Quarteroni and Rozza (2013*a*), then

$$J(\boldsymbol{v},\Omega)=\int_0^{\mathrm{T}}\int_{\Omega_{\mathrm{obs}}}\max(0,\det(\nabla\boldsymbol{v}))\,\mathrm{d}\omega\,\mathrm{d}t$$

can be used when dealing with vortex suppression.

- A WSS gradient-based functional is given by

$$J(\boldsymbol{v},\Omega)=\int_0^{\mathrm{T}}\int_{\Gamma_{\mathrm{obs}}}WSSG(t)\,\mathrm{d}\gamma\,\mathrm{d}t,$$
$$WSSG(t)=\left(\left(\frac{\partial\boldsymbol{w}_p}{\partial\boldsymbol{\tau}_p}\right)^2+\left(\frac{\partial\boldsymbol{w}_n}{\partial\boldsymbol{\tau}_n}\right)^2\right),$$

that is, by a time-averaged WSS gradient, measured over the portion $\Gamma_{\mathrm{obs}}\subset\partial\Omega$ of the boundary in the anastomosis region. Here, *WSSG* denotes the WSS gradient, where $\boldsymbol{w}=\boldsymbol{w}(t,\boldsymbol{x})$ is the WSS vector of components $w^{(j)}=\mu\nabla\boldsymbol{v}\boldsymbol{n}(t,\boldsymbol{x})\cdot\boldsymbol{\tau}^{(j)}$, and $\boldsymbol{\tau}_p$ and $\boldsymbol{\tau}_n$ are the unit vectors parallel and normal to the direction of the time-averaged WSS vector $\boldsymbol{w}$, respectively. Only a linear combination of the *normal* components $\partial\boldsymbol{x}_j/\partial\boldsymbol{\tau}_j$, $j=p,n$ is considered as an index to quantify the tension yielding intimal thickening. Moreover, the time-averaged WSS is relatively insensitive to changes in the anastomosis configuration, whereas the time-averaged WSS gradient is highly sensitive, and has been linked to localized mechanobiological responses in tissues (see Lei *et al.* 1997 and the discussion therein). Using *WSSG* rather than *WSS* can be understood as filtering the WSS by removing its component induced by the steady mean flow and considering only the spatially fluctuating term as part of the indicator. For the sake of numerical efficiency of the whole optimization process, a steady flow simulation (*e.g.* corresponding to the systolic peak) can be considered, and the WSS gradient of the steady flow can be taken as an approximation of the time-averaged WSS gradient. The interested reader can refer to Kleinstreuer (2006), for example, for further details.

Many works of the past few decades have focussed on the optimal shape design of end-to-side anastomoses, typically by acting on the wall shape near the anastomosis by local shape variation. If a simpler parametric optimization approach is considered, the three most significant design variables (see Loth *et al.* 2008) are the anastomosis angle, the graft-to-host diameter ratio (Keynton *et al.* 2001, Do, Owida, Yang and Morsi 2011) and the toe shape, that is, the profile of the bypass junction. Optimizing a complex configuration in terms of few design variables is more advantageous since it is known that grafts usually have an extended patch or cuff that effectively provides a hood to ease the flow transition from the graft to the artery. Further, improved anastomosis design must comply with the constraints set by surgical realization. For a more comprehensive review of bypass graft design results, we refer to Migliavacca and Dubini (2005), Loth *et al.* (2008), Owida, Do and Morsi (2012) and Marsden (2014).

Concerning the objective to be minimized, each cost functional involves suitable observations, obtained as functions of the state variables over the entire domain or some boundary portions, and over a given time interval and, possibly, data acquired from measurements, as in the case of a tracking-type functional. There are of course other parameters affecting the cost functional, such as the Reynolds number, or the flow split between the proximal host artery and the graft, *i.e.* the ratio of the corresponding flow rates (Giordana *et al.* 2005). All these parameters should be considered as uncertainties within a robust optimization framework, in order to characterize the optimal shape of the graft in a range of possible operating conditions. Examples of optimal design in the presence of uncertainty in cardiovascular applications were considered by Sankaran and Marsden (2010).

As a concluding remark, we point out that the coupling of optimization algorithms to blood flow simulations is computationally challenging, since each evaluation of the cost functional requires the solution of an unsteady, three-dimensional Navier–Stokes problem. If relying on the adjoint approach to characterize the gradient of the cost functional, a further linearized Navier–Stokes (Oseen) problem has to be solved at every iteration. For this reason, the majority of works related to applications in surgery and device optimization have focussed, so far, on small-scale and/or two-dimensional problems, or on steady-flow problems, usually relying on gradient-free methods.

For the sake of illustration, we report some numerical results for the optimal design of a femoropopliteal bypass graft. This surgery is used to bypass diseased blood vessels above or below the knee, and is one of the most common surgical treatments of chronic lower-extremity ischaemia. We model the blood flow across a bypass graft via a steady Navier–Stokes model, and

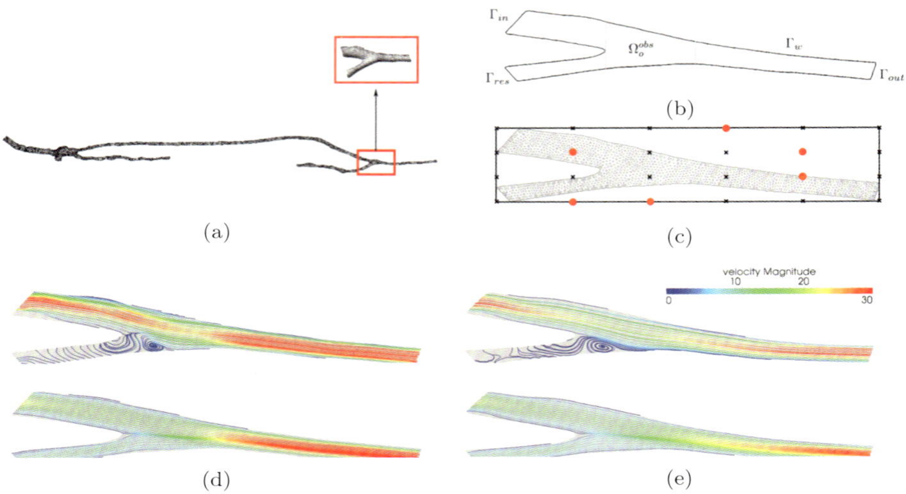


Figure 8.2 Optimal design of bypass grafts. (a) A tract of femoral artery with a bypass graft. (b) Computational domain, boundaries and observation region; (c) FFD shape parametrization used to generate admissible shapes. Global shape deformations are induced by the displacement of a few selected control points (shown in red) in the $6 \times 4$ FFD lattice. These control points are selected by a preliminary screening procedure based on sensitivity analysis. (d) Initial and (e) optimal bypass configurations in the case of total (above) or partial (below) occlusion. Numerical results were obtained using the MATLAB finite element library MLife.

consider a vorticity cost functional

$$J(\boldsymbol{v}, \Omega) = \int_{\Omega_{\text{obs}}} |\nabla \times \boldsymbol{v}|^2 \, \mathrm{d}\omega,$$

where $\Omega_{\text{obs}} \subset \Omega$ is the observation region. Initial and optimal shapes are shown in Figure 8.2 for the case of a stenosed host artery; its occlusion, either total or partial, is expressed via a Dirichlet boundary condition on the incoming velocity field on $\Gamma_{\text{res}}$, homogeneous for the completely occluded case and non-homogeneous otherwise. See Figure 8.2(b) for the definition of $\Omega_{\text{obs}}$ and $\Gamma_{\text{ref}}$. A shape parametrization technique based on free-form deformations (FFDs) is very suitable for describing admissible shapes via deformation of a reference configuration by acting on a small set of control points: see *e.g.* Manzoni (2012) and Manzoni *et al.* (2012*b*).

### *8.3.2 Optimal control of electrical defibrillation*

Whereas in healthy conditions the electrical activation of the heart is an extremely organized (and efficient) process, some disturbances in the formation and/or propagation of electrical signals may induce re-entrant activation patterns which lead to tachycardia, that is, a noticeable increase in the heart's activation rate. In the worst cases, this may turn into an even less organized activation pattern, called fibrillation. A common therapy to terminate fibrillation and restore regular cardiac rhythm is electrical defibrillation, consisting in the delivery of a strong electrical shock by injecting external currents through a set of electrodes. This restores a spatially uniform activation pattern, recovering an extracellular potential distribution showing damped voltage gradients. Today, electrical defibrillation is carried out by implanting devices (so-called cardioverter defibrillators) able to monitor the heart rhythm and then deliver electrical discharges when needed.

This process can be modelled by considering the monodomain equation (6.11) as the state system, for which the extracellular stimulation current $I_e = I_e(t)$ to be applied plays the role of a distributed control function, and has to be determined in order to minimize the cost functional

$$J(V_m, I_e) = \frac{1}{2}\int_0^T \int_{\Omega_{\text{obs}}} |V_m - v_d|^2 \,\mathrm{d}\Omega\,\mathrm{d}t + \frac{\alpha}{2}\int_0^T \int_{\Omega_{\text{con}}} |I_e|^2 \,\mathrm{d}\Omega\,\mathrm{d}t. \quad (8.14)$$

Here $V_m$ is the trans-membrane potential, $\Omega_{\text{obs}} \subseteq \Omega_{\text{mus}}$ is the observation domain, $\Omega_{\text{con}} \subseteq \Omega_{\text{mus}}$ is the control domain, and $v_d$ is the target potential distribution. For instance, if $v_d = 0$, the minimum of $J(V_m, I_e)$ corresponds to the case of an excitation wave which is suppressed in the region $\Omega_{\text{obs}}$: see *e.g.* Nagaiah, Kunisch and Plank (2011). The trans-membrane potential $V_m$ can be obtained by solving the monodomain equations

$$\begin{aligned}
&\chi_m C_m \frac{\partial V_m}{\partial t} - \nabla\cdot(\boldsymbol{\Sigma}\nabla V_m) + \chi_m I_{\text{ion}} = I_e && \text{in } \Omega_{\text{mus}} \times (0,T), && (8.15\text{a})\\
&\frac{\partial w}{\partial t} = g(V_m, w) && \text{in } \Omega_{\text{mus}} \times (0,T), && (8.15\text{b})\\
&V_m|_{t=0} = V_{m,0} && \text{in } \Omega_{\text{mus}}, && (8.15\text{c})\\
&w|_{t=0} = w_0 && \text{in } \Omega_{\text{mus}}, && (8.15\text{d})\\
&\boldsymbol{\Sigma}\nabla V_m \cdot \mathbf{n} = 0 && \text{on } \Sigma_{\text{epi}} \cup \Sigma_{\text{endo}} && (8.15\text{e})
\end{aligned}$$

(see Section 6.1.3), where $I_{\text{ion}}$ is provided, for example, by the FitzHugh–Nagumo model (see Section 6.1.2):

$$I_{\text{ion}} = f(V_m, w) = -kV_m(V_m - a)(V_m - 1) - w, \quad g(V_m, w) = \epsilon(V_m - \gamma w).$$

An analysis of this optimal control problem can be found in Nagaiah *et al.* (2011), for example. We can exploit the Lagrangian approach to derive a system of first-order optimality conditions, by introducing the Lagrangian

$$\begin{aligned}
&\mathcal{L}(V_m, w, I_e, z, q) \\
&\quad = J(V_m, I_e) + \langle \mathcal{E}(V_m, w, I_e), (z, q)\rangle_{V,V^*} \\
&\quad = J(V_m, I_e) \\
&\qquad + \int_0^T \int_{\Omega_{\text{mus}}} \left( \chi_m C_m \frac{\partial V_m}{\partial t} - \nabla \cdot (\boldsymbol{\Sigma} \nabla V_m) + \chi_m I_{\text{ion}} - I_e \right) z \, \mathrm{d}\Omega \, \mathrm{d}t \\
&\qquad + \int_0^T \int_{\Omega_{\text{mus}}} \left( \frac{\partial w}{\partial t} - g(V_m, w) \right) q \, \mathrm{d}\Omega \, \mathrm{d}t,
\end{aligned}$$

where $(z, q)$ denote the dual variables of $V_m$, $w$, respectively. Here $(V_m, w) \in V = L^2(0, T; \mathcal{V}) \times W^{1,2}(0, T; \mathcal{H})$, where $\mathcal{V} = H^1(\Omega_{\text{mus}})$ and $\mathcal{H} = L^2(\Omega_{\text{mus}})$; the control space can be chosen as $U = L^2(0, T; L^2(\Omega))$, and the initial conditions can be kept as explicit constraints. By setting the partial derivatives of $\mathcal{L}$ equal to zero, we find the following expression for the adjoint problem:

$$\begin{aligned}
&-\chi_m C_m \frac{\partial z}{\partial t} - \nabla \cdot (\boldsymbol{\Sigma} \nabla z) + \chi_m \frac{\partial I_{\text{ion}}}{\partial V_m} z - \frac{\partial g}{\partial V_m} q \\
&\qquad\qquad = v_d - V_m \quad \text{in } \Omega_{\text{mus}} \times (0, T), && (8.16\text{a}) \\
&-\frac{\partial q}{\partial t} - \frac{\partial g}{\partial w} q + \frac{\partial I_{\text{ion}}}{\partial w} z = 0 \quad \text{in } \Omega_{\text{mus}} \times (0, T), && (8.16\text{b}) \\
&z|_{t=T} = 0 \quad \text{in } \Omega_{\text{mus}}, && (8.16\text{c}) \\
&q|_{t=T} = 0 \quad \text{in } \Omega_{\text{mus}}, && (8.16\text{d}) \\
&\boldsymbol{\Sigma} \nabla z \cdot \mathbf{n} = 0 \quad \text{on } \Sigma_{\text{epi}} \cup \Sigma_{\text{endo}} && (8.16\text{e})
\end{aligned}$$

and the optimality condition

$$z + \alpha I_e = 0 \quad \text{on } \Omega_{\text{con}}. \tag{8.17}$$

The optimal control problem (8.14, 8.15) can be solved by an *optimize-then-discretize* strategy, where both spatial and temporal discretizations are required because of the time-dependent nature of the problem. After discretization, we can employ an iterative method, by computing at each step the solution of the (coupled) state problem (8.15) over $(0, T)$, and the solution of the adjoint problem (8.16), which is a linear problem, backward in time, where the adjoint variables are coupled similarly to $(V_m, w)$ in the state problem. Note that the data of the adjoint problem are related to the Fréchet derivative of the cost functional with respect to the state variables, and that the adjoint problem depends on the control function only through the state variable. Moreover, the adjoint operator calls into play the linearization of the state operator around the computed state solution; that is, the derivatives $\partial I_{\text{ion}}/\partial V_m$, $\partial g/\partial V_m$, $\partial I_{\text{ion}}/\partial w$, $\partial g/\partial w$ have to be evaluated, at each step, around the computed solution of the state system. The optimality condition (8.17) then allows us to determine the gradient $\tilde{J}'(I_e)$ of the cost functional $\tilde{J}(I_e) = J(V_m(I_e), I_e)$, required to update the control function at each step.

To simplify the optimal control problem, we can for instance look for control functions of the form

$$I_e(t,\mathbf{x}) = \sum_{k=1}^{N_{el}} u_k(t)\mathcal{I}_{\Omega_{\text{con},k}}(\mathbf{x})\mathcal{I}_{(0,T_{\text{def}})}(t),$$

where the location of $N_{el}$ electrodes through which the current is delivered is prescribed, and only its time intensity has to be controlled over time. Here $\mathcal{I}_{\Omega_{\text{con},k}}(\mathbf{x})$ denotes the indicator function of the region $\Omega_{\text{con},k}$ where the $k$th electrode is located. Additional inequality constraints of the form $u_{\min} \leq u_k(t) \leq u_{\max}$ can also be taken into account in order to limit current amplitude.

Further extensions of this framework consider, for example, the bidomain model (Nagaiah *et al.* 2013*b*), the case of boundary controls (Nagaiah, Kunisch and Plank 2013*a*), and a different Mitchell–Schaeffer model to describe ionic currents, together with the presence of a conductive bath medium outside the heart effects and experimentally based fibre and sheet orientations (Nagaiah, Kunisch and Plank 2016). Moreover, the case where the shock duration itself is also optimized has been considered by Kunisch and Rund (2015). The reason to consider this further effect is that after applying a defibrillation shock, the muscle tissue needs a suitable amount of time to reach a non-fibrillatory state, so that a successful defibrillation can only be assessed at a time $T \gg T_{\text{def}}$, where $T_{\text{def}}$ is the end time of the defibrillation shock and $T$ the final observation time, at which the tissue should have reached a non-excited state. In this context, the cost functional

$$J(V_m, u, T_{\text{def}}) = T_{\text{def}} + \frac{\mu}{2}\int_{\Omega_{\text{obs}}} |V_m(\cdot, T)|^2 \,\mathrm{d}\Omega + \frac{\alpha}{2}\sum_{k=1}^{N_{el}}\int_0^T |u_k|^2 \,\mathrm{d}t$$

can be minimized, accounting for (i) a minimum time term, (ii) a final time observation at $t = T$, and (iii) the amplitude of the applied currents, subject to the state system (8.15) to be solved over $(0,T)$. Indeed, the shock duration and its energy have to be minimized to avoid negative side effects of the applied shock, while the final time observation term is taken into account to quantify defibrillation, thus requiring that the tissue reaches a non-excited state at $T \gg T_{\text{def}}$.

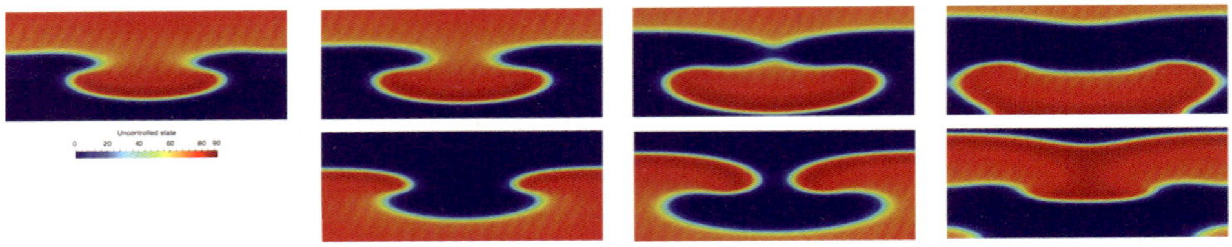


(a)

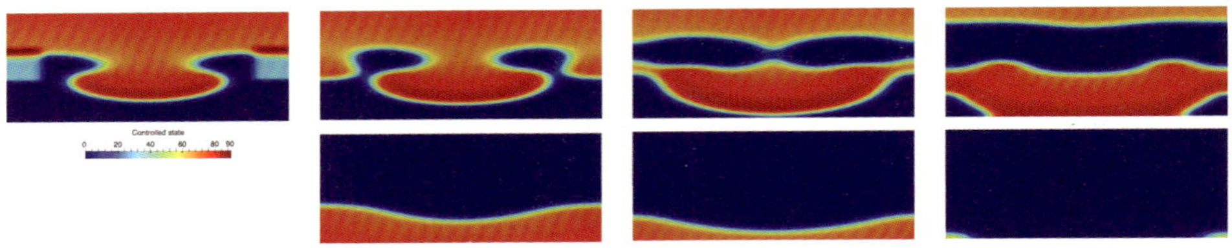


(b)

Figure 8.3 Electric trans-membrane potential at times $t = 0, 4, 12, 20, 40, 52, 64$ ms in the uncontrolled case (a) and in the controlled case (b). The re-entry wave appearing in the uncontrolled case is damped by the control acting on $\Omega_{\text{con}}$.

For illustration, we consider the case of an axially symmetric domain $\Omega_{\text{mus}} = (0, 2) \times (0, 0.8)$, where a constant pulse of intensity $u$ is delivered in the control domain $\Omega_{\text{con}} = (0, 0.25) \times (0.3, 0.55) \cup (1.75, 2) \times (0.3, 0.55)$, until time $T_{\text{def}}$. Here $\boldsymbol{U} = (u, T_{\text{def}})^{\text{T}}$ is the control variable, with $1 \leq u \leq 100$ mV and $0.1 \leq T_{\text{def}} \leq 4$ ms; the final time is $T = 64$ ms. The initial condition $(V_{m,0}, w_0)^{\text{T}}$ describes a re-entry wave of the 'figure of eight' type, obtained following the procedure described by Kunisch and Rund (2015), who also took into account more general optimal control problems. For the case at hand, a planar wavefront travelling from the bottom to the top can be damped by imposing an optimal control of intensity $u \approx 95$ mV until $T_{\text{def}} \approx 1.2$ ms on the control region. The successful defibrillation – resulting from a trade-off between a large intensity and a short duration of the pulse – is clearly visible in Figure 8.3, where in the controlled case at the final time the tissue is almost completely unexcited. Indeed, the pulse acts on the excitable region of the tissue adjacent to the wavefront, bringing it to a non-excitable state.

**Remark 8.3** We point out that choosing the cost functional and, if necessary, imposing suitable constraints on the control and/or the state variable, are two extremely hard, problem-dependent tasks. Moreover, very often control functions are described in terms of (possibly few) relevant parameters, which play the role of design variables. However, in the case of complex, patient-dependent geometries, for example, their automatic selection can result in a fairly involved procedure. Last but not least, in the case where a target state to be reached depends on acquired data, the effect of uncertainty has to be considered in the formulation (and then solution) of the problem. This leads to robust optimization problems, for example, or PDE-constrained optimization problems under uncertainty, an active research field, where very few applications to cardiovascular modelling have yet been considered.

# 9

# Parameter estimation from clinical data

When dealing with the mathematical and numerical modelling of the circulatory system, initial conditions, boundary conditions or physical coefficients, for example tissue properties, might be (partially) unknown (Veneziani and Vergara 2013): see Chapters 2 and 5. From here on we refer to any of these quantities as input parameters, independent of their mathematical nature (they could be scalars or vectors, or even parametric fields varying in space) and we refer to the issue of making inferences about unknown parameters from data as *parameter estimation* (or *identification*). To perform parameter estimation for a system of PDEs, we need to combine state observations and additional data that are not strictly required for solving the PDE problem, and have to be acquired from measurements.

Parameter estimation for PDEs can be done according to several techniques, which can be roughly classified depending on their outcome (Tarantola 2004, Le Dimet and Talagrand 1986). *Point estimates* rely on either *variational* or *sequential* methods (Ide, Courtier, Ghil and Lorenc 1997). Both methods provide optimal least-squares estimates by minimizing a cost functional accounting for the misfit between measured data and state observations. A second class of techniques instead yields *confidence regions* or, more generally speaking, the possibility of characterizing the probability distribution of the unknown parameters provided they are described in terms of random variables; this is the goal of statistical inversion theory relying for example on *Bayesian inference*, which will be the main focus of Section 10.2.

In the context of cardiovascular modelling, parameter estimation is necessary for *model calibration/personalization*, for the purpose of diagnosis or treatment. Indeed, parameters that are not directly measurable (*e.g.* for tissue conductivity or vessel compliance) are tuned so that the outcome of the numerical model is able to reproduce patient-specific data (Krishnamurthy *et al.* 2013). Difficulties arise because of data sparsity (Konukoglu *et al.*

2011). Indeed, spatial resolution and temporal frequency are typically undersampled; experimental data, on the other hand, are always contaminated by measurement noise.

**Remark 9.1** Data assimilation (DA) is the process by which a numerical model of a given system, usually affected by noise or model uncertainties, is improved by incorporating system observations. Although data assimilation relies on the same variational or filtering approaches addressed in this chapter, in the case of geophysical fluids, for example, its main goal often goes beyond parameter estimation; indeed, it is more often related to *state estimation*, namely, to improving the outcome of the numerical model and of its initial state to correctly initialize forecasts, by assimilating available measurements into the numerical model itself. Data assimilation is intrinsically related to time-varying phenomena and deals with highly non-linear dynamical systems, very often far from being periodical (such as in the case of meteorological models) and ill-posed: see *e.g.* Blum, Le Dimet and Navon (2009), Voss, Timmer and Kurths (2004) and Le Dimet and Talagrand (1986) for a detailed discussion. In the past decade several works dealing with cardiovascular applications have focussed on *data assimilation* (Sermesant *et al.* 2006, Delingette *et al.* 2012, Bertagna, D'Elia, Perego and Veneziani 2014, Lal, Mohammadi and Nicoud 2017), which has been considered, in many cases, as synonymous with *parameter estimation.*

In this chapter we provide an overview of both variational and sequential approaches for parameter estimation in time-dependent systems. Parameter estimation problems dealing with stationary systems in cardiovascular applications have also been solved: see *e.g.* D'Elia, Perego and Veneziani (2012), Bertagna *et al.* (2014), MacLachlan, Nielsen, Lysaker and Tveito (2006), Nielsen, Cai and Lykaser (2007*a*), Lassila, Manzoni, Quarteroni and Rozza (2013*b*) and Manzoni, Lassila, Quarteroni and Rozza (2014). For the sake of space and relevance, we will focus on time-dependent problems.

## 9.1 Variational approach: PDE-constrained optimization

The variational approach recasts parameter estimation in the framework of PDE-constrained optimization, by considering the equations governing the problem at hand as the state system, and the discrepancy between the observation of the state and the measured data as the cost functional to be minimized (Banks and Kunisch 1989, Chavent 2010). The parameters to be estimated (often involving the initial condition) play the role of optimization variables, just like control variables in the case of optimal control problems;

however, unlike the optimal control case, the parameters to be estimated are quantities which no one can actually control. They are often coefficients of the operator appearing in the PDE problem.

Here we provide an abstract formulation of the variational approach, following Bertoglio, Moireau and Gerbeau (2012) and Blum *et al.* (2009); for more details see *e.g.* Nichols (2010), Chapelle, Fragu, Mallet and Moireau (2013*a*) and Sermesant *et al.* (2006). We assume that the state problem has already been discretized in space. We let $\boldsymbol{X}(t) \in \mathbb{R}^{n_x}$ denote the semi-discrete state, $\boldsymbol{\theta} \in \mathbb{R}^p$ the parameters of the model to be estimated, and $\boldsymbol{A}(t, \boldsymbol{X}(t), \boldsymbol{\theta})$ the (semi-discretized in space) state operator; note that usually $p \ll n_x$. The state variable then solves the dynamical system

$$\dot{\boldsymbol{X}}(t) = \boldsymbol{A}(t, \boldsymbol{X}(t), \boldsymbol{\theta}), \quad t \in (0, T), \tag{9.1a}$$

$$\boldsymbol{X}(0) = \boldsymbol{G}. \tag{9.1b}$$

For instance, in the case of the FSI system (3.19), $\boldsymbol{X} = (\boldsymbol{v}, p, \boldsymbol{d})$ contains fluid velocity and pressure, and structure displacement, and $\boldsymbol{\theta}$ may contain the value of the Young's modulus (here assumed to be piecewise constant) in different patches of the arterial wall.

We consider the case where the parameter vector $\boldsymbol{\theta}$ is unknown, and for which the estimation problem consists in finding $\widehat{\boldsymbol{\theta}}$ such that the discrepancy between the observation and a set of measurements $\boldsymbol{Z}(t) \in \mathbb{R}^{n_z}$, $t \in (0, T)$, is minimized, for example in a least-squares sense. The case of unknown initial data $\boldsymbol{G}$ to be estimated can be treated in essentially the same way. We usually assume that measurements $\boldsymbol{Z}(t)$ are related to observations of the true state through an *additive noise* model; that is,

$$\boldsymbol{Z}(t) = H(t)\boldsymbol{X}(t) + \varepsilon(t), \quad t \in (0, T),$$

where $H = H(t) \in R^{n_z \times n_x}$ is an observation operator which maps the state space into the observation space $R^{n_z}$, and $\varepsilon = \varepsilon(t)$ is a *noise* term accounting for measurement errors. The following minimization problem is then solved:

$$J(\boldsymbol{X}, \boldsymbol{\theta}) = \frac{1}{2} \int_0^{\mathrm{T}} \|\boldsymbol{Z}(t) - H(t)\boldsymbol{X}(t)\|_M^2 \, \mathrm{d}t + \frac{\alpha_\theta}{2} \|\boldsymbol{\theta} - \boldsymbol{\theta}_0\|_{P_\theta^{-1}}^2 \to \min_{\boldsymbol{\theta} \in \mathcal{P}}, \tag{9.2}$$

where $\boldsymbol{X} = \boldsymbol{X}(t)$ is the solution of (9.1). Here $\mathcal{P} \subset R^p \times R^{n_x}$ denotes the set of admissible parameters. Additional information is usually added to the least-squares objective expressed by the first term in (9.2), via a background estimate $\boldsymbol{\theta}_0$ of $\boldsymbol{\theta}$; $M$ and $P_\theta^{-1}$ are suitable symmetric positive definite matrices (the reason why we consider an inverse matrix to define this latter norm will be clarified in the following). This procedure goes by the name of *Levenberg–Marquardt–Tikhonov regularization*. For a discussion of classical regularization methods for inverse problems, see Kaipio and Somersalo (2005); note that the usual penalization coefficients are embedded in the definition of the matrix $P_\theta^{-1}$.

The minimization problem (9.2) can be solved by an optimization algorithm based on the evaluation of the gradient of $J$ with respect to $\boldsymbol{\theta}$. As shown in Section 8.1, this latter can be computed by relying on the solution of a suitable *adjoint problem*. This is a *four-dimensional variational* (4D-Var) assimilation; a three-dimensional variational (3D-Var) assimilation would arise in the case of steady-state systems. See Section 9.3.1 for further details on a relevant example in cardiovascular modelling, and Blum *et al.* (2009) and Chapelle *et al.* (2013*a*) for more on 4D-Var assimilation problems.

Since measurements $\boldsymbol{Z}$ are only available at a discrete number of times $\tau^1, \ldots, \tau^K$, we formulate the identification problem by replacing the dynamical system (9.1) with its time-discretized version:

$$\boldsymbol{X}^{k+1} = \boldsymbol{A}_{k|k+1}(\boldsymbol{X}^k, \boldsymbol{\theta}), \quad k = 0, \ldots, K-1, \tag{9.3a}$$

$$\boldsymbol{X}^0 = \boldsymbol{G} \tag{9.3b}$$

where $\boldsymbol{A}_{k|k+1}$ is a non-linear function describing the evolution of the state from time $\tau^k$ to time $\tau^{k+1}$ and $\boldsymbol{X}^k \approx \boldsymbol{X}(k\Delta\tau)$ denotes the state vector at time $\tau^k$. Note that the length $\Delta\tau = \tau^{k+1} - \tau^k$ of the time window between two subsequent measurements is usually larger than the time step $\Delta t$ used for time discretization, and that $\boldsymbol{\theta}$ does not depend on $k$. From here on $k$ will denote the temporal index of system evolution, thus using a different notation from that introduced in Parts 1 and 2 (where the temporal index was denoted by $n$).

We then formulate an optimal time-discretized minimization criterion and, finally, determine the corresponding adjoint problem, rather than discretizing the adjoint problem in time. This yields the minimization problem

$$J_K(\boldsymbol{X}, \boldsymbol{\theta}) = \frac{1}{2}\sum_{k=1}^{K} \|\boldsymbol{Z}^k - H\boldsymbol{X}^k\|^2_{M_k} + \frac{1}{2}\|\boldsymbol{\theta} - \boldsymbol{\theta}_0\|^2_{P_\theta^{-1}} \rightarrow \min_{\boldsymbol{\theta}\in\mathcal{P}}, \tag{9.4}$$

where $\boldsymbol{X} = (\boldsymbol{X}^1, \ldots, \boldsymbol{X}^k)$, and we set

$$\boldsymbol{Z}^k = H_k\boldsymbol{X}^k + \boldsymbol{\varepsilon}^k. \tag{9.5}$$

Here $\boldsymbol{\varepsilon}^k$ denotes the noise of the measurement device at $\tau^k = k\Delta\tau$; a possible choice for $M_k$ is $M_k = \Delta\tau M$, whereas $H_k \approx H(k\Delta\tau)$. Also in this case a gradient-based optimization procedure can be used to solve the constrained optimization problem (9.3, 9.4) with gradients evaluated by introducing a suitable adjoint problem.

## 9.2 Sequential approach: Kalman filter and extensions

A drawback of the variational approach is the need to wait until the whole set of measurements has been acquired in order to perform an optimization step. A sequential approach instead performs the assimilation of acquired measurements *on the fly*, and updates the estimate of the unknown quantities accordingly.

A numerical milestone for the solution of sequential estimation problems, the Kalman filter (KF) (Kalman 1960), was introduced as a recursive filter for the estimation of the state of a noisy dynamical system from a set of measurements, that is, to improve the prediction of the state dynamics by taking into account additional data. An augmented form of the Kalman filter can be easily adapted to the problem of estimating unknown parameters, as we will see. Originally designed for linear dynamical systems, the Kalman filter has severe memory requirements. To mitigate these two limitations, several improvements and extensions have been proposed in the past few decades, most notably the extended Kalman filter (EKF), the unscented Kalman filter (UKF) and the ensemble Kalman filter (EnKF); detailed reviews can be found, for example, in Kaipio and Somersalo (2005), Simon (2006), Humphreys, Redd and West (2012) and Asch, Bocquet and Nodet (2017). In this section we recall the formulation of the basic Kalman filter and provide some hints about its extensions, with a special focus on the field of cardiovascular modelling where these techniques have been applied.

The literature offers many possible derivations of the Kalman filter; following Humphreys *et al.* (2012) and Chapelle *et al.* (2013*a*), we will exploit the analogy with the solution of a recursive least-squares problem yielding the best linear unbiased estimator for a linear model; alternative derivations can be obtained, for example, by relying on the so-called push-forward and subsequent conditioning of Gaussian measures (Sullivan 2015) or a sequential Bayesian estimation framework (Law, Stuart and Zygalakis 2015).

### *9.2.1 The Kalman filter algorithm*

The KF algorithm sequentially generates an estimate of the unknown quantity by means of a linear combination of the current estimate and the acquired measurement. Let us first consider the case where there is no dynamics, and data are generated by the linear model

$$\boldsymbol{Z} = H\boldsymbol{X} + \boldsymbol{\varepsilon}, \tag{9.6}$$

where $H$ is a given $n_z \times n_x$ matrix of rank $n_x$, $\boldsymbol{\varepsilon}$ is an $n_z$-dimensional random variable with zero mean and known positive definite covariance $Q = \mathbb{E}[\boldsymbol{\varepsilon}\boldsymbol{\varepsilon}^{\mathrm{T}}] > 0$, and $\boldsymbol{Z}$ denotes known, but inexact, measurements with errors given by $\boldsymbol{\varepsilon}$. The vector $\boldsymbol{X} \in R^{n_x}$ is the quantity to be estimated from the observation $\boldsymbol{Z}$; $\mathbb{E}[\cdot]$ denotes the expected value.

Among all linear estimators of $\boldsymbol{X}$, that is, estimators of the form $\widehat{\boldsymbol{X}} = K\boldsymbol{Z}$ for some matrix $K \in R^{n_x \times n_z}$, which are unbiased (*i.e.* $\mathbb{E}[\widehat{\boldsymbol{X}}] = \boldsymbol{X}$), the best choice is the one that minimizes the mean-square error $\mathbb{E}[(\widehat{\boldsymbol{X}}-\boldsymbol{X})^{\mathrm{T}}(\widehat{\boldsymbol{X}}-\boldsymbol{X})]$; by the Gauss–Markov theorem (see *e.g.* Sullivan 2015, Chapter 7), the best or minimum variance linear unbiased estimator for (9.6) is given by

$$\widehat{\boldsymbol{X}} = (H^{\mathrm{T}}Q^{-1}H)^{-1}H^{\mathrm{T}}Q^{-1}\boldsymbol{Z}. \tag{9.7}$$

In that case, $E[(\widehat{\boldsymbol{X}} - \boldsymbol{X})(\widehat{\boldsymbol{X}} - \boldsymbol{X})^{\mathrm{T}}] = (H^{\mathrm{T}}Q^{-1}H)^{-1}$. Equivalently, (9.7) can also be obtained by solving the weighted least-squares problem

$$\widehat{\boldsymbol{X}} = \frac{1}{2}\|H\boldsymbol{X} - \boldsymbol{Z}\|^2_{Q^{-1}} \to \min_{\boldsymbol{X}}, \tag{9.8}$$

again resorting to a variational argument. In the slightly different case where we want to combine the observation and a background estimate $\boldsymbol{X}_0$ of $\boldsymbol{X}$ with covariance matrix $P^-$, (9.8) becomes

$$\widehat{\boldsymbol{X}} = \frac{1}{2}\|H\boldsymbol{X} - \boldsymbol{Z}\|^2_{Q^{-1}} + \frac{1}{2}\|\boldsymbol{X} - \boldsymbol{X}_0\|^2_{(P^-)^{-1}} \to \min_{\boldsymbol{X}},$$

and instead of (9.7) we find

$$\widehat{\boldsymbol{X}} = \boldsymbol{X}_0 + K(\boldsymbol{Z} - H\boldsymbol{X}_0), \quad K = P^+H^{\mathrm{T}}Q^{-1}, \tag{9.9}$$

upon defining the matrix playing the role of *updated* covariance as

$$P^+ = ((P^-)^{-1} + H^{\mathrm{T}}Q^{-1}H)^{-1}. \tag{9.10}$$

Note that this estimate is given by a linear combination of the background estimate $\boldsymbol{X}_0$ and the so-called *innovation* $\boldsymbol{Z} - H\boldsymbol{X}_0$. $K$ is usually referred to as the *Kalman gain matrix*; it can also be evaluated by exploiting the prior covariance $P^-$ instead of the updated covariance $P^+$, according to the equivalence

$$P^+H^{\mathrm{T}}Q^{-1} = P^-H^{\mathrm{T}}(HP^-H^{\mathrm{T}} + Q)^{-1}. \tag{9.11}$$

We now consider the case of a time-discretized linear system, with data acquired over a time interval. Then the model (9.6) is replaced by

$$\begin{aligned} \boldsymbol{X}^k &= A_{k-1|k}\boldsymbol{X}^{k-1} + \boldsymbol{v}^k, \quad k = 1, \dots, K, \ \boldsymbol{X}^0 = \boldsymbol{G}, \\ \boldsymbol{Z}^k &= H_k \boldsymbol{X}^k + \boldsymbol{w}^k, \end{aligned} \tag{9.12}$$

where $\boldsymbol{X}^k \in \mathbb{R}^{n_x}$ denotes the state and $\boldsymbol{Z}^k \in \mathbb{R}^{n_z}$ are the measurements; $\boldsymbol{v}_k$ and $\boldsymbol{w}_k$ are uncorrelated zero-mean random noise processes with positive-definite covariances $Q_k$ and $R_k$, modelling the uncertainty of the model and the additive noise in the observation, respectively. The state estimation problem is the problem of finding the state $\boldsymbol{X}^k$ given $k$ known observations $\boldsymbol{Z}^1, \dots, \boldsymbol{Z}^k$.

The Kalman filter is a recursive algorithm that provides the best linear unbiased estimate $\boldsymbol{X}_a^k$ of $\boldsymbol{X}^k$ in terms of both the previous estimate $\boldsymbol{X}_a^{k-1}$ and the latest data $\boldsymbol{Z}^k$ up to that point in time. It is based on a *predictor-corrector* strategy, consisting of the following steps.

(1) A *prediction* step (called the forecast or the time update) consists in letting the system dynamics evolve from $\boldsymbol{X}_a^{k-1}$ without taking into account the observations, yielding the *forecast* state $\boldsymbol{X}_f^k$.
(2) A *correction* step (called the analysis or the measurement update) updates the forecast state $\boldsymbol{X}_f^k$ by *assimilating* the measurements into the model, yielding the *assimilated* state $\boldsymbol{X}_a^k$.

To derive the expression of the correction step, let us suppose that the current prediction based on observations $\boldsymbol{Z}^1, \dots, \boldsymbol{Z}^{k-1}$ is $\boldsymbol{X}_f^k$, with covariance matrix $P_k^f$. If the true state is $\boldsymbol{X}_k$, model (9.6) becomes

$$\begin{bmatrix} \boldsymbol{X}_f^k \\ \boldsymbol{Z}^k \end{bmatrix} = \begin{bmatrix} I \\ H_k \end{bmatrix} \boldsymbol{X}^k + \boldsymbol{\varepsilon},$$

where $\boldsymbol{\varepsilon}$ is an $(n_x + n_z)$-dimensional random variable with zero mean and covariance $Q_k = \operatorname{diag}(P_k^f, R_k)$. The best linear unbiased estimator of this system (see (9.7)) is given by

$$\boldsymbol{X}_a^k = P_k^a \begin{bmatrix} I & H_k^{\mathrm{T}} \end{bmatrix} \begin{bmatrix} (P_k^f)^{-1} & 0 \\ 0 & R_k^{-1} \end{bmatrix} \begin{bmatrix} \boldsymbol{X}_f^k \\ \boldsymbol{Z}^k \end{bmatrix} = P_k^a\big((P_k^f)^{-1}\boldsymbol{X}_f^k + H_k^{\mathrm{T}} R_k^{-1} \boldsymbol{Z}^k\big), \tag{9.13}$$

and results from the linear combination of the current estimate and the *last* observation $\boldsymbol{Z}^k$, where

$$P_k^a = \left( \begin{bmatrix} I & H_k^{\mathrm{T}} \end{bmatrix} \begin{bmatrix} (P_k^f)^{-1} & 0 \\ 0 & R_k^{-1} \end{bmatrix} \begin{bmatrix} I \\ H_k \end{bmatrix} \right)^{-1} = ((P_k^f)^{-1} + H_k^{\mathrm{T}} R_k^{-1} H_k)^{-1}.$$

Note the formal analogy with (9.10), where $P_k^f$ and $P_k^a$ now play the role of $P^-$ and $P^+$, respectively. Equation (9.13) can be written in the more convenient form

$$\begin{aligned}\boldsymbol{X}_a^k &= P_k^a\big[(P_k^a)^{-1} - H_k^{\mathrm{T}} R_k^{-1} H_k)) \boldsymbol{X}_f^k + H_k^{\mathrm{T}} R_k^{-1} \boldsymbol{Z}^k\big] \\ &= \boldsymbol{X}_f^k + P_k^a H_k^{\mathrm{T}} R_k^{-1}(\boldsymbol{Z}^k - H_k \boldsymbol{X}_f^k) = \boldsymbol{X}_f^k + K_k(\boldsymbol{Z}^k - H_k \boldsymbol{X}_f^k)\end{aligned}$$

as a function of the innovation $\boldsymbol{Z}^k - H_k \boldsymbol{X}_f^k$. Similarly to (9.11), we obtain

$$K_k = P_k^a H_k^{\mathrm{T}} R_k^{-1} = P_k^f H_k^{\mathrm{T}} (H_k P_k^f H^{\mathrm{T}} + R_k)^{-1}, \tag{9.14}$$

so it is possible to evaluate the Kalman gain matrix $K_k$ as a function of $P_k^f$, and then correct the covariance:

$$\begin{aligned}P_k^a &= ((P_k^f)^{-1} + H_k^{\mathrm{T}} R_k^{-1} H_k)^{-1} \\ &= (I - K_k H_k) P_k^f (I - K_k H_k)^{\mathrm{T}} + K_k R_k K_k^{\mathrm{T}} = (I - K_k H_k) P_k^f.\end{aligned}$$

The prediction step instead exploits the dynamical system to propagate the state, yielding

$$\boldsymbol{X}_f^{k+1} = A_{k|k+1} \boldsymbol{X}_a^k$$

for the time update of the state, and

$$\begin{aligned}P_{k+1}^f &= \mathbb{E}[(\boldsymbol{X}_f^{k+1} - \boldsymbol{X}^{k+1})(\boldsymbol{X}_f^{k+1} - \boldsymbol{X}^{k+1})^{\mathrm{T}}] \\ &= \mathbb{E}[(A_{k|k+1} \boldsymbol{X}_a^k - A_{k|k+1} \boldsymbol{X}_k - \boldsymbol{w}_k)(A_{k|k+1} \widehat{\boldsymbol{X}}_a^k - A_{k|k+1} \boldsymbol{X}_k - \boldsymbol{w}_k)^{\mathrm{T}}] \\ &= A_{k|k+1} P_k^a A_{k|k+1}^{\mathrm{T}} + Q_{k+1}\end{aligned}$$

for the time update of the covariance.

Grouping the prediction and the correction steps together, we finally obtain the $k$th step of the KF algorithm:

$$\boldsymbol{X}_f^k = A_{k-1|k} \boldsymbol{X}_a^{k-1} \qquad \text{state prediction,} \tag{9.15a}$$

$$P_k^f = A_{k-1|k} P_{k-1}^a A_{k-1|k}^{\mathrm{T}} + Q_k \qquad \text{error covariance prediction,} \tag{9.15b}$$

$$K_k = P_f^k H_k^{\mathrm{T}} (H_k P_k^f H_k^{\mathrm{T}} + R_k)^{-1} \qquad \text{Kalman gain evaluation,} \tag{9.15c}$$

$$\boldsymbol{X}_a^k = \boldsymbol{X}_f^k + K_k(\boldsymbol{Z}^k - H_k \boldsymbol{X}_f^k) \qquad \text{state correction,} \tag{9.15d}$$

$$P_k^a = (I - K_k H_k) P_k^f \qquad \text{error covariance correction.} \tag{9.15e}$$

Note that from (9.15d) only, the estimated state from the above step and the current measurement are needed to compute the estimate of the current state. The two prediction and correction steps alternate: the prediction advances the state until the next measurement is acquired, and then the correction incorporates this measurement.

**Remark 9.2** The Kalman gain $K_k$ defined in (9.14) can also be expressed as $K_k = P_k^{X_f Z}(P_k^Z)^{-1}$. Here

$$P_k^{X_f Z} = \mathbb{E}[\boldsymbol{X}_f^k(\boldsymbol{Z}^k - H_k\boldsymbol{X}_f^k)^{\mathrm{T}}] = P_k^f H_k^{\mathrm{T}}$$

is the cross-covariance between $\boldsymbol{X}_f^k$ and the innovation $\boldsymbol{Z}^k - H_k\boldsymbol{X}_f^k$, and

$$P_k^Z = \mathbb{E}[(\boldsymbol{Z}^k - H_k\boldsymbol{X}_f^k)(\boldsymbol{Z}^k - H_k\boldsymbol{X}_f^k)^{\mathrm{T}}] = H_k P_k^f H_k + R_k$$

is the innovation covariance. Similarly, (9.15e) can be rewritten as $P_k^a = P_k^f - K_k P_k^Z K_k^{\mathrm{T}}$. This interpretation is useful when dealing with the unscented Kalman filter (see Section 9.2.3).

**Remark 9.3** In the linear case, the variational and the sequential approaches yield the same result at the end of a time window, provided the following assumptions are made: the same background estimation and the same covariance matrices are used, and the same measurements are acquired – that is, both algorithms are optimal from a least-squares or minimum variance standpoint.

Let us now return to our problem of estimating the parameter $\boldsymbol{\theta}$. We apply the KF algorithm to the system

$$\begin{aligned}
&\boldsymbol{X}^k = A_{k-1|k}\boldsymbol{X}^{k-1} + B_k\boldsymbol{\theta}^k + \boldsymbol{v}^k, \quad k = 1, \ldots, K, \quad \boldsymbol{X}^0 = \boldsymbol{G}, \\
&\boldsymbol{\theta}^k = \boldsymbol{\theta}^{k-1}
\end{aligned}$$

with observations

$$\boldsymbol{Z}^k = H_k\boldsymbol{X}^k + \boldsymbol{w}^k, \quad k = 1, \ldots, K.$$

Here $\boldsymbol{\theta}_k \in \mathbb{R}^p$ denotes the parameter vector and (under the linearity assumption) $B_k \in \mathbb{R}^{n_x \times p}$, and we assume that no random error is associated with model parameters. This is the so-called *state augmentation* technique. In order to exploit the KF algorithm, we consider $\widetilde{\boldsymbol{X}}^k = (\boldsymbol{X}^k, \boldsymbol{\theta}^k)^{\mathrm{T}}$ as state vector instead of $\boldsymbol{X}^k$, thus yielding the *augmented* KF algorithm

$$\begin{aligned}
\widetilde{\boldsymbol{X}}_f^k &= \widetilde{A}_{k-1|k}\widetilde{\boldsymbol{X}}_a^{k-1} && \text{state prediction,} && (9.16a)\\
\widetilde{P}_k^f &= \widetilde{A}_{k-1|k}\widetilde{P}_{k-1}^a\widetilde{A}_{k-1|k}^{\mathrm{T}} + \widetilde{Q}_k && \text{error covariance prediction,} && (9.16b)\\
K_k &= \widetilde{P}_f^k\widetilde{H}_k^{\mathrm{T}}(\widetilde{H}_k\widetilde{P}_k^f H_k^{\mathrm{T}} + \widetilde{R}_k)^{-1} && \text{Kalman gain evaluation,} && (9.16c)\\
\widetilde{\boldsymbol{X}}_a^k &= \widetilde{\boldsymbol{X}}_f^k + K_k(\widetilde{\boldsymbol{Z}}^k - \widetilde{H}_k\widetilde{\boldsymbol{X}}_f^k) && \text{state correction,} && (9.16d)\\
\widetilde{P}_k^a &= (I - K_k\widetilde{H}_k)\widetilde{P}_k^f && \text{error covariance correction,} && (9.16e)
\end{aligned}$$

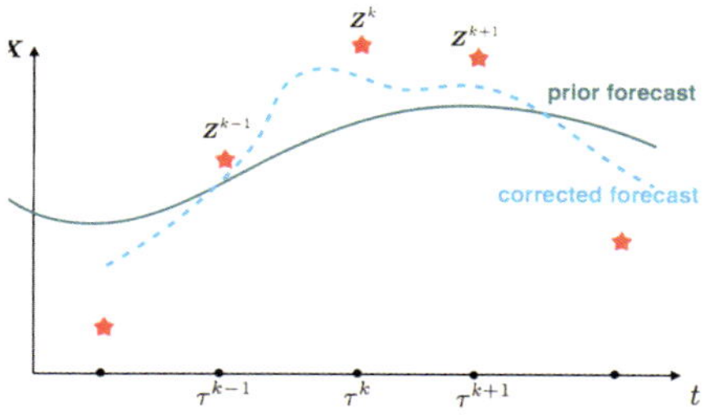


(a)

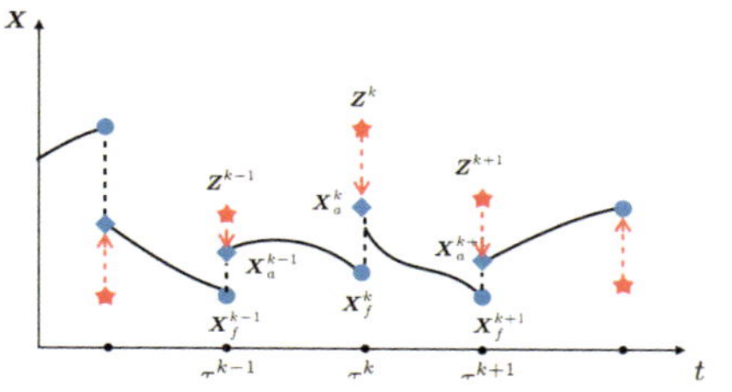


(b)

Figure 9.1 Variational approach (a) versus Kalman filter (b) approach: in the former, at each optimization stage the whole state dynamics has to be computed, whereas in the latter each measurement is sequentially used for the state (and parameter) correction.

where

$$\widetilde{A}_{k-1|k} = \begin{bmatrix} A_{k-1|k} & B_k \\ 0 & I \end{bmatrix}, \quad \widetilde{\boldsymbol{Z}}^k = \begin{bmatrix} \boldsymbol{Z}^k \\ 0 \end{bmatrix},$$

$$\widetilde{H}_k = \begin{bmatrix} H_k & 0 \\ 0 & 0 \end{bmatrix}, \quad \widetilde{Q}_k = \begin{bmatrix} Q_k \\ 0 \end{bmatrix}, \quad \widetilde{R}_k = \begin{bmatrix} R_k & 0 \\ 0 & 0 \end{bmatrix}.$$

We point out that, by construction of the filtering procedure, the estimated parameter values evolve along the simulation period and the actual estimation is achieved with the final values; that is, the estimated parameter vector is $\widehat{\boldsymbol{\theta}} = \boldsymbol{\theta}_a^K$. (Note that in the current formulation $\theta$ is independent of time.) Hence, we expect these estimation *trajectories* to fluctuate less and less during the course of the simulation (see *e.g.* Figure 10.3 in Section 10.3.2); the non-converging case would therefore denote the presence of persistent modelling errors.

We conclude this section by pointing out that when a sequential approach like the Kalman filter is used for parameter estimation, the dynamical system has to be solved only once, by updating the parameter value after each assimilation of new measurements. On the other hand, a variational approach would require us to solve the dynamical system on the whole time interval several times, assuming that an iterative approach is used to perform the optimization: see the sketch in Figure 9.1.

### 9.2.2 The extended Kalman filter

The classical Kalman filter formulation is well suited to low-dimensional, linear dynamical systems, although in real applications these assumptions are seldom verified. The extended Kalman filter (EKF) was introduced for non-linear dynamical systems, where (9.12) is replaced by

$$\boldsymbol{X}^k = \mathbf{f}(\boldsymbol{X}^{k-1}, \tau^k) + \boldsymbol{\varepsilon}^k, \quad \boldsymbol{Z}^k = \mathbf{h}(\boldsymbol{X}^k, \tau^k) + \boldsymbol{\eta}^k, \tag{9.17}$$

where $\mathbf{f}$ and $\mathbf{h}$ are two non-linear functions. Non-linearity here involves both the system dynamics and the observation model. The EKF consists in applying the KF algorithm (9.15) to a linearized version of (9.17) around the previous state, so that at each step we set

$$A_{k-1|k} = \left.\frac{\partial \mathbf{f}}{\partial \boldsymbol{X}}\right|_{\boldsymbol{X}_a^{k-1}, \boldsymbol{\theta}^k}, \qquad H_k = \left.\frac{\partial \mathbf{h}}{\partial \boldsymbol{X}}\right|_{\boldsymbol{X}_f^k}.$$

At each step two Jacobian matrices have to be evaluated at the current predicted state/parameters. A similar extension of the algorithm (9.16) provides the EKF for parameter estimation. Although feasible in principle, the EKF suffers from several drawbacks. For instance, it entails prohibitive computational costs to invert large matrices and to propagate the covariance matrix in time. Even more importantly, the EKF may lack stability, meaning that as the estimated state deviates from the true state, the linearized model becomes inaccurate, which may lead to an even larger error in state estimation. To mitigate these shortcomings, several strategies have been put in place: low-rank approximation of the covariance matrices have been considered, and other extensions of the original Kalman filter such as the UKF and EnKF have been introduced.

### *9.2.3 The unscented Kalman filter*

While the EKF exploits the differentiation of non-linear operators, modelling both the state dynamics and the observation process, to evaluate the propagation of means and covariances, the unscented Kalman filter (UKF), introduced by Julier, Uhlmann and Durrant-Whyte (1995), relies on a set of well-chosen deterministic points (or *sigma points*) whose propagation via the non-linear operators yields the empirical means and covariances required in the Kalman prediction-correction formulas. The rationale goes by the name of *unscented transformation*, whose goal is to map a set of points so that their sample distribution approximates the true distribution (Julier, Uhlmann and Durrant-Whyte 2000).

Supposing that we know the mean $\mathbb{E}[\boldsymbol{X}]$ and the covariance $\Sigma$ of a random vector $\boldsymbol{X} \in \mathbb{R}^{n_x}$, the simplest choice is to select $2n_x$ (symmetric) sigma points $x_{(i)}$ as

$$x_{(i)} = \mathbb{E}[\boldsymbol{X}] + \left(\sqrt{n_x \Sigma}\right)_i, \quad x_{(n_x+i)} = \mathbb{E}[\boldsymbol{X}] - \left(\sqrt{n_x \Sigma}\right)_i, \quad i = 1, \dots, n_x,$$

where $\left(\sqrt{n_x \Sigma}\right)_i$ is the $i$th column of the Cholesky factor of $n_x \Sigma$. Different options for the sigma points selection are however possible: see *e.g.* Julier and Uhlmann (2004).

The prediction-correction strategy of the Kalman filter is then performed. Referring to the same notation used in Section 9.2.1 and supposing that the current forecast based on $\boldsymbol{Z}^1, \dots, \boldsymbol{Z}^{k-1}$ is $\widehat{\boldsymbol{X}}_f^k$, with covariance matrix $P_k^f$, the following *correction step* is performed.

- From the estimated mean $\widehat{\boldsymbol{X}}_f^k$ and covariance $P_k^f$ at time $\tau^k$, select a set of $2n_x$ sigma points

$$x_{f,(i)}^k = \widehat{\boldsymbol{X}}_f^k + \left(\sqrt{n_x P_k^f}\right)_i, \quad x_{f,(n_x+i)}^k = \widehat{\boldsymbol{X}}_f^k - \left(\sqrt{n_x P_k^f}\right)_i, \quad i = 1, \dots, n_x,$$

  centred around $\widehat{\boldsymbol{X}}_f^k$ at a distance given by the standard deviation extracted from the covariance matrix, and obtain the predicted measurement

$$\widehat{\boldsymbol{Z}}^k = \frac{1}{2n_x} \sum_{i=1}^{2n_x} \widehat{\boldsymbol{Z}}_{(i)}^k, \quad \text{where } \widehat{\boldsymbol{Z}}_{(i)}^k = \mathbf{h}(x_{f,(i)}^k, \tau^k), \quad i = 1, \dots, 2n_x.$$

- Estimate the covariance of the predicted measurement,

$$P_k^Z = \frac{1}{2n_x} \sum_{i=1}^{2n_x} \left(\widehat{\boldsymbol{Z}}_{(i)}^k - \widehat{\boldsymbol{Z}}^k\right)\left(\widehat{\boldsymbol{Z}}_{(i)}^k - \widehat{\boldsymbol{Z}}^k\right)^{\mathrm{T}} + R_k,$$

  and the cross-covariance between $\boldsymbol{X}_f^k$ and $\widehat{\boldsymbol{Z}}^k$:

$$P_k^{X_f Z} = \frac{1}{2n_x} \sum_{i=1}^{2n_x} \left(\widehat{\boldsymbol{X}}_f^k - x_{f,(i)}^k\right)\left(\widehat{\boldsymbol{Z}}^k - \widehat{\boldsymbol{Z}}_{(i)}^k\right)^{\mathrm{T}}.$$

- Perform the Kalman gain evaluation, state correction and the error covariance correction similarly to (9.16c–9.16e) (recall Remark 9.2),

$$\begin{aligned} K_k &= P_k^{X_f Z} (P_k^Z)^{-1}, \\ \widehat{\boldsymbol{X}}_a^k &= \widehat{\boldsymbol{X}}_f^k + K_k(\boldsymbol{Z}^k - \widehat{\boldsymbol{Z}}^k), \\ P_k^a &= P_k^f - K_k P_k^Z K_k^{\mathrm{T}}. \end{aligned}$$

In the *prediction step*, a set of sigma points is selected as

$$x_{a,(i)}^k = \widehat{\boldsymbol{X}}_a^k + \left(\sqrt{n_x P_k^a}\right)_i, \quad x_{a,(n_x+i)}^k = \widehat{\boldsymbol{X}}_a^k - \left(\sqrt{n_x P_k^a}\right)_i, \quad i = 1, \dots, n_x$$

and a forward computation of one time window is performed to get the state prediction at step $k+1$:

$$\widehat{\boldsymbol{X}}_f^{k+1} = \frac{1}{2n_x}\sum_{i=1}^{2n_x} x_{f,(i)}^{k+1}, \quad \text{where } x_{f,(i)}^{k+1} = \mathbf{f}(x_{a,(i)}^k, \tau^{k+1})$$

(note that each sigma point is treated independently). Finally, the covariance is updated as

$$P_{k+1}^f = \frac{1}{2n_x}\sum_{i=1}^{2n_x}\big(\widehat{\boldsymbol{X}}_f^{k+1} - x_{f,(i+1)}^k\big)\big(\widehat{\boldsymbol{X}}_f^{k+1} - x_{f,(i+1)}^k\big)^{\mathrm{T}} + Q_{k+1}.$$

Provided the analysis step is performed in parallel, the cost of the whole estimation procedure is comparable to that of a simple forward simulation. By contrast, a variational estimation would require a significant number of successive iterations (typically, of the order of hundreds) of both forward and adjoint simulations.

An augmented formulation of the UKF can be easily obtained, similarly to (9.16), in order to treat the case where the system depends on a set of $p$ parameters affected by uncertainty, which need to be estimated. Nevertheless, the very large dimension of the state vector (depending on the spatial discretization of the state variable) makes this filter intractable in practice. In those cases where uncertainty only affects the parameters, and $p \ll n_x$, a much more feasible version yielding a reduced-order UKF limits the computations of the filter operator to a subspace of small dimension and is much more efficient. The reduction to the parametric space as regarding the choice of the sigma points for the sake of parameter estimation was originally introduced by Pham (2001) and Hoteit, Pham and Blum (2002); an initial application to the estimation of electrophysiology parameters can be found in Wang, Zhang, Wong and Shi (2009) and Wang *et al.* (2011). A detailed analysis of the reduced-order UKF can be found in Moireau and Chapelle (2011), for example. A possible alternative, recently explored by Pagani, Manzoni and Quarteroni (2017) and Pagani (2016), is to perform a *state reduction* (rather than a reduction of the parameter space) relying on a reduced-order model, and then consider the problem of simultaneous state/parameter estimation.

## 9.3 Applications to cardiovascular modelling

In the past decade, parameter identification problems have been considered in several applications to cardiovascular modelling. In this section we describe some relevant contributions; two substantive examples will be more specifically discussed in Sections 9.3.1 and 9.3.2.

The problem of identifying a set of parameters of one-dimensional models for the arterial circulation was first considered by Martin, Clément, Decoene and Gerbeau (2005), who considered a non-linear least-squares approach based on the optimization of a cost function and the introduction of a suitable adjoint problem. A relevant application in this context is the estimation of the elastic coefficient of a subject-specific vessel based on measurements of its displacement recovered from medical images. A *variational approach* based on the minimization of suitable functionals was proposed by Perego, Veneziani and Vergara (2011) and, more recently, by Bertagna and Veneziani (2014); we present this technique in Section 9.3.1. A different approach based on an unscented Kalman filter has been proposed by Bertoglio *et al.* (2012) and further explored by Moireau *et al.* (2013) to estimate modelling parameters pertaining to vessel wall boundary conditions. Similar strategies based on the unscented Kalman filter have been considered by Lombardi (2014), for example, to solve inverse problems in large one-dimensional arterial networks, and by Pant, Fabrèges, Gerbeau and Vignon-Clementel (2014) to estimate lumped (*e.g.* windkessel) model parameters by using the pressure curve in the ascending aorta.

Other approaches have been considered, for example in Blanco, Watanabe and Feijóo (2012), for characterizing the terminal peripheral resistances in a network describing one-dimensional arterial blood flow, or, in Spilker and Taylor (2010), for adjusting the parameters of windkessel outflow boundary conditions of three-dimensional blood flow models, in order to match some desired features of pressure and flow waveforms.

Several recent works have focussed on parameter identification and, more generally speaking, on the solution of inverse problems in heart modelling. The classical *inverse problem in electrocardiology* has been considered by many authors in recent decades. It consists in recovering the electrical potential at the epicardial surface by using a number of remote, non-invasive or minimally invasive potential recordings, such as those acquired along the body surface (Rudy and Messinger-Rapport 1988, Pullan *et al.* 2001, Cheng, Bodley and Pullan 2003), usually referred to as *body surface-potential data.* In its original formulation, this problem involves the pure (linear) diffusion model for the torso as a direct problem (Colli Franzone, Taccardi and Viganotti 1978, Colli Franzone, Guerri, Viganotti and Taccardi 1985, Yamashita 1982): see Section 6.1.5. This inverse problem is mathematically ill-posed, and several regularization strategies have been proposed; see *e.g.* the reviews by Pullan *et al.* (2010) and Colli Franzone *et al.* (2014). Another method for solving the inverse electrocardiology problem relies on measurements of the electrical potential within one of the heart chambers (ventricles and atria) by means of non-contact multi-electrode catheter arrays, and tries to estimate the endocardial surface potential from them. Since the measurements are recorded closer to the endocardial surface than those acquired on the body surface, this problem is less ill-conditioned than the former. If the problem is recast in the form of a parameter estimation problem, that is, where the epicardial potential distribution is described in terms of a set of parameters, the inverse problem can be more easily tackled.

More generally speaking, inverse and parameter estimation problems have been considered in several works in order to approximately reconstruct the cardiac electrical activity in the myocardium, for example, and to provide indications of the presence of ischaemic or infarcted zones by estimating conductibility parameters. Concerning *variational approaches*, we can mention a level-set framework for identifying heart infarctions (Lykaser and Nielsen 2006) by relying on a least-squares formulation and an adjoint problem to determine the gradient of the cost functional. In this case, the infarcted region in a simplified two-dimensional domain has been described in terms of a discrete level-set function, involving a set of parameters to be identified from synthetic ECG boundary measurements, and a Tikhonov regularization procedure. MacLachlan *et al.* (2006) and Nielsen *et al.* (2007*a*) considered the solution of a parameter identification problem to locate (in terms of size and position) ischaemic regions, where a simplified state elliptic system models the electrical potential in both the heart and the torso in the resting phase. In all these papers, the PDE-constrained optimization problem was solved using an iterative method, following an optimize-then-discretize approach. Nielsen, Lykaser and Tveito (2007*b*) instead considered an all-at-once approach for a similar problem, also taking into account anisotropic cardiac conductivities and fibre orientation. A more involved version of this problem, still focussing on the inverse electrocardiographic source localization of ischaemias, has been considered more recently by Wang, Kirby, MacLeod and Johnson (2013).

The personalization of an eikonal model, via the identification of local conduction velocities and parameters related to the action potential duration restitution curve, was addressed by Chinchapatnam *et al.* (2008) and Relan *et al.* (2011). More recently, Yang and Veneziani (2015) proposed a variational approach for the estimation of cardiac conductivities in a bidomain model, from measurements of the trans-membrane and extracellular potentials available at some locations in the tissue. Boulakia, Fernández, Gerbeau and Zemzemi (2008) have considered parameter estimation in a problem where the bidomain model for the heart is coupled with the Laplace equation for the passive conduction in the torso, in order to estimate the torso conductivity parameters.

The unscented Kalman filter was exploited by Wang *et al.* (2011) and by Marchesseau *et al.* (2013) and Talbot *et al.* (2015) to identify scar locations and their size from body surface-potential and MRI data, using a monodomain two-variable Aliev–Panfilov model. A reduced-order UKF was used by Corrado, Gerbeau and Moireau (2015) to estimate electrical parameters within a coupled electromechanical model, by taking advantage of observations from both electrocardiograms and myocardium displacements.

Another inverse problem in electrophysiology has been studied by Vergara *et al.* (2014) and Palamara *et al.* (2015). Measurements of the electrical activation time on the endocardium, acquired via NavX (see Section 5.2), were used to find the optimal Purkinje network configuration. For this problem, the parameters to be estimated are the coordinates of the network. In particular, starting from an initial network with a fractal shape, a functional accounting for the discrepancy between measured and computed activation times is minimized in order to find the patient-specific location of the Purkinje muscle junctions (see Section 4.3). This methodology has been successfully applied to real pathological scenarios: see Palamara *et al.* (2014).

Regarding cardiac biomechanics, Moireau, Chapelle and Le Tallec (2009) and Moireau and Chapelle (2011) addressed the estimation of contractility parameters using the unscented Kalman filter, where the degree of damage in cardiac tissues caused by an infarct is estimated using velocity measurements from tagged MRI; see also Moireau, Chapelle and Le Tallec (2008). A reduced-order UKF was used by Xi *et al.* (2011) to identify material parameters in a transversally isotropic mechanical model; further details concerning this application will be provided in Section 9.3.2. Subsequently, the same technique was exploited by Chabiniok *et al.* (2012) to estimate contractility values in a more complex cardiac model, where the tissue is described by combining an active constitutive law in the muscle fibre direction and a visco-hyperelastic material, using actual clinical data consisting of *in vivo* cine-MRI image sequences and pressure measurements.

Finally, for the coupled electromechanical problem, very few numerical results are now available. The personalization of a 3D electromechanical model has been tackled by variational approaches, for example by Sermesant *et al.* (2006), who estimated local ventricular myocardium contractility using MRI in an electromechanical model. Similarly, Delingette *et al.* (2012) estimated both the parameters of a Mitchell–Schaeffer model and cardiac contractilities from catheterized electrophysiology data and cine-MRI images, respectively. Marchesseau, Delingette, Sermesant and Ayache (2012) performed the calibration of mechanical parameters of a complete electromechanical model of the heart involving the eikonal model for electrophysiology and an isotropic Mooney–Rivlin material model for cardiac mechanics, relying on the unscented Kalman filter.

Although several works have made a big step forward, the solution of parameter estimation problems remains an open computational challenge if complex, coupled models and patient-specific data are taken into account. Further, when UKF and EnKF techniques are exploited – which exhibit natural parallelism to a high degree – the need to evaluate the state dynamics for several different scenarios (given by the elements of the ensemble, for example) makes the computational effort exorbitant. For this reason, simplified physical models have been considered in many contexts; on the other hand, reduced-order strategies, such as the reduced-order unscented Kalman filter, have recently been proposed as a possible way of overcoming the computational complexity arising from these problems. Dramatic progress is expected in this field in the next few years.

### 9.3.1 A variational approach for estimating the tissue compliance

In this section we illustrate a variational approach introduced by Perego *et al.* (2011) for estimating the Young's modulus $E$ of a cardiovascular tissue from displacement data. Indeed, this parameter – and, more generally speaking, the deformability of a soft tissue – is an important index for detecting diseases: low compliance may indicate atherosclerosis or hypertension in the case of an artery, or a marker of diastolic dysfunction in the case of the left ventricle wall. The basic steps are (i) to retrieve the vessel displacement $\boldsymbol{d}_{\text{meas}}$ by image registration procedures on time frames of the vessel of interest, and then (ii) to minimize the difference between $\boldsymbol{d}_{\text{meas}}$ and the displacement computed by solving the coupled 3D blood vessel problem, in order to estimate Young's modulus. Here the structure is assumed to be linearly elastic, and the only parameter to be estimated is $E$, which is generally a function of space (*e.g.* an atherosclerotic plaque has a different modulus to healthy tissue) but not of time.

The former step consists of data acquisition, image segmentation and reconstruction, and finally registration; see Perego *et al.* (2011) for further details. The latter, which we will address, is an example of an *inverse fluid–structure interaction* (IFSI) problem, and results in a constrained optimization problem, where the constraint is the FSI problem and the functional to be minimized is a measure of the mismatch between the data and the computed solution.

An initial formulation of the IFSI problem is obtained by assuming that the displacement data $\boldsymbol{d}_{\text{meas}}(\boldsymbol{x}, \tau_k)$ for $\boldsymbol{x} \in \Sigma^{\tau_k}$ retrieved from the image registration process are available within the interval $[0, T]$ in some instants denoted by $\tau^k$, $k = 1, \ldots, K$. Here $K$ is the number of instants when image registration is performed, $\Delta\tau$ is the time step between two measurements, driven by the sampling frequency of the image devices, and $\Sigma^{\tau_k}$ denotes the interface between the fluid and the structure domain. Following the formulation of problem (9.4), we consider the functional

$$\begin{aligned} \mathcal{J}_K(\boldsymbol{d}, E) = \frac{1}{2} \sum_{k=1}^{K} \int_{\Sigma^{\tau_k}} \left(\boldsymbol{d}_{\text{meas}}(\boldsymbol{x}, \tau^k) - \boldsymbol{d}(\boldsymbol{x}, \tau^k)\right)^2 \mathrm{d}\sigma \\ + \frac{\alpha_E}{2} \sum_{k=1}^{K} \int_{\Omega_s} \left(E(\boldsymbol{x}, \tau^k) - E_{\text{ref}}\right)^2 \mathrm{d}\boldsymbol{x}, \end{aligned} \tag{9.18}$$

where $\boldsymbol{d}(\boldsymbol{x}, \tau^k)$ denotes the solution of the FSI system (3.44) in the ALE formulation, at $t = \tau^k$ and the second term is a non-negative *Tikhonov* regularization term. Here $E_{\text{ref}}$ is a prior estimate (available from *ex vivo* specimens, for example), so that the regularization forces $E$ to be close to its reference value. Given an admissible set $\mathcal{E}_{\text{ad}}$ where we seek the parameter $E$, a possible formulation of the IFSI problem reads as follows. For $t > 0, \boldsymbol{x} \in \Omega_s$, find $E = E(\boldsymbol{x}, t) \in \mathcal{P}$ that minimizes (9.18) under the constraint (3.44). A possible choice for $\mathcal{P}$ is

$$\mathcal{P} = \{E : E \in L^\infty(\Omega_s),\, 0 < E_{\min} \leq E \leq E_{\max}, \quad \text{with } E_{\min}, E_{\max} \in \mathbb{R}\}. \tag{9.19}$$

Such a problem entails the solution of a time-dependent minimization problem, for which a classical KKT system can be obtained using the Lagrange multiplier method. In this setting the parameter $E$ plays the role of the control variable. However, this approach is rather involved, since the adjoint problem results in a final-value problem which would involve differentiation with respect to the deformable domain as well: the so-called *shape derivative*. Moreover, it requires a massive memory occupancy as the solution at all the time steps needs to be stored due to the back-in-time nature of the adjoint problem.

A more convenient alternative numerical approach proposed by Perego *et al.* (2011) first considers the time-discretization of the forward problem, and formulates a minimization problem at each time step. For simplicity a constant time step $\Delta t = \Delta\tau/m$ is assumed, for a suitable $m \in \mathbb{N}$, $m \geq 1$, that is, the instants $\tau^k$ in which measurements are acquired are a subset of the time discretization of (3.44); for simplicity, we will consider $m = 1$. For the time discretization of (3.44), we consider implicit methods with a semi-implicit treatment of the convective term and of the fluid domain, whereas the fluid viscous term is treated implicitly. As in Section 3.6.1, we use the superscript $*$ to identify fluid quantities extrapolated from corresponding quantities at previous time steps. Moreover, we introduce the spaces

$$\boldsymbol{V}^* = \{\boldsymbol{v} \in \boldsymbol{H}^1(\Omega_f^*) : \boldsymbol{v}|_{\Gamma_{D,f}^*} = \boldsymbol{0}\}, \quad Q^* = L^2(\Omega_f^*),$$
$$\boldsymbol{W} = \{\boldsymbol{\psi} \in \boldsymbol{H}^1(\Omega_s) : \boldsymbol{\psi}_{\Gamma_{D,s}} = \boldsymbol{0}\},$$

where $\Gamma_{D,f}^*$ and $\Gamma_{D,s}$ are the portions of the boundary where a Dirichlet condition is prescribed. Further, we let

$$\boldsymbol{Z}^* = \{(\boldsymbol{v}, \boldsymbol{\psi}) \in \boldsymbol{V}^* \times \boldsymbol{W} : \boldsymbol{v}|_{\Sigma^*} - \widehat{\boldsymbol{\psi}}|_{\Sigma^*}/\Delta t = \boldsymbol{0}\},$$

and introduce the following bilinear forms:

$$\begin{aligned} a(\boldsymbol{v}, \boldsymbol{d}; \boldsymbol{w}, \boldsymbol{\psi})^* &= \frac{\rho_f}{\Delta t}(\boldsymbol{v}, \boldsymbol{w})_f^* + (\boldsymbol{T}_f(\boldsymbol{v}, p), \nabla \boldsymbol{w})_f^* \\ &\quad + \rho_f(((\boldsymbol{v}^* - \boldsymbol{v}_f^*) \cdot \nabla)\boldsymbol{v}, \boldsymbol{w})_f^* + \rho_s\left(\frac{\boldsymbol{d}}{\Delta t^2}, \frac{\boldsymbol{\psi}}{\Delta t}\right)_s, \\ b(q; \boldsymbol{w})^* &= -(q, \nabla \cdot \boldsymbol{w})_f^*, \end{aligned}$$

where

$$(\boldsymbol{v}, \boldsymbol{w})_f^* = \int_{\Omega_f^*} \boldsymbol{v} \cdot \boldsymbol{w} \, \mathrm{d}\boldsymbol{x} \quad \text{and} \quad (\boldsymbol{\psi}, \boldsymbol{\chi})_s = \int_{\Omega_s} \boldsymbol{\psi} \cdot \boldsymbol{\chi} \, \mathrm{d}\boldsymbol{x}.$$

Then, for any given $E \in \mathcal{E}_{\mathrm{ad}}$, at each time $t^{n+1}$, the time-discretized forward FSI problem consists of the following steps.

(1) Compute extrapolations $\Omega_f^*$, $\boldsymbol{v}^*$ and $\boldsymbol{v}_f^*$ to approximate $\Omega_f^{n+1}$, $\boldsymbol{v}^{n+1}$ and $\boldsymbol{v}_f^{n+1}$.

(2) Given $\boldsymbol{f}_f^{n+1} \in \boldsymbol{L}^2(\Omega_f^*)$ and $\boldsymbol{f}_s^{n+1} \in \boldsymbol{L}^2(\Omega_s)$, find $(\boldsymbol{v}^{n+1}, \boldsymbol{d}^{n+1}) \in \boldsymbol{Z}^*$ and $p^{n+1} \in Q^*$ such that

$$\begin{aligned} & a(\boldsymbol{v}^{n+1}, \boldsymbol{d}^{n+1}; \boldsymbol{w}, \boldsymbol{\psi})^* + \left(E\, \boldsymbol{S}_s(\boldsymbol{d}^{n+1}), \frac{1}{\Delta t}\nabla \boldsymbol{\psi}\right)_s + b(p^{n+1}; \boldsymbol{v})^* \\ & \quad = F_f^{n+1}(\boldsymbol{w}) + F_s^{n+1}\left(\frac{\boldsymbol{\psi}}{\Delta t}\right) - a(\boldsymbol{R}_f^{n+1}, \boldsymbol{0}; \boldsymbol{w}, \boldsymbol{\psi})^* \quad \text{for all } (\boldsymbol{w}, \boldsymbol{\psi}) \in \boldsymbol{Z}^* \\ & b(q; \boldsymbol{v}^{n+1})^* = 0 \quad \text{for all } q \in Q^*. \end{aligned} \tag{9.20}$$

(3) Update the fluid domain to obtain $\Omega_f^{n+1}$.

We used the notation

$$\boldsymbol{S}_s(\boldsymbol{d}) = \frac{1}{2(1+\nu)}(\nabla\boldsymbol{d} + (\nabla\boldsymbol{d})^{\mathrm{T}}) + \frac{\nu}{(1+\nu)(1-2\nu)}(\nabla\cdot\boldsymbol{d})\boldsymbol{I}$$

so that we can write $\boldsymbol{T}_s = E\,\boldsymbol{S}_s$. Moreover, given $\boldsymbol{g} \in \boldsymbol{H}^{1/2}(\Sigma^*)$, we let

$$\boldsymbol{R}_f(\boldsymbol{g}) \in \boldsymbol{H}^{\mathrm{div}}(\Omega_f^*) = \{\boldsymbol{v} \in \boldsymbol{H}^1(\Omega_f^*) : \nabla\cdot\boldsymbol{v} = 0\} \quad \text{and} \quad \boldsymbol{R}_s(\boldsymbol{g}) \in \boldsymbol{H}^1(\Omega_s)$$

denote two lifting functions for the fluid–structure interface continuity, given by

$$\boldsymbol{R}_f(\boldsymbol{g}) - \boldsymbol{R}_s(\boldsymbol{g}) = -\boldsymbol{g}/\Delta t \quad \text{on } \Sigma^*.$$

Due to the arbitrariness of one of these functions, in what follows we set $\boldsymbol{R}_s(\boldsymbol{g}) = \boldsymbol{0}$. Moreover, when applied to function $\boldsymbol{d}^{n-1}$, it is possible to set $\boldsymbol{R}_f^n = \boldsymbol{R}_f(\boldsymbol{d}^{n-1})$. Finally, the functionals $F_f^{n+1}$ and $F_s^{n+1}$ in (9.20) account for forcing terms, boundary data on $\partial\Omega_f^* \setminus \Sigma^*$ and $\partial\Omega_s \setminus \Sigma$ and terms coming from the time discretization at previous time steps.

Regarding the parameter estimation problem, once the problem has been discretized in time, the minimization of the cost functional

$$\widetilde{\mathcal{J}}_k(\boldsymbol{d}, E) = \int_\Sigma (\boldsymbol{d}_{\mathrm{meas}}(\boldsymbol{x}, \tau^k) - \boldsymbol{d}(\boldsymbol{x}, \tau^k))^2\, \mathrm{d}\sigma + \frac{\alpha_E}{2}\int_{\Omega_s}(E(\boldsymbol{x}, \tau^k) - E_{\mathrm{ref}})^2\, \mathrm{d}\boldsymbol{x}$$

for each $k = 1, 2, \ldots, K$, was considered by Perego *et al.* (2011), under the constraint (9.20). Hence, a system of KKT conditions can be derived relying on the standard Lagrange multiplier approach (see Section 8.1.2). With this aim we introduce the Lagrangian functional at time $\tau^k$:

$$\begin{aligned}\mathcal{L}(\boldsymbol{v}, p, \boldsymbol{d}; \boldsymbol{\lambda}_v, \lambda_p, \boldsymbol{\lambda}_d; E) &= \widetilde{\mathcal{J}}_k(\boldsymbol{d}, E) + a(\boldsymbol{v}, \boldsymbol{d}; \boldsymbol{\lambda}_v, \boldsymbol{\lambda}_d)^* + \left(E\,\boldsymbol{S}_s(\boldsymbol{d}), \frac{1}{\Delta t}\nabla\boldsymbol{\lambda}_d\right)_s \\ &+ b(p; \boldsymbol{\lambda}_v)^* + b(\lambda_p; \boldsymbol{v})^* - F_f(\boldsymbol{\lambda}_v) - F_s\left(\frac{\boldsymbol{\lambda}_d}{\Delta t}\right) + a(\boldsymbol{R}_f, \boldsymbol{0}; \boldsymbol{\lambda}_v, \boldsymbol{\lambda}_d)^*.\end{aligned}$$

The dependence on the superscript $k$ is omitted. By the requirement that the gradient of $\mathcal{L}$ vanishes, we obtain the following.

- The *adjoint problem*, by forcing to zero the (Gâteaux) derivatives of the Lagrangian functional with respect to $(\boldsymbol{v}, p, \boldsymbol{d})$, which in fact is a time-discretized FSI problem (see below for the interface condition). Find

$(\boldsymbol{\lambda}_v, \boldsymbol{\lambda}_d) \in \boldsymbol{Z}^*$, $\lambda_p \in Q^*$ such that

$$a(\boldsymbol{v}, \boldsymbol{\psi}; \boldsymbol{\lambda}_v, \boldsymbol{\lambda}_d)^* + \left( E\,\boldsymbol{S}_s\left(\frac{\boldsymbol{\psi}}{\Delta t}\right), \nabla \boldsymbol{\lambda}_d \right)_s + b(\lambda_p; \boldsymbol{w})^*$$
$$+ \int_\Sigma (\boldsymbol{d} - \boldsymbol{d}_{\text{meas}}) \cdot \boldsymbol{\psi} \, \mathrm{d}\sigma = 0,$$
$$b(q; \boldsymbol{\lambda}_v)^* = 0 \quad \text{for all } (\boldsymbol{w}, \boldsymbol{\psi}) \in \boldsymbol{Z}^*, q \in Q^*. \tag{9.21}$$

- The *optimality condition*

$$(\varphi\, \boldsymbol{S}_s(\boldsymbol{d}), \nabla \boldsymbol{\lambda}_d)_s = 0 \quad \text{for all } \varphi \in L^\infty(\Omega_s),$$

  by forcing to zero the derivative with respect to $E$.
- We also require the following state problem. Find $(\boldsymbol{v}, \boldsymbol{d}) \in \boldsymbol{Z}^*$, $p \in Q^*$ such that

$$a(\boldsymbol{v}, \boldsymbol{d}; \boldsymbol{w}, \boldsymbol{\psi})^* + \left( E\,\boldsymbol{S}_s(\boldsymbol{d}), \frac{1}{\Delta t} \nabla \boldsymbol{\psi} \right)_s + b(p; \boldsymbol{w})^*$$
$$= F_f(\boldsymbol{w}) + F_s\left(\frac{\boldsymbol{\psi}}{\Delta t}\right) - a(\boldsymbol{R}_f, \boldsymbol{0}; \boldsymbol{w}, \boldsymbol{\psi})^*$$
$$b(q; \boldsymbol{v})^* = 0 \quad \text{for all } (\boldsymbol{w}, \boldsymbol{\psi}) \in \boldsymbol{Z}^*, q \in Q^*,$$

  formally obtained by deriving the Lagrangian with respect to $(\boldsymbol{\lambda}_v, \lambda_p, \boldsymbol{\lambda}_d)$.

The adjoint problem, the optimality condition and the state problem yield the system of KKT conditions at each $\tau^k$, which couples two linearized FSI problems and a scalar equation.

In particular, for the adjoint problem the interface velocity condition reads

$$\boldsymbol{\lambda}_v = \frac{\boldsymbol{\lambda}_d}{\Delta t} \quad \text{on } \Sigma^*,$$

whereas the interface stress condition is

$$\boldsymbol{T}_s(\boldsymbol{\lambda}_d)\,\boldsymbol{n} - \boldsymbol{T}_f(\boldsymbol{\lambda}_v, \lambda_p)\,\boldsymbol{n} = -(\boldsymbol{d} - \boldsymbol{d}_{\text{meas}}) \quad \text{on } \Sigma^*, \tag{9.22}$$

taking into account the mismatch between the data and the solution, and modifying the homogeneous interface stress condition (3.19d) accordingly.

The same strategies described in Section 8.2 (*e.g.* gradient-based methods) can be exploited to solve the KKT system numerically. To take into account the constraint $E > 0$ in the case at hand, it is possible to transform the parameter as $\psi = \log(E)$, so that $E = \exp(\psi) > 0$ for every $\psi \in L^\infty(\Omega_s)$, and then optimize with respect to $\psi$. Finally, a finite element discretization in space is required to solve the state and the adjoint problem numerically.

By construction, this approach provides an estimate for $E$ at each time;

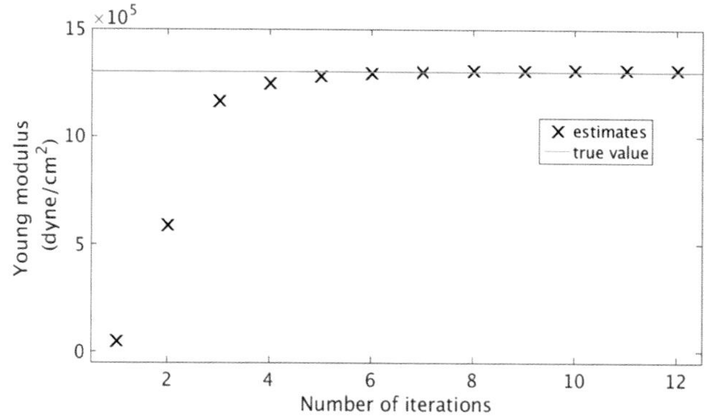


Figure 9.2 Convergence history for the estimation of Young's modulus by means of the algorithm proposed by Perego *et al.* (2011). Rectangular fluid and structure domains are used, with synthetic measurements generated by means of forward FSI simulations. Numerical results were obtained using the MATLAB finite element library MLife.

a possible option is then to average them to obtain a unique estimate, although this may suffer from instabilities in the presence of highly noisy data. A more robust approach is to solve the minimization problem over time. In this case, however, the complexity of the problem would increase, due to the inclusion of the shape derivatives in the minimization problem. In Figure 9.2 we show the number of iterations and the convergence history for the algorithm described above for the estimation of Young's modulus.

### 9.3.2 A Kalman filter approach for estimating material parameters in cardiac mechanics

In this section we illustrate a Kalman filter approach introduced by Xi *et al.* (2011) for estimating material parameters occurring in the mechanical model describing myocardial contractility. Only passive mechanics is modelled, making a quasi-static assumption, and without taking into account the electromechanical coupling. A transversely isotropic Guccione's constitutive law (Guccione *et al.* 1991) is used, and four parameters are estimated *in silico* from noisy displacement measurements of material points located on the myocardial surface. In principle, a similar approach can also be used, for example, to identify the material parameters affecting the orthotropic model (6.24).

The transversely isotropic strain energy function in the Guccione law can be expressed as

$$\Theta(\boldsymbol{E}) = \frac{1}{2}\theta_1(\mathrm{e}^{Q} - 1),$$

where

$$Q = \theta_2 E_{ff}^2 + \theta_3(E_{ss}^2 + E_{nn}^2 + 2E_{sn}^2) + \theta_4(2E_{fs}^2 + 2E_{fn}^2).$$

Here $\boldsymbol{\theta} = (\theta_1, \ldots, \theta_4) \in \mathbb{R}^p$ denotes a vector of $p = 4$ material parameters, and $E_{ij}$ is the $(i,j)$th component of the Green–Lagrange strain tensor $\boldsymbol{E} = \frac{1}{2}(\boldsymbol{F}^{\mathrm{T}}\boldsymbol{F} - I) = \frac{1}{2}(\boldsymbol{C} - I)$, with $i, j \in \{f, s, n\}$ denoting fibre, sheet and sheet-normal directions, respectively. After performing spatial discretization, at each time step the augmented state $\widetilde{\boldsymbol{X}}^k = (\boldsymbol{X}^k, \boldsymbol{\theta}^k)^{\mathrm{T}} \in \mathbb{R}^{n_x+p}$, made up of the deformed configuration $\boldsymbol{X}^k$ and the material parameter vector $\boldsymbol{\theta}^k$, has to be determined by solving a non-linear problem of the form

$$\widetilde{\boldsymbol{X}}^k = \mathbf{f}(\widetilde{\boldsymbol{X}}^{k-1}, \boldsymbol{u}^{k-1}) + \boldsymbol{\varepsilon}^k, \quad \mathbf{f}(\widetilde{\boldsymbol{X}}^{k-1}, \boldsymbol{u}^{k-1}) = \begin{bmatrix} G(\boldsymbol{\theta}^{k-1}, \boldsymbol{u}^{k-1}) \\ \boldsymbol{\theta}^{k-1} \end{bmatrix},$$

where the input vector $\boldsymbol{u}^{k-1}$ at time $k-1$ is given by the external forces, with observations

$$\boldsymbol{Z}^k = \boldsymbol{h}(\widetilde{\boldsymbol{X}}^k + \boldsymbol{w}^k), \quad k = 1, \ldots, K.$$

Xi *et al.* (2011) take $\boldsymbol{h} : \mathbb{R}^{n_x+p} \to \mathbb{R}^{n_z}$ to be a linear (interpolation) matrix $H \in \mathbb{R}^{(n_x+p)\times n_z}$, mapping the augmented state vector to the coordinates of the points where measurements are acquired. These measurements are assumed to be contaminated by a noise term $\boldsymbol{w}^k$ with zero mean and covariance $R_k$; note that the material parameter has no explicit time dependence. Nevertheless, as already pointed out, the filter will provide recursively updated estimates of $\boldsymbol{\theta}^k$. The goal is thus to compute the estimate $\boldsymbol{\theta}^K$ at the final time $t = t^K$.

Moreover, since the augmented state vector $\widetilde{\boldsymbol{X}}^k$ does not depend on the deformed configuration $\widetilde{\boldsymbol{X}}^{k-1}$, the rank of the error covariance matrix $\widetilde{P}_k$ at each step will be equal to $p$. This is a crucial point in order to devise a reduced-order UKF, making it possible to (i) store a covariance matrix of dimension $(n_x + p) \times p$, (ii) perform inversion of $p \times p$ matrices and, even more importantly, (iii) decrease the number of model evaluations required by the filter at each time step from $O(n_x + p)$ to $O(p)$.

Slight differences arise with respect to the UKF formulation addressed in Section 9.2.3, due to the reduction of the estimation process to the subset of $\widetilde{\boldsymbol{X}}^k$ corresponding to the $p$ parameter components. The filtering algorithm consists of three steps.

- *Initialization.* A singular value decomposition $P_0^a = L_0^a \Lambda_0^a (L_0^a)^{\mathrm{T}}$ of the initial error covariance $P_0^a \in \mathbb{R}^{(n_x+p)\times(n_x+p)}$ is performed. For instance, $P_0^a$ can be given by a diagonal matrix with $p$ non-zero entries representing the variances of the initial (or background) parameter estimates. Letting $L_{0,p}^a$ be the matrix whose columns are the first $p$ singular vectors of $L_0^a$ and $\Lambda_{0,p}^a$, the $p \times p$ diagonal matrix of the singular values, the reduced-rank square-root approximation $S_0^a \in \mathbb{R}^{(n_x+p)\times p}$ can be obtained as

$$S_0^a = L_{0,p}^a \sqrt{\Lambda_{0,p}^a}.$$

- *Prediction* (*or time update*). At each step $k = 1, \ldots,$ starting from the assimilated state $\widehat{\boldsymbol{X}}_a^{k-1}$ at step $k-1$, a set of sigma points is selected as

$$\widetilde{x}_{a,(i)}^{k-1} = \widehat{\boldsymbol{X}}_a^{k-1} + (S_{k-1}^a)_i, \quad \widetilde{x}_{a,(p+i)}^{k-1} = \widehat{\boldsymbol{X}}_a^{k-1} - (S_{k-1}^a)_i, \quad i = 1, \ldots, p.$$

The sigma points are then transformed via the state dynamics to obtain

$$\widetilde{x}_{f,(i)}^{k} = \mathbf{f}\big(\widetilde{x}_{a,(i)}^{k-1}, \boldsymbol{u}^{k-1}\big), \quad i = 1, \ldots, 2p,$$

and the mean $\widehat{\boldsymbol{X}}_f^k$ and the error covariance $P_k^f$ are estimated as

$$\widehat{\boldsymbol{X}}_f^k = \sum_{i=1}^{2p} \widetilde{x}_{f,(i)}^k, \quad P_k^f = \sum_{i=1}^{2p} (\widehat{\boldsymbol{X}}_f^k - \widetilde{x}_{f,(i)}^k)(\widehat{\boldsymbol{X}}_f^k - \widetilde{x}_{f,(i)}^k)^{\mathrm{T}}.$$

To preserve the low-rank structure of the correlation matrix $P_k^f$, a singular value decomposition $P_k^f = L_k^f \Lambda_0^f (L_k^f)^{\mathrm{T}}$ is performed, thus yielding

$$P_k^f = S_k^f (S_k^f)^{\mathrm{T}}, \quad S_k^f = L_{k,p}^f \sqrt{\Lambda_{k,p}^f}.$$

- *Correction* (*or measurement update*). At each step $k = 1, \ldots,$ the observation $\boldsymbol{Z}^k$ is assimilated into the forecast $\widehat{X}_f^k$ yielding the corrected state

$$\widehat{\boldsymbol{X}}_a^k = \widehat{\boldsymbol{X}}_f^k + K_k(\boldsymbol{Z}^k - H\widehat{\boldsymbol{X}}_f^k).$$

In this case the Kalman gain can be shown to be

$$K_k = S_k^f (I + (HS_k^f)^{\mathrm{T}} R_k^{-1} H S_k^f)^{-1} (HS_k^f)^{\mathrm{T}} R_k^{-1}$$

along with the square-root of the error covariance, given by

$$S_k^a = S_k^f (I + (HS_k^f)^{\mathrm{T}} R_k^{-1} H S_k^f)^{-1/2}.$$

Note that here, compared to the UKF formulation of Section 9.2.3, update formulas for the Kalman gain and the error covariance are directly obtained for the square-root of the covariance matrix. For further details see Simon (2006) or Xi *et al.* (2011).

Xi *et al.* (2011) show that such a reduced-order UKF is able to estimate $p = 4$ (and subsequently $p = 12$) material parameters, starting from a set of synthetic measurements generated by adding Gaussian noise to a set of noise-free measurements, obtained via model simulation for a chosen ground truth parameter vector. Myocardial dilatation is considered by loading the structure with a given ventricular pressure on the endocardium, and $n_z = 600$ material points located on the epicardium and endocardium.

We have chosen to describe this example to illustrate how to take advantage of a Kalman filter strategy in a *relatively* simple cardiovascular application; further details and more involved cases can be found in Moireau and Chapelle (2011), Bertoglio *et al.* (2012), Chabiniok *et al.* (2012), Moireau *et al.* (2013) and Corrado *et al.* (2015), for example. Numerical results related to parameter identification in electrophysiology by means of an ensemble Kalman filter – a technique that indeed shares several similarities with the UKF – will be shown in Section 10.2.2.

# 10
# Accounting for uncertainty

Moving towards model personalization – that is, the adaptation of model inputs to subject-specific conditions – the question immediately arises as to the sensitivity of model predictions to errors and uncertainties in the model inputs. The inputs to be personalized may include the computational domain (*e.g.* vascular networks), physical parameters (*e.g.* vascular material properties) and boundary conditions. Because of noise in input measurements, as well as their large biological variability, model inputs are inevitably hampered by uncertainty. Furthermore, as already seen in Section 9, not all model inputs are directly measurable, as in the case of the local mechanical properties of the arterial wall, thus calling into play the need to solve parameter estimation problems. The uncertainties carried by patient-specific features should then be incorporated into the computational model, to quantify their impact on the computed results and to obtain more reliable predictions or best/worst-case scenarios (Eck *et al.* 2016). These are the main reasons behind the very rapid growth of applications of sensitivity analysis and uncertainty quantification (UQ) to cardiovascular problems in the past decade. Since UQ is a very active field (and less mature than PDE-constrained optimization or parameter estimation) from both a mathematical and computational viewpoint, in this chapter we only touch on some basic, yet relevant, issues related to UQ techniques; see *e.g.* Sullivan (2015), Kaipio and Somersalo (2005) and Le Maître and Knio (2010) for a more in-depth overview of numerical aspects of UQ.

Typically, UQ problems involve a mathematical model for a process of interest, subject to some uncertainty about the correct form of this model or, more frequently, about some of its parameters. Although exhibiting substantial overlap with the field of parameter estimation and data assimilation, UQ problems also involve the propagation of uncertainty on outputs of interest, reliability or certification problems, prediction problems and, very often, consist of several of these aspects coupled together. For instance, after estimating some model parameters, we may use them to forward-propagate other uncertainties. Often, though not always, uncertainties are treated probabilistically, thus calling into play probabilistic and statistical methods. Here we focus on basic aspects related to *forward propagation* and *backward propagation* of uncertainty, for the latter case focussing on statistical inversion methods within a Bayesian framework.

## 10.1 Forward uncertainty quantification

The goal of forward UQ is to derive information about the uncertainties in system outputs of interest, given information about the uncertainties in the system inputs. The goal is to obtain the probability density function (PDF) of some output of interest $\boldsymbol{Z} = \boldsymbol{f}(\boldsymbol{\theta}) \in \mathbb{R}^{n_z}$ given the probability distribution of the input $\boldsymbol{\theta} \in \mathbb{R}^p$, or evaluate moments (*e.g.* the expected value and the variance), correlation functions, confidence regions or quantiles.[1] Here $\boldsymbol{f} : \mathbb{R}^p \to \mathbb{R}^{n_z}$ denotes an input/output map. For instance, Sankaran and Marsden (2011) take the radius of an abdominal aortic aneurysm, the radii and the inflow velocity of the carotid artery bifurcation, and the flow split of the left and right pulmonary arteries as random variables to account for the uncertainty impact on blood flows modelled by three-dimensional Navier–Stokes equations with rigid arterial walls, by considering as outputs blood velocity and wall shear stresses.

Once a probabilistic description of the random inputs has been provided, a suitable strategy is needed to propagate uncertainties through the model. The simplest case is one where the PDE system depends on a set of random inputs that are constant with respect to space and time. In this case, they can be described by means of a finite-dimensional random vector, with a given probability distribution. A more involved case is one where input data may vary randomly from one point of the physical domain to another (and possibly from one time instant to another); in this case, they are described in terms of random fields. Two popular strategies for describing correlated random fields include Karhunen–Loève expansions, and expansions in terms of global orthogonal polynomials (Ghanem and Spanos 2003, Xiu and Karniadakis 2002*b*). Made up of infinitely many terms, these expansions are usually truncated to approximate random fields: the milder the varia-

[1] Sensitivity analysis (see *e.g.* Saltelli *et al.* 2008 for a detailed review) may be seen as a precursor of forward UQ, sharing the need to provide a quantitative description of the dependence of the solution of a model on input parameters. See Donders, Huberts, van de Vosse and Delhaas (2015) for the application of sensitivity analysis to a pulse wave propagation model of arterial flows.

tions in space and time of the random field realizations, the fewer the terms retained in the expansion.

Several approaches are available for solving PDE problems with random input data. Monte Carlo (MC) methods are the most popular. These are based on independent realizations $\boldsymbol{\theta}_1, \ldots, \boldsymbol{\theta}_M$ of the random variable $\boldsymbol{\theta}$ (whose probability distribution is denoted by $\mu$) yielding approximations of the expectation by averaging over the corresponding realizations of that quantity; that is,

$$\mathbb{E}[\boldsymbol{f}(\boldsymbol{\theta})] = \int_{\mathbb{R}^p} f(\boldsymbol{\theta})\mu(\mathrm{d}\boldsymbol{\theta}) \approx \frac{1}{M}\sum_{i=1}^{M} \boldsymbol{f}(\boldsymbol{\theta}_i), \tag{10.1}$$

where the sample $\boldsymbol{\theta}_1, \ldots, \boldsymbol{\theta}_M$ is generated randomly from the probability distribution of $\boldsymbol{\theta}$. Such a method requires a deterministic PDE query for each realization and a very large number of queries to achieve a small error, this latter being proportional to $1/\sqrt{M}$. This entails an excessive computational burden, especially for systems which are already computationally expensive in their deterministic setting. See, for example, Fishman (1996), Robert and Casella (2004) and Voss (2013) for more on Monte Carlo methods, and Dick, Kuo and Sloan (2013) and Giles (2015) for quasi-Monte Carlo and multilevel Monte Carlo methods, respectively.

When the solution depends analytically on the random input parameters, other approaches exhibit much faster convergence rates. These include spectral (global) stochastic Galerkin (SG) methods (Ghanem and Spanos 2003, Xiu and Karniadakis 2002*a*, Babuška, Tempone and Zouraris 2004) and stochastic collocation (SC) methods (Babuška, Nobile and Tempone 2007, Xiu and Hesthaven 2005, Nobile, Tempone and Webster 2008); for a mathematical and numerical discussion, see the detailed review by Gunzburger, Webster and Zhang (2014) and the recent books by Le Maître and Knio (2010) and Sullivan (2015). These methods are based on the discretization of a PDE system, not only with respect to spatial variables but also with respect to the random inputs. Stochastic Galerkin methods are intrusive approaches since the physical and the probabilistic variables are coupled; stochastic sampling (SS) and interpolatory-type stochastic collocation methods are instead non-intrusive. Furthermore, stochastic Galerkin methods require the solution of discrete systems that couple all spatial and probabilistic variables, whereas stochastic collocation methods can combine standard approximations in physical space with globally defined polynomial approximation in the probability domain, either by full polynomial spaces, tensor product polynomial spaces or sparse tensor product polynomials. The

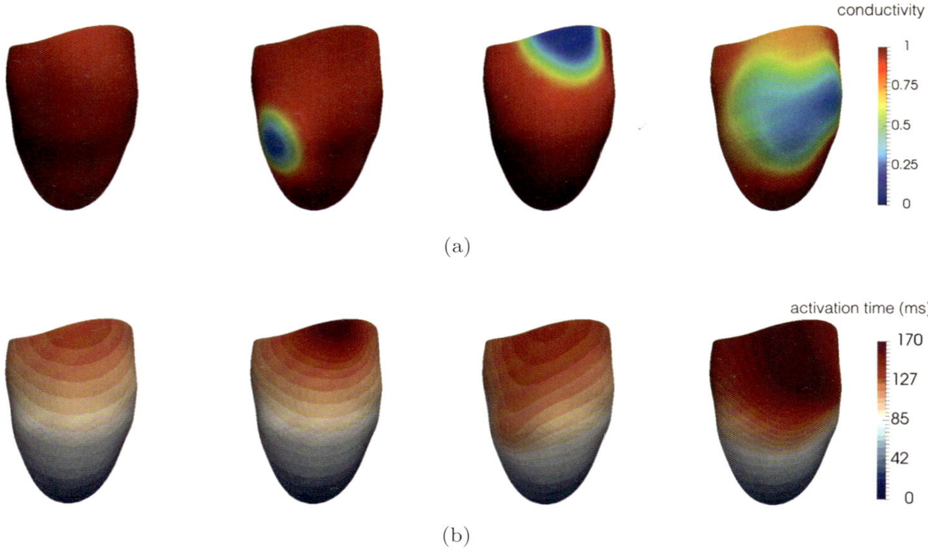


Figure 10.1 Different degrees of tissue damage in terms of relative conductivity (a) and activation times in milliseconds (b) for a healthy case (left) and different ischaemic regions on the myocardium. The patient-specific geometry of the left ventricle has been reconstructed using the semi-automatic segmentation method proposed by Fedele *et al.* (2015). Numerical results were obtained using the finite element library redbKIT v2.1 (github.com/redbKIT/redbKIT/releases).

stochastic space can then be queried at any point in order to construct the PDF of the output, the interpolation in the stochastic space being built on top, and independently, of the PDE solver.

By way of illustration, Figure 10.1 gives the activation times obtained using the monodomain model coupled with the Aliev–Panfilov cell model. This computation is carried out on a patient-specific left ventricle geometry, obtained by considering different levels of tissue damage (or ischaemia), caused by an insufficient blood perfusion of the myocardium. In this case, each component of the conductivity $\mathbf{\Sigma}$ is multiplied by a spatial field $\sigma(\boldsymbol{x};\boldsymbol{\theta})$ ranging from 0 (lack of conductivity, damaged tissue) to 1 (regular conductivity, healthy tissue), which we refer to as relative conductivity; as soon as the position and size of the ischaemia are unknown, $\sigma$ is a random field, depending on (a finite number $p$ of) random inputs $\theta_1,\ldots,\theta_p$. We emphasize that in this case input uncertainty yields significant variability in the output, thus making uncertainty propagation a problem of interest in this context.

## 10.2 Inverse uncertainty quantification

Inverse UQ (or backward uncertainty propagation) problems refer to those situations in which input quantities are inferred starting from observed system outputs. Variational or sequential methods described in Sections 9.1 and 9.2 provide point estimates of the quantities of interest, given a set of observations. The *statistical inversion* approach provides a well-established framework for better characterization of the uncertainty in the data and the resulting uncertainty in the computed estimates, adopting a Bayesian formulation. In this setting, all the model inputs included in the model are described by random variables, where randomness accounts for the available degree of information concerning their realizations, and is expressed in terms of probability distributions; as a result, the solution of the inverse UQ problem is the *posterior* PDF of the unknown inputs. Compared with the variational methods of Section 9.1, where classical regularization methods yield point estimates by curing the ill-posedness of the problem, statistical inversion aims at removing ill-posedness by recasting the inverse problem in a larger space of probability distributions (Kaipio and Somersalo 2005). This strategy also enables better characterization of the prior information contained in the regularization terms in (9.2), in the form of a *prior* PDF of the unknown inputs. The task of Bayesian inversion is to improve the knowledge of the unknown system features starting from the prior belief and exploiting information from a set of model realizations. For more on this topic, see Stuart (2010) and Sullivan (2015), for example.

### *10.2.1 Static problems*

Assume that we are measuring an output $\boldsymbol{z} = \boldsymbol{f}(\boldsymbol{\theta}, \boldsymbol{\varepsilon}) \in \mathbb{R}^{n_z}$ in order to get information on the unknown input $\boldsymbol{\theta} \in \mathbb{R}^p$, and that the measured quantity is contaminated by noise $\boldsymbol{\varepsilon}$. By treating input and output as random quantities, let us denote by $\boldsymbol{Z} \in \mathbb{R}^{n_z}$ and $\boldsymbol{\Theta} \in \mathbb{R}^p$ two random variables, of which $\boldsymbol{z}$ and $\boldsymbol{\theta}$ denote the corresponding realizations. Very often, the noise is modelled as additive and mutually independent of $\boldsymbol{\Theta}$, so that the input/output map takes the form

$$\boldsymbol{Z} = \boldsymbol{f}(\boldsymbol{\Theta}) + \boldsymbol{\varepsilon},$$

where $\boldsymbol{Z}, \boldsymbol{\varepsilon} \in \mathbb{R}^{n_z}$, $\boldsymbol{\Theta} \in \mathbb{R}^p$ are random variables. Here $\boldsymbol{Z}$ is called the *measurement*, and its realization $\boldsymbol{Z} = \boldsymbol{z}$ in the actual measurement process is called the *data*. Moreover, let $\pi_{\text{noise}}(\boldsymbol{\varepsilon})$ denote the PDF of the noise $\boldsymbol{\varepsilon}$, usually encoding experimental errors. Before performing output measurements, all the information (*e.g.* structure or regularity) about the distribution of the input $\boldsymbol{\Theta}$ are encapsulated in the *prior* PDF $\pi_{\text{prior}}(\boldsymbol{\theta})$, to be selected according to problem-specific considerations.

The conditional probability $\pi(\boldsymbol{z} \mid \boldsymbol{\theta})$ of $\boldsymbol{Z} \mid \boldsymbol{\Theta} = \boldsymbol{\theta}$ (*i.e.* of $\boldsymbol{Z}$ conditioned on $\boldsymbol{\Theta} = \boldsymbol{\theta}$) is the so-called (*conditional*) *likelihood function*, and expresses the likelihood of different measurement outcomes $\boldsymbol{z}$ given $\boldsymbol{\Theta} = \boldsymbol{\theta}$. In our case the input/output map $\boldsymbol{f} : \mathbb{R}^p \to \mathbb{R}^{n_z}$ requires the solution of a PDE problem, and the evaluation of the output $\boldsymbol{f}(\boldsymbol{\theta})$. Thanks to the assumption of mutual independence of $\boldsymbol{\Theta}$ and $\boldsymbol{\varepsilon}$, $\boldsymbol{Z} \mid \boldsymbol{\Theta} = \boldsymbol{\theta}$ is distributed like $\boldsymbol{\varepsilon}$, that is, the likelihood function is

$$\pi(\boldsymbol{z} \mid \boldsymbol{\theta}) = \pi_{\text{noise}}(\boldsymbol{z} - \boldsymbol{f}(\boldsymbol{\theta})).$$

Assuming that the measurement data $\boldsymbol{Z} = \boldsymbol{z}$ is given, in the Bayesian framework the inverse problem is to find the conditional PDF $\pi(\boldsymbol{\theta} \mid \boldsymbol{z})$ of $\boldsymbol{\Theta}$. This latter is the *posterior* PDF of $\boldsymbol{\Theta}$ given the data $\boldsymbol{Z} = \boldsymbol{z}$ and can be expressed via Bayes' theorem as

$$\pi(\boldsymbol{\theta} \mid \boldsymbol{z}) = \frac{\pi_{\text{prior}}(\boldsymbol{\theta})\pi(\boldsymbol{z} \mid \boldsymbol{\theta})}{\pi(\boldsymbol{z})},$$

where

$$\pi(\boldsymbol{z}) = \int_{\mathbb{R}^{n_z}} \pi(\boldsymbol{z} \mid \boldsymbol{\theta})\pi_{\text{prior}}(\boldsymbol{\theta})\, \mathrm{d}\boldsymbol{\theta}$$

plays the role of a normalization constant, and often has little importance from a computational standpoint.

Solving an inverse UQ problem in the static case – alternatively, in the literature such a problem is referred to as the *stationary inverse problem* – thus consists in finding a prior PDF $\pi_{\text{prior}}(\boldsymbol{\theta})$, expressing the likelihood function $\pi(\boldsymbol{z} \mid \boldsymbol{\theta})$ using the interplay between the observation and the unknown, and finally developing suitable numerical techniques to explore the posterior PDF. Each of these tasks is a challenging problem from a computational standpoint; here we provide some hints on how to use this framework for a wide range of applications related to backward uncertainty quantification in cardiovascular modelling.

In the case where the unknown is a random variable with few components, the posterior PDF can also be visualized in the form of a non-negative function of these variables. Most applications, however, yield larger-scale inverse UQ problems, and resulting PDFs in high-dimensional spaces, for which it is much more effective to evaluate suitable *point estimators*, such as the *maximum a posteriori* estimator

$$\boldsymbol{\theta}_{\text{MAP}} = \arg\max_{\boldsymbol{\theta} \in \mathbb{R}^p} \pi(\boldsymbol{\theta} \mid \boldsymbol{z})$$

or the *conditional mean*

$$\boldsymbol{\theta}_{\mathrm{CM}} = \mathbb{E}[\boldsymbol{\theta} \mid \boldsymbol{z}] = \int_{\mathbb{R}^p} \boldsymbol{\theta}\, \pi(\boldsymbol{\theta} \mid \boldsymbol{z})\, \mathrm{d}\theta.$$

Evaluating the former requires the solution of an optimization problem, for example using iterative, gradient-based methods; computing the latter involves a numerical quadrature problem in high-dimensional spaces. The evaluation of variability estimators such as the *conditional covariance*

$$\mathrm{Cov}\,(\boldsymbol{\theta} \mid \boldsymbol{z}) = \int_{\mathbb{R}^p} (\boldsymbol{\theta} - \boldsymbol{\theta}_{\mathrm{CM}})(\boldsymbol{\theta} - \boldsymbol{\theta}_{\mathrm{CM}})^{\mathrm{T}}\, \pi(\boldsymbol{\theta} \mid \boldsymbol{z})\, \mathrm{d}\theta \in \mathbb{R}^{p \times p},$$

or *confidence regions*, also provides further indicators for uncertainty quantification.

The simplest probabilistic model that can be used to describe experimental uncertainties is the Gaussian model, for which the noise $\boldsymbol{\varepsilon} \sim \mathcal{N}(\mathbf{0}, \Sigma_\varepsilon)$ is normally distributed, with mean $\mathbf{0}$ and covariance matrix $\Sigma_\varepsilon$. In this case, the likelihood function is

$$\pi(\boldsymbol{z} \mid \boldsymbol{\theta}) \propto \exp\Big( -\frac{1}{2} \|\boldsymbol{z} - \boldsymbol{f}(\boldsymbol{\theta})\|^2_{\Sigma_\varepsilon^{-1}} \Big).$$

If we can also assume a Gaussian model on the *prior* knowledge of the parameter distributions, that is, $\pi_{\mathrm{prior}} \sim \mathcal{N}(\boldsymbol{\theta}_p, \Sigma_p)$, then the posterior PDF will be normally distributed as well, that is,

$$\pi(\boldsymbol{\theta} \mid \boldsymbol{z}) \propto \exp\Big( -\frac{1}{2} \|\boldsymbol{z} - \boldsymbol{f}(\boldsymbol{\theta})\|^2_{\Sigma_\varepsilon^{-1}} - \frac{1}{2} \|\boldsymbol{\theta} - \boldsymbol{\theta}_p\|^2_{\Sigma_p^{-1}} \Big). \tag{10.2}$$

In this case, the maximum *a posteriori* estimator is

$$\boldsymbol{\theta}_{\mathrm{MAP}} = \arg \min_{\boldsymbol{\theta} \in \mathbb{R}^p} \Big( \frac{1}{2} \|\boldsymbol{z} - \boldsymbol{f}(\boldsymbol{\theta})\|^2_{\Sigma_\varepsilon^{-1}} + \frac{1}{2} \|\boldsymbol{\theta} - \boldsymbol{\theta}_p\|^2_{\Sigma_p^{-1}} \Big);$$

that is, it coincides with the estimator obtained by solving the (static version, with $K = 1$ of the) regularized least-squares problem (9.4), as long as we choose $\boldsymbol{\theta}_0 = \boldsymbol{\theta}_p$, $P_\theta = \Sigma_p$ and $M = \Sigma_\varepsilon^{-1}$. If we assume instead that no information is available about the parameter distribution except that it resides in a subset $\mathcal{D}$ of the parameter space $\mathbb{R}^p$, then $\pi_{\mathrm{prior}}(\boldsymbol{\theta}) \sim \mathcal{U}(\mathcal{D})$ is a uniform distribution over $\mathcal{D}$.

**Remark 10.1** The parameter estimation techniques of Section 9.1 can be seen as strategies yielding point estimates without any reference to underlying statistical models. However, when a Gaussian assumption is made in the Bayesian framework, the regularization term and the norms $\|\cdot\|_{\Sigma_\varepsilon^{-1}}$, $\|\cdot\|_{\Sigma_p^{-1}}$ and the value $\boldsymbol{\theta}_p$ have a clear interpretation in terms of measurement noise and prior probability distribution. Hence, a prior that carries sufficient information about the true underlying structure of the parameters often provides more meaningful estimates and regularizes the inverse problem in a more natural way than relying on abstract regularization terms, as in (9.4), that might not have any interpretation. The benefit of casting parameter estimation problems in the form of inverse UQ problems is that one is also able to characterize the variance of the prediction due to measurement and model errors more precisely than from the single-point estimates.

Exploring the posterior distribution in the case where the input space $\mathcal{D}$ has a larger dimension than $p = 2$ or 3 calls into play suitable *sampling methods*, among which the Markov chain Monte Carlo (MCMC) techniques are the most relevant example. Instead of evaluating the posterior PDF at a single point, an MCMC technique is a systematic way of generating a sample which can be used to *explore* the distribution, as well as to perform Monte Carlo integration as in (10.1) in order to compute the conditional mean or conditional covariance, for example. In the former case, the posterior $\pi(\boldsymbol{\theta} \mid \boldsymbol{z})$ plays the role of target probability distribution that we want to explore, and is obtained as a realization of a Markov chain by relying on the following *Metropolis–Hastings algorithm*, for example.

(1) Pick an initial $\boldsymbol{\theta}_1$.
(2) For $m = 1, \dots, M$:
   1. Compute $\pi(\boldsymbol{\theta}_m \mid \boldsymbol{z})$.
   2. Draw $\boldsymbol{w} \sim \mathcal{N}(\mathbf{0}, \Sigma_\varepsilon)$ and take a random step to find the next candidate $\widehat{\boldsymbol{\theta}} = \boldsymbol{\theta}_k + \boldsymbol{w}$.
   3. Compute $\pi(\widehat{\boldsymbol{\theta}} \mid \boldsymbol{z})$.
   4. Define the acceptance ratio
$$\alpha_m = \min\left\{1, \frac{\pi(\widehat{\boldsymbol{\theta}} \mid \boldsymbol{z})}{\pi(\boldsymbol{\theta}_m \mid \boldsymbol{z})}\right\}.$$
   5. Let $u \sim \mathcal{U}([0,1])$. If $u \le \alpha_m$, then accept, set $\boldsymbol{\theta}_{m+1} = \widehat{\boldsymbol{\theta}}$, and add to the set of samples $\Xi$; otherwise reject, and keep $\boldsymbol{\theta}_{m+1} = \boldsymbol{\theta}_m$.

After $M$ steps of the algorithm, the set $\Xi$ of samples contains realizations of the probability distribution $\pi(\boldsymbol{\theta} \mid \boldsymbol{z})$. The random step in point (b) from the current sample to the next candidate is distributed as white noise; its covariance should be chosen as large as possible while still maintaining a reasonable acceptance rate. Moreover, the initial points of the generated set usually represent the distribution to be explored poorly, and are then removed from the sample. To learn more on MCMC algorithms we refer to

Kaipio and Somersalo (2005), Robert and Casella (2004) and Voss (2013), and references therein.

### 10.2.2 Dynamical problems

Backward UQ problems whose forward system is stationary, or with observations that are not acquired sequentially in time, cannot be cast in the form of a Bayesian inverse problem, as shown in the previous section. In these cases, backward UQ can be formulated in the Bayesian framework by means of *Bayesian filtering methods*, among which the Kalman filter can be seen as a particular instance. These problems are also referred to as *non-stationary inverse problems*. As in Section 9.2, depending on the quantities that have to be estimated, the problem can be formulated as a state estimation or a joint state/parameter estimation problem. We will treat both these cases but will limit our discussion to finite-dimensional models (which usually arise from space and time discretization of unsteady PDEs) and using time-discretized evolution models. Further discussion can be found in Kaipio and Somersalo (2005), Särkkä (2013), Sullivan (2015) and Houtemaker and Zhang (2016), for example.

Let $\{\boldsymbol{X}^k\}_{k=0}^K$ and $\{\boldsymbol{Z}^k\}_{k=1}^K$ denote two stochastic processes; the former is related to the quantity we are interested in, whereas the latter represents the measurement. In particular, the random vector $\boldsymbol{X}^k \in \mathbb{R}^{n_x}$ is referred to as the *state vector*, whereas the random vector $\boldsymbol{Z}^k \in \mathbb{R}^{n_z}$ is referred to as the *observation*, both considered at the $k$th time $\tau^k$. From a Bayesian standpoint, the goal is to use the observations until time $k$ to get information about the state $\boldsymbol{X}^k$ and quantify the uncertainty related to this estimate. To frame this problem in the Bayesian setting, we assume that $\{\boldsymbol{X}^k\}_{k=0}^K$ and $\{\boldsymbol{Z}^k\}_{k=1}^K$ are an *evolution/observation model*, as follows.

(1) $\{\boldsymbol{X}^k\}_{k=0}^K$ and $\{\boldsymbol{Z}^k\}_{k=1}^K$ are Markov processes, that is,

$$\pi(\boldsymbol{x}^{k+1} \mid \boldsymbol{x}^0, \boldsymbol{x}^1, \ldots, \boldsymbol{x}^k) = \pi(\boldsymbol{x}^{k+1} \mid \boldsymbol{x}^k), \quad k = 0, 1, \ldots,$$
$$\pi(\boldsymbol{z}^k \mid \boldsymbol{x}^0, \boldsymbol{x}^1, \ldots, \boldsymbol{x}^k) = \pi(\boldsymbol{z}^k \mid \boldsymbol{x}^k), \qquad k = 1, 2, \ldots.$$

(2) $\{\boldsymbol{X}^k\}_{k=0}^K$ depends on the past observations only through its own history, that is,

$$\pi(\boldsymbol{x}^{k+1} \mid \boldsymbol{x}^k, \boldsymbol{z}^1, \ldots, \boldsymbol{z}^k) = \pi(\boldsymbol{x}^{k+1} \mid \boldsymbol{z}^k), \quad k = 0, 1, \ldots.$$

Here $\boldsymbol{x}^k$, $\boldsymbol{z}^k$ denote the realizations of the processes $\{\boldsymbol{X}^k\}_{k=0}^K$ and $\{\boldsymbol{Z}^k\}_{k=1}^K$, respectively. In order to characterize such a model, we need to specify the PDF of the initial state $\boldsymbol{X}^0$, $\pi_{\text{prior}}(\boldsymbol{x}^0)$, the so-called *transition kernel* $\pi(\boldsymbol{x}^{k+1} \mid \boldsymbol{x}^k)$, $k = 0, 1, \dots$ and the conditional probability $\pi(\boldsymbol{z}^k \mid \boldsymbol{x}^k)$, $k = 1, 2, \dots,$ the so-called (conditional) likelihood function. We assume a *state evolution equation* of the form

$$\boldsymbol{X}^{k+1} = \boldsymbol{f}^{k+1}(\boldsymbol{X}^k, \boldsymbol{V}^{k+1}), \quad k = 0, 1, \dots \tag{10.3}$$

and an *observation equation* of the form

$$\boldsymbol{Z}^k = \boldsymbol{h}^k(\boldsymbol{X}^k, \boldsymbol{W}^k), \quad k = 1, 2, \dots. \tag{10.4}$$

Here $\boldsymbol{f}^{k+1}$ and $\boldsymbol{h}^k$ are known functions, whereas $\boldsymbol{V}^{k+1} \in \mathbb{R}^{n_x}$ and $\boldsymbol{W}^k \in \mathbb{R}^{n_z}$ denote the *state noise* and the *observation noise*, respectively. We want to determine the conditional PDF $\pi(\boldsymbol{x}^k \mid \boldsymbol{D}^k)$ of the state at the $k$th time instant given the observations $\boldsymbol{D}^k = (\boldsymbol{z}^1, \dots, \boldsymbol{z}^k)$ up to the same time instant; this procedure is usually referred to as *filtering problem*. By recursive application of Bayes' theorem, we have the following.

- The *time-evolution updating*, *i.e.*, the problem of determining $\pi(\boldsymbol{x}^{k+1} \mid \boldsymbol{D}^k)$ given $\pi(\boldsymbol{x}^k \mid \boldsymbol{D}^k)$ and the transition kernel $\pi(\boldsymbol{x}^{k+1} \mid \boldsymbol{x}^k)$, provides

$$\pi(\boldsymbol{x}^{k+1} \mid \boldsymbol{D}^k) = \int_{\mathbb{R}^{n_x}} \pi(\boldsymbol{x}^{k+1} \mid \boldsymbol{x}^k)\pi(\boldsymbol{x}^k \mid \boldsymbol{D}^k)\, \mathrm{d}\boldsymbol{x}^k. \tag{10.5}$$

- The *observation updating*, *i.e.*, the problem of determining the posterior distribution $\pi(\boldsymbol{x}^{k+1} \mid \boldsymbol{D}^{k+1})$ of $\boldsymbol{X}^k \mid \boldsymbol{D}^k$ based on the new observation $\boldsymbol{Z}^{k+1}$ given $\pi(\boldsymbol{x}^{k+1} \mid \boldsymbol{D}^k)$ and the likelihood function $\pi(\boldsymbol{z}^{k+1} \mid \boldsymbol{x}^{k+1})$, provides

$$\pi(\boldsymbol{x}^{k+1} \mid \boldsymbol{D}^{k+1}) = \frac{\pi(\boldsymbol{z}^{k+1} \mid \boldsymbol{x}^{k+1})\pi(\boldsymbol{x}^{k+1} \mid \boldsymbol{D}^k)}{\pi(\boldsymbol{z}^{k+1} \mid \boldsymbol{D}^k)}, \tag{10.6}$$

where

$$\pi(\boldsymbol{z}^{k+1} \mid \boldsymbol{D}^k) = \int_{\mathbb{R}^{n_x}} \pi(\boldsymbol{z}^{k+1} \mid \boldsymbol{x}^{k+1})\pi(\boldsymbol{x}^{k+1} \mid \boldsymbol{D}^k)\, \mathrm{d}\boldsymbol{x}^{k+1}.$$

Formula (10.6) is Bayes' formula, where $\pi(\boldsymbol{x}^{k+1} \mid \boldsymbol{D}^k)$ is considered as the prior distribution for $\boldsymbol{x}^{k+1}$.

The Kalman filter introduced in Section 9.2.1 is a remarkable instance of Bayesian filter method. Indeed, let us assume that the state and the observation equations are linear with additive noise processes; that is,

$$\boldsymbol{f}^{k+1}(\boldsymbol{x}^k, \boldsymbol{v}^k) = A_{k|k+1}\boldsymbol{x}^k + \boldsymbol{v}^k, \quad \boldsymbol{h}^k = H_k\boldsymbol{x}^k + \boldsymbol{w}^k,$$

for given matrices $A_{k|k+1}$, $H_k$, that the noise vectors $\boldsymbol{V}^{k+1}$ and $\boldsymbol{W}^k$ are mutually independent, Gaussian, with zero mean and known covariances $Q_{k+1}$

and $R_k$, respectively, and that the prior PDF of $\boldsymbol{X}^0$ is Gaussian with mean $\boldsymbol{m}^0$ and covariance $P^0$. Under these assumptions, the time evolution and the observation updating formulas (10.3, 10.4) involve Gaussian distributions, whose means and covariances can be updated at each step according to prediction formulas (9.15a, 9.15b) and correction formulas (9.15d, 9.15e), respectively. In particular, we have that

$$\begin{aligned}
\pi(\boldsymbol{x}^{k+1} \mid \boldsymbol{x}^k) &\sim N(A_{k|k+1}\boldsymbol{x}^k, Q^k), \\
\pi(\boldsymbol{z}^k \mid \boldsymbol{x}^k) &\sim N(H_k\boldsymbol{x}^k, R_k).
\end{aligned}$$

The Bayesian filtering equations can be evaluated in closed form, yielding the following Gaussian distributions:

$$\begin{aligned}
\pi(\boldsymbol{x}^k \mid \boldsymbol{D}^{k-1}) &\sim \mathcal{N}(\boldsymbol{m}_f^k, P_k^f), \\
\pi(\boldsymbol{x}^k \mid \boldsymbol{D}^k) &\sim \mathcal{N}(\boldsymbol{m}_a^k, P_k^a), \\
\pi(\boldsymbol{z}^k \mid \boldsymbol{D}^{k-1}) &\sim \mathcal{N}(H_k\boldsymbol{m}_f^k, H_k P_k^f H_k^{\mathrm{T}} + R_k),
\end{aligned}$$

where the means and the variances can be computed with the Kalman filter prediction step

$$\begin{aligned}
\boldsymbol{m}_f^k &= A_{k-1|k}\boldsymbol{m}^{k-1}, \\
P_k^f &= A_{k-1|k}P_{k-1}^a A_{k-1|k}^{\mathrm{T}} + Q_{k-1}
\end{aligned} \tag{10.7}$$

and the consequent correction step

$$\begin{aligned}
K_k &= P_k^f H_k^{\mathrm{T}}(H_k P_k^f H_k^{\mathrm{T}} + R_k)^{-1}, \\
\boldsymbol{m}_a^k &= \boldsymbol{m}_f^k + F_k(\boldsymbol{z}^k - H_k\boldsymbol{m}_f^k), \\
P_k^a &= (I - K_k H_k)P_k^f.
\end{aligned} \tag{10.8}$$

In other words, under the Gaussian assumption, the density is updated only through the mean and the covariance. A similar interpretation also holds for the EKF, as soon as a Gaussian approximation of the densities is considered, and the evolution of these densities is taken into account. In this respect, Bayesian filtering can be seen as a generalization of deterministic filters, such as the KF, EKF and UKF introduced in Section 9.2.

As already remarked in Section 9.2.2, when the evolution model is fully non-linear, the EKF, which can be seen as a particular instance of an approximate Gaussian filter, may perform badly: this can be explained by considering that the push-forward of the previous state estimate (which has a Gaussian distribution) by a non-linear map is poorly approximated by a Gaussian distribution. To avoid the linearization of the evolution and the observation models, one can rely on Monte Carlo methods to simulate the distributions by random samples, similarly to what has been done in the static case. This strategy yields the so-called *particle filters* (also referred to as *sequential Monte Carlo methods*), now very popular for complex backward UQ problems.

The goal of a particle filter is to produce an ensemble $\{\boldsymbol{x}_1^{k|k}, \ldots, \boldsymbol{x}_{N_e}^{k|k}\}$ of $N_e$ *particles* sequentially, that is, a random sample distributed according to the conditional probability distribution $\pi(\boldsymbol{x}^k \mid \boldsymbol{D}^k)$. The ensemble Kalman filter (EnKF), introduced by Evensen (1994, 2003), is a particle filter exploiting the idea of approximating the means and the covariances of the current estimate involved in the Kalman filter prediction-correction strategy by a set of particles sampled from the distribution. Unlike the Kalman filter itself, we evaluate the error covariance predictions and corrections by the ensemble covariance matrices around the corresponding ensemble mean, instead of classical covariance equations (9.15b–9.15e) given in the KF algorithm. The covariance matrices of the state vector $\boldsymbol{X}$ need not be evolved, thus eliminating the costs associated with storing, multiplying and inverting the matrices appearing in the equations (9.15b–9.15e).

The ensemble is initialized by drawing $N_e$ independent particles from, say, a Gaussian distribution with mean $\boldsymbol{m}^0$ and covariance $P_0$.

- At each *prediction step*, each particle is evolved using the Kalman filter prediction step,

$$\boldsymbol{x}_e^{k|k-1} = A_{k-1|k}\boldsymbol{x}_e^{k-1|k-1} + \boldsymbol{v}^{k-1}$$

  if the system is linear, or

$$\boldsymbol{x}_e^{k|k-1} = \boldsymbol{f}^k(\boldsymbol{x}_e^{k-1|k-1}, \boldsymbol{v}^{k-1})$$

  if the system is non-linear.
- At each *correction step*, the observation $\boldsymbol{z}^k$ is replicated $N_e$ times, obtaining

$$\boldsymbol{d}_e^k = \boldsymbol{z}^k + \boldsymbol{\eta}_e^k, \quad \boldsymbol{\eta}_e^k \sim N(\boldsymbol{0}, R_k).$$

  Then, the empirical mean

$$\bar{\boldsymbol{x}}_e^{k|k-1} = \frac{1}{N_e}\sum_{e=1}^{N_e} \boldsymbol{x}_e^{k|k-1}$$

  and the empirical covariance

$$C_{k|k-1}^E = \frac{1}{N_e - 1}\sum_{e=1}^{N_e}\left(\boldsymbol{x}_e^{k|k-1} - \bar{\boldsymbol{x}}_e^{k|k-1}\right)\left(\boldsymbol{x}_e^{k|k-1} - \bar{\boldsymbol{x}}_e^{k|k-1}\right)^{\mathrm{T}}$$

of the particles set $\{\boldsymbol{x}_e^{k|k-1}\}_{e=1}^{N_e}$ are computed. The exact Kalman gain is then approximated by

$$K_k^E = C_{k|k-1}^E H_k^{\mathrm{T}} (H_k C_{k|k-1}^E H_k^{\mathrm{T}} + R_k)^{-1}$$

and, finally, the state correction is obtained by applying the formula (9.15d) to each particle; that is,

$$\boldsymbol{x}_e^{k|k} = \boldsymbol{x}_e^{k|k-1} + K_k^E(\boldsymbol{d}_e^k - H_k \boldsymbol{x}_e^{k|k-1}).$$

Several alternative implementations can be found, for example in Evensen (1994, 2009); for more on the ensemble Kalman filter, see also Iglesias, Law and Stuart (2013), Kelly, Law and Stuart (2014), Ernst, Sprungk and Starkloff (2014) and Houtemaker and Zhang (2016).

If the backward UQ problem also involves random inputs (as in the case of model parameters $\boldsymbol{\theta}$, which can also be time-varying), the problem of state estimation and parameter estimation simultaneously arises. Generally speaking, there is no unique optimal solution for this problem. Similarly to the *state augmentation* technique presented in Section 9.2, a possible way of facing this problem is to treat the unknown parameters $\boldsymbol{\theta}$ as part of the state, and use conventional filtering technique to infer the parameter and state simultaneously. This strategy goes by the name of joint estimation: see *e.g.* Moradkhani, Sorooshian, Gupta and Houser (2005), Ching, Beck and Porter (2006) and Evensen (2009) for more details. An example related to cardiovascular modelling where an EnKF can be exploited to deal with state and parameter estimation is addressed in Section 10.3.2.

## 10.3 Applications to cardiovascular modelling

Until recently, UQ has not been a priority for cardiovascular modelling. Today, a growing number of works focus on both forward and inverse UQ problems, taking into account uncertainties related to (i) measurement errors in experimental data (also referred to as observational uncertainty), (ii) model parameters, which may result from observational uncertainty as well as from variability, or lack of information, (iii) boundary and/or initial conditions and, possibly, (iv) the computational model itself, because of model limitations (model uncertainty) or systematic approximation errors (which can be seen as a form of *epistemic uncertainty*) introduced, for example, when the original high-fidelity model is replaced by a cheaper surrogate model or a reduced-order model. The list of contributions we mention is inevitably incomplete.

The effect of uncertain parameters in one-dimensional models of the arterial network was first considered by Xiu and Sherwin (2007), who exploited a high-order stochastic collocation method based on the generalized polynomial chaos expansion, combined with a discontinuous Galerkin spectral/hp element discretization in physical space, in order to analyze the effects of parametric uncertainties related to material properties and the initial cross-sectional area of the arterial vessel in pulse wave propagation, in a network of up to 37 vessels connected via 16 bifurcations. Chen, Quarteroni and Rozza (2013) have considered a more general setting, taking into account a wider network and many more sources of parametric uncertainties, including parameter-dependent boundary conditions in each distal boundary site and geometric parameters describing the cross-section area in each arterial segment. Similar problems, involving both sensitivity analysis and uncertainty propagation for networks built over patient-specific datasets, can be found in Leguy *et al.* (2011), Huberts *et al.* (2013*a*, 2013*b*) and Brault, Dumas and Lucor (2017).

The use of an adaptive stochastic collocation framework to deal with UQ in haemodynamic simulations was considered by Sankaran and Marsden (2011), who extracted relevant haemodynamic features – and quantified their uncertainty – for two idealized problems, namely an abdominal aortic aneurysm and a carotid artery bifurcation, and for a patient-specific problem, a Fontan procedure for congenital heart defects. In the former case, for instance, the radius of the abdominal aortic aneurysm, the radius and inflow velocity of the carotid artery bifurcation, and the flow split of the left and right pulmonary arteries were treated as random variables, following either Gaussian or uniform distributions, to account for the uncertainty impact on blood flows described by three-dimensional Navier–Stokes equations with rigid walls in small arterial portions. More detailed versions of this methodology have recently been exploited by Sankaran, Grady and Taylor (2015) and Sankaran, Kim, Choi and Taylor (2016) to analyze the impact of geometric uncertainties (*i.e.* anatomic uncertainties resulting in errors in the reconstructed geometry) and physiological uncertainties (yielding errors in boundary conditions or blood viscosity) for the blood flow and pressures in the coronary arteries.

The problem of calibrating outflow boundary conditions of blood flow simulations in truncated arterial domains has been cast in a Bayesian framework by D'Elia and Veneziani (2013) and Perdikaris and Karniadakis (2015), with the goal of quantifying the uncertainty affecting velocity and flow-related variables of interest, all treated as random variables.

A complete uncertainty propagation pipeline from clinical data to computational results was considered by Schiavazzi *et al.* (2016), focussing on an example of single ventricle palliation surgery. After determining the probability density functions of right pulmonary artery flow split and average pulmonary pressures from clinical measurements, Bayesian parameter estimation is carried out in order to characterize the distributions of boundary conditions yielding the observed flow splits and average pressure distributions. Then, uncertainties in the boundary conditions are propagated to simulation predictions by employing sparse grid stochastic collocation to statistically characterize model predictions of post-operative haemodynamics in models with and without pulmonary artery stenosis, in order to quantify the statistical variability in virtual surgery predictions. Finally, the impact of uncertainty on the optimal design of idealized bypass graft models has been considered by Sankaran and Marsden (2010) and Lassila *et al.* (2013*a*, 2013*b*), for example.

As to cardiac electrophysiology, a systematic application of UQ techniques to the forward problem of electrocardiography (*i.e.* the characterization of the torso potential given the electrical conductivity inside the heart and the torso) has been considered by Geneser, Kirby and MacLeod (2008), focussing on a simplified 2D configuration representing a geometric model of a slice through the human thorax. The forward UQ propagation problem yielding the standard deviation of the resulting stochastic torso potentials depending on several uncertainties affecting, for example, the electrical conductivities of the organs and the representation of cardiac sources, was tackled by a stochastic Galerkin method based on the generalized polynomial chaos expansion. Model personalization in cardiac electrophysiology was considered by Konukoglu *et al.* (2011), who applied an efficient Bayesian method exploiting polynomial chaos and compressed sensing to an eikonal–diffusion model involving a large ($> 10$) number of parameters, by integrating uncertainty on data and parameters.

Johnstone *et al.* (2016) have addressed a UQ framework for cardiac action potential models, focussing on (i) the inverse UQ problem of inferring the maximal conductance of ionic channels from noisy experimental recordings, and (ii) the forward UQ problem of propagating the uncertainty in maximal ion channel conductances to suitable outputs of interest, such as the action potential duration. To solve the inverse UQ problem a Bayesian framework, such as that described in Section 10.2, has been successfully employed, whereas the UQ propagation problem has been tackled by means of a Monte Carlo approach exploiting suitable surrogate models, such as Gaussian process emulators, to speed up the evaluation of the system model under analysis. A detailed analysis of the mechanisms underlying physiological variability in cardiac electrophysiology and pro-arrhythmic risks under a variety of conditions can be found in Muszkiewicz *et al.* (2016).

Concerning heart electromechanics, Osnes and Sundnes (2012) have addressed the quantification of the effect of uncertainties in the fibre orientation and the elasticity parameters included in the strain energy function on global output quantities such as the increase in cavity volume, the elongation of the ventricle, the increase in the inner radius, the decrease in wall thickness, and the rotation at the apex during the passive filling phase. Wallman, Smith and Rodriguez (2014) have estimated cardiac tissue properties by integrating structural information with electrophysiological data from electro-anatomical mapping systems, for example. By means of Bayesian inference tools, they obtained a simultaneous description of clinically relevant electrophysiological conduction properties and their associated uncertainty for various levels of noise, together with suitable design strategies to optimize the location and number of measurements required to maximize information and reduce uncertainty. A relevant application of UQ techniques to non-linear biomechanics has been considered by Biehler, Gee and Wall (2015), where parametric uncertainties related to the constitutive law for the artery wall of an AAA are modelled as random fields. In particular, Biehler *et al.* use a lognormal three-dimensional random field to describe the inter- and intra-patient variations of one constitutive parameter of a hyperelastic constitutive model, and sampling-based approaches such as Monte Carlo to solve the resulting stochastic mechanical problem. A multi-fidelity Bayesian framework incorporating information from different low-fidelity models was developed to speed up the intensive approximation of the resulting problem, following some general ideas reported by Kennedy and O'Hagan (2000) and Koutsourelakis (2009). Employment of surrogate models or more reliable reduced-order models (for more on this subject, see Section 11) to speed up the numerical solution of direct and inverse UQ problems is indeed a powerful alternative to stochastic collocation and stochastic Galerkin methods. However, they have only been partially touched on in the case of simple problems, for example in the works of Cui, Marzouk and Willcox (2015), Chen and Schwab (2015), Dihlmann and Haasdonk (2016), Manzoni, Pagani and Lassila (2016) and Pagani *et al.* (2017).

### *10.3.1 Backward uncertainty propagation in a simplified blood flow model*

We want to compare the solution of a parameter estimation problem in a variational framework and in a Bayesian setting, on a simplified blood

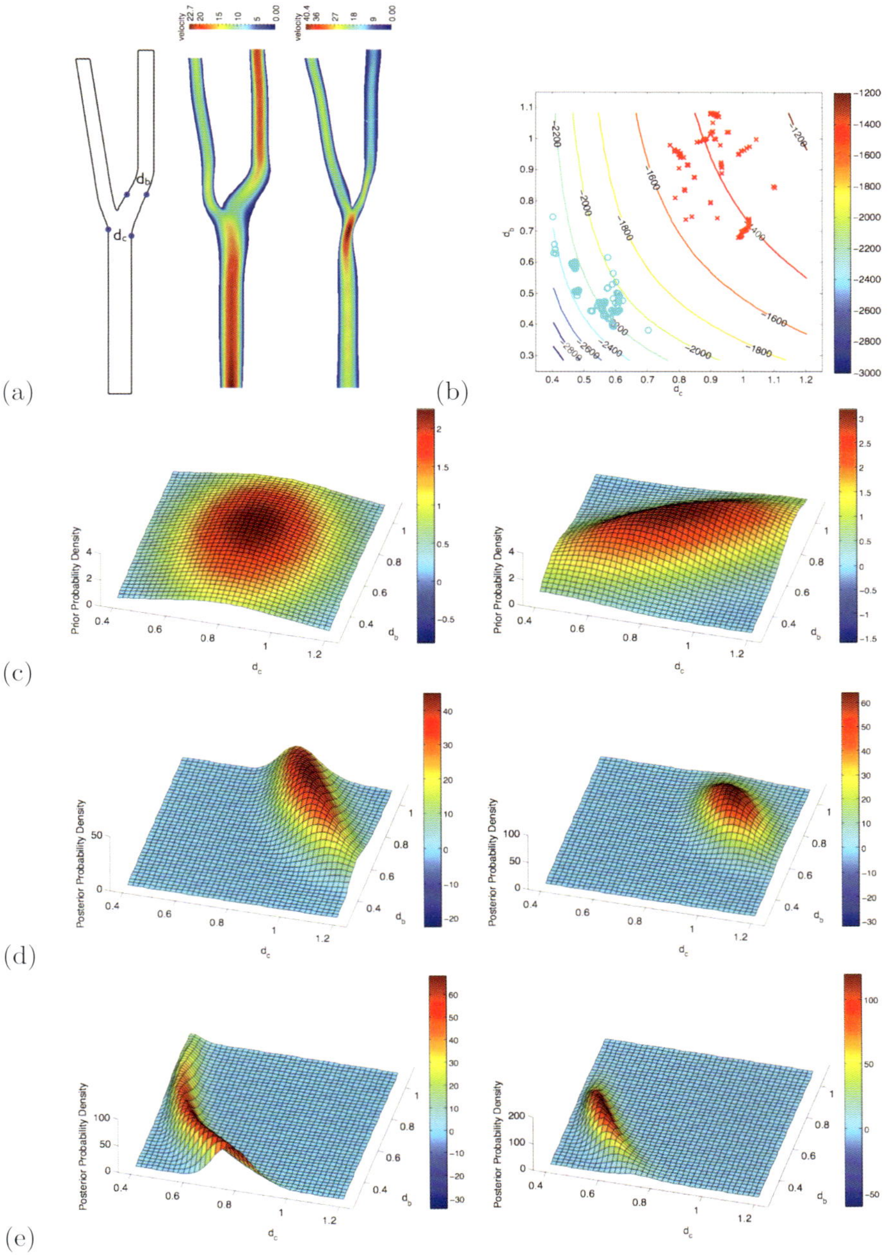


Figure 10.2 (a) Velocity profiles (cm $s^{-1}$) for different carotid bifurcations parametrized with respect to the diameters $d_c, d_b$. (b) Variational parameter estimation and isolines of the pressure drop. (c) Two different choices of the prior distribution on diameters $\boldsymbol{\theta} = (d_c, d_b)^{\mathrm{T}}$. (d, e) Results of the backward UQ problem obtained with the priors in (c) with observed pressure drop $\boldsymbol{z}_{\mathrm{obs}} = -1400$ and $\boldsymbol{z}_{\mathrm{obs}} = -2200$ (dyn $\mathrm{cm}^{-2}$), respectively. Numerical results were obtained using the MATLAB finite element library MLife.

flow problem. We consider a two-dimensional section of a carotid artery bifurcation where the diameters $d_c, d_b$ of the common carotid artery (CCA) at the bifurcation and of the mid-sinus level of the internal carotid artery (ICA) are the input parameters, assumed to be uncertain. In this idealized setting, our goal is to identify $\boldsymbol{\theta} = (d_c, d_b)^{\mathrm{T}}$ from the observation of the mean pressure drop)

$$\boldsymbol{z} = \frac{1}{|\Gamma_{\mathrm{in}}|} \int_{\Gamma_{\mathrm{in}}} p \,\mathrm{d}\gamma - \frac{1}{|\Gamma_{\mathrm{ICA}}|} \int_{\Gamma_{\mathrm{ICA}}} p \,\mathrm{d}\gamma$$

between the internal carotid outflow $\Gamma_{\mathrm{ICA}}$ and the inflow $\Gamma_{\mathrm{in}}$: see Figure 10.2(a). For simplicity, a steady incompressible Navier–Stokes model is employed to model the blood flow, although the same approach concerning the solution of the inverse UQ problem can be applied to the case of an unsteady fluid model, as soon as a peak (or time average) pressure drop is evaluated. Although presented here in a very simplified way for the sake of illustration, the problem of recovering information about vessel features by evaluating physical indices related to flow variables is of general interest for diagnostic purposes too. For instance, fractional flow reserve is a procedure exploited in coronary catheterization to measure pressure differences across a coronary artery stenosis in order to determine the degree of stenosis.

The parameter estimation problem is first solved by minimizing a least-squares functional for different observations of the pressure drop, $z = -1400$ and $z = -2200$, by assuming 5% relative additive noise in the measurements. The results of the inverse identification problem are represented in Figure 10.2(b) for 100 realizations of random noise in both cases. The recovered diameter values are shown to be quite sensitive to small noise variations. This is due to the fact that several geometric configurations – in terms of diameters $(d_c, d_b)$ – may correspond to the same output observation. The backward UQ propagation problem is then solved in a Bayesian setting, characterizing the posterior PDF of $\boldsymbol{\theta} = (d_c, d_b)$ starting from a Gaussian prior and assuming a Gaussian model to describe experimental noise. In particular, we can assume that the two diameters are either *a priori* independent (case (c), left), or correlated (case (c), right)). The two corresponding posterior distributions, obtained for the observations $z = -1400$ and $z = -2200$ of the pressure drop, are shown in Figure 10.2(d, e).

### *10.3.2 Backward uncertainty propagation in cardiac electrophysiology*

We finally consider the problem of identifying the size and the position of an ischaemic region in the myocardial tissue, as a remarkable instance of a backward UQ problem dealing with cardiovascular applications. Such a problem case can be cast in the form of a joint state/parameter estimation problem, and can be tackled efficiently by an EnKF technique.

The state evolution equation is given by the (space and time discretization of the) monodomain equation for the trans-membrane potential $V_m$, coupled with an Aliev–Panfilov cellular model involving a single gating variable $w$; the state variable is thus $\boldsymbol{u} = (V_m, w)^{\mathrm{T}}$. Similarly to the example in Section 10.1, in order to represent lack of conductivity in the tissue we introduce the relative conductivity $\sigma = \sigma(\boldsymbol{x}; \boldsymbol{\theta}) \in [0, 1]$; here $\sigma = 1$ and $\sigma = 0$ correspond to proper electrical conduction or total lack of conductivity, respectively.

Because the position and the extension of the ischaemic region is unknown, $\sigma(\boldsymbol{x}; \boldsymbol{\theta})$ is a random field. In order to make its representation low-dimensional, we parametrize the field $\sigma(\boldsymbol{x}; \boldsymbol{\theta})$ in terms of $p = 20$ random inputs
$\boldsymbol{\theta} = (\theta_1, \ldots, \theta_{20})^{\mathrm{T}}$ entering into a linear combination of $p = 20$ radial basis functions (RBFs), around $p$ given centres $\{\boldsymbol{x}_i\}_{i=1}^{20}$,

$$\sigma(\boldsymbol{x}; \boldsymbol{\theta}) = \frac{1}{\nu(\boldsymbol{x})} \sum_{i=1}^{p} \theta_i \exp\biggl(-\frac{\|\boldsymbol{x} - \boldsymbol{x}_i\|^2}{\lambda^2}\biggr), \quad \nu(\boldsymbol{x}) = \sum_{i=1}^{p} \exp\biggl(-\frac{\|\boldsymbol{x} - \boldsymbol{x}_i\|^2}{\lambda^2}\biggr),$$

where $\nu(\boldsymbol{x})$ is a normalization factor so that $\sigma(\boldsymbol{x}; \boldsymbol{\theta}) \in [0, 1]$. We consider a patient-specific left-ventricle geometry, and assume that a dataset $\boldsymbol{z}^1, \ldots, \boldsymbol{z}^K$ is acquired sequentially over a time interval. In particular, at each time $\tau^k$, $k = 1, \ldots, K$, data are given by the trans-membrane potential values computed at a set of nine points located on the endocardium, contaminated by Gaussian noise with zero mean and known covariance, to simulate the effect of experimental noise while evaluating the so-called *simultaneous endocardial mapping* in the human left ventricle; these invasive measurements are usually obtained using a non-contact catheter (see *e.g.* Schilling, Peters and Davies 1998, Álvarez *et al.* 2012). For the sake of the computational experiment, we assume that the data $\boldsymbol{z}^k$, $k = 1, \ldots, K$, are generated by the monodomain model with relative conductivity $\sigma^* = \sigma^*(\boldsymbol{x}; \boldsymbol{\theta}^*)$ for a particular choice $\boldsymbol{\theta} = \boldsymbol{\theta}^*$ of the input vector, that is,

$$\boldsymbol{z}^k = \boldsymbol{h}(\boldsymbol{u}(\boldsymbol{\theta}^*)) + \boldsymbol{\eta}^k, \quad \boldsymbol{\eta}^k \sim N(\boldsymbol{0}, R_k).$$

The goal is thus to recover the (posterior) PDF of $\boldsymbol{\theta}^K \mid \boldsymbol{D}^k$ given the observations $\boldsymbol{D}^k = (\boldsymbol{z}^1, \ldots, \boldsymbol{z}^k)$, evaluate the conditional mean $\boldsymbol{\theta}_{\mathrm{CM}}^K = \mathbb{E}[\boldsymbol{\theta}^K \mid \boldsymbol{D}^k]$, and finally estimate the conductivity field as $\sigma(\boldsymbol{x}; \boldsymbol{\theta}_{\mathrm{CM}}^K)$.

Starting from a prior distribution for the input vector $\boldsymbol{\theta}^0 \sim \mathcal{U}([0, 1]^{20})$, reflecting the lack of information about the possible presence and position of the ischaemic region, we rely on the EnKF to produce sequentially an ensemble $\{\boldsymbol{\theta}_e^k\}_{e=1}^{N_e}$ of $N_e$ particles distributed according to the conditional distribution $\pi(\boldsymbol{\theta}^k \mid \boldsymbol{D}^k)$, and the associated ensemble of $N_e$ states $\{\boldsymbol{u}^{k|k}(\boldsymbol{\theta}_e^k)\}_{e=1}^{N_e}$. Hence, starting from the initial ensemble $\{\mathcal{P}^{(0)}, \mathcal{U}^{(0)}\}$ sampled from the prior distribution, the *prediction-analysis* procedure of the EnKF is given by the following two-stage recursion.

(1) At each *prediction step*, compute the solution $\boldsymbol{u}^{k|k-1}(\boldsymbol{\theta}_e^{k-1})$ of the state system over $[\tau^{k-1}, \tau^k)$ with initial datum $\boldsymbol{u}^{k|k-1}(\boldsymbol{\theta}_e^{k-1})$.

(2) At each *correction step*, the observation $\boldsymbol{z}^k$ is replicated $N_e$ times, obtaining

$$\boldsymbol{d}_e^k = \boldsymbol{z}^k + \boldsymbol{\eta}_e^k, \quad \boldsymbol{\eta}_e^k \sim N(\mathbf{0}, R_k).$$

Then, compute the sample means

$$\begin{aligned} \overline{\boldsymbol{u}}^{k|k-1} &= \frac{1}{N_e}\sum_{e=1}^{N_e} \boldsymbol{u}^{k|k-1}(\boldsymbol{\theta}_e^{k-1}), \\ \overline{\boldsymbol{s}}_e^{k|k-1} &= \frac{1}{N_e}\sum_{e=1}^{N_e} \boldsymbol{h}(\boldsymbol{u}^{k|k-1}(\boldsymbol{\theta}_e^{k-1})), \\ \overline{\boldsymbol{\theta}}_e^{k-1} &= \frac{1}{N_e}\sum_{e=1}^{N_e} \boldsymbol{\theta}_e^{k-1}, \end{aligned} \tag{10.9}$$

and the sample covariances

$$\mathbf{C}_{ss}^k = \frac{1}{N_e - 1}\sum_{e=1}^{N_e} \boldsymbol{v}_e \boldsymbol{v}_e^{\mathrm{T}} \in \mathbb{R}^{n_z \times n_z}, \tag{10.10}$$

$$\mathbf{C}_{\theta s}^k = \frac{1}{N_e - 1}\sum_{e=1}^{N_e} (\boldsymbol{\theta}_e^{k-1} - \overline{\boldsymbol{\theta}}_e^{k-1})\boldsymbol{v}_e^{\mathrm{T}} \in \mathbb{R}^{p \times n_z}, \tag{10.11}$$

$$\mathbf{C}_{us}^k = \frac{1}{N_e - 1}\sum_{e=1}^{N_e} (\boldsymbol{u}^{k|k-1}(\boldsymbol{\theta}_e^{k-1}) - \overline{\boldsymbol{u}}^{k|k-1})\boldsymbol{v}_e^{\mathrm{T}} \in \mathbb{R}^{n_x \times n_z}, \tag{10.12}$$

where $\boldsymbol{v}_e = \boldsymbol{h}(\boldsymbol{u}^{k|k-1}(\boldsymbol{\theta}_e^{k-1}))$. Finally, the state/parameter ensembles are updated via the *Kalman formula*

$$\begin{bmatrix} \boldsymbol{\theta}_e^k \\ \boldsymbol{u}^{k|k}(\boldsymbol{\theta}_e^k) \end{bmatrix} = \begin{bmatrix} \boldsymbol{\theta}_e^{k-1} \\ \boldsymbol{u}^k(\boldsymbol{\theta}_e^{k-1}) \end{bmatrix} + \begin{bmatrix} \mathbf{C}_{\theta z}^k \\ \mathbf{C}_{uz}^k \end{bmatrix} (R_k + \mathbf{C}_{zz}^k)^{-1}(\boldsymbol{d}_e^k - \boldsymbol{h}(\boldsymbol{u}^{k|k-1}(\boldsymbol{\theta}_e^{k-1}))), \tag{10.13}$$

for $e = 1, \ldots, N_e$.

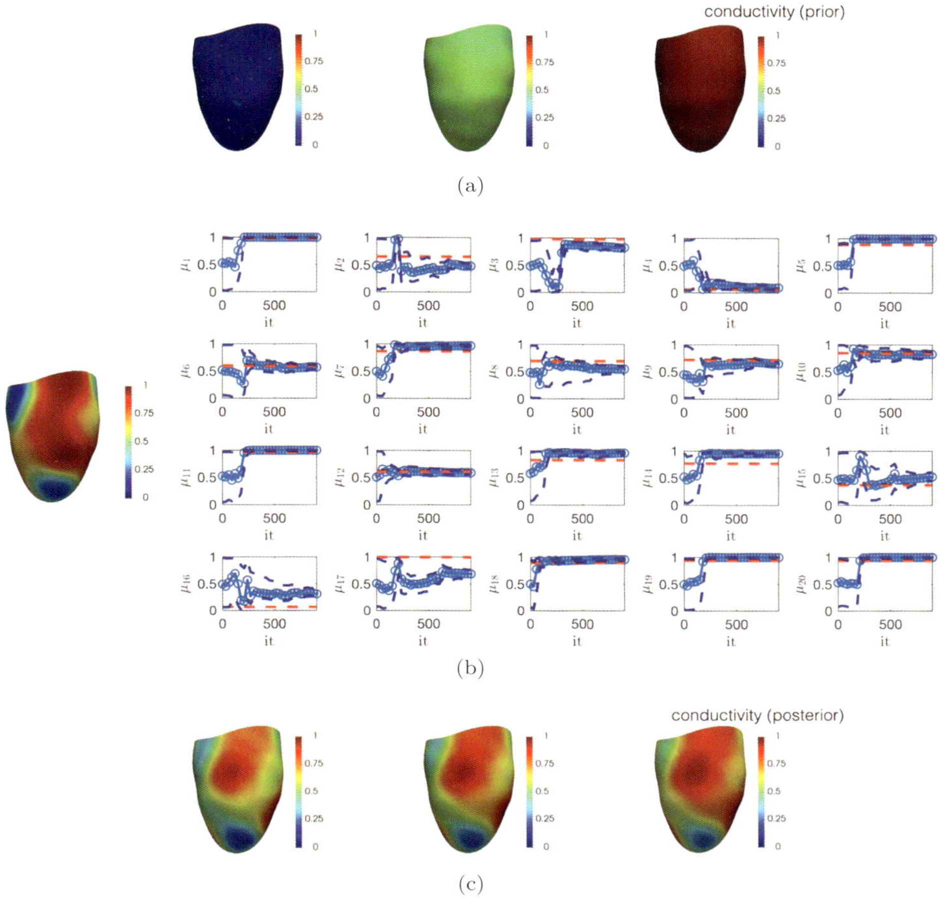


Figure 10.3 (a) 5% quantile, mean and 95% quantile of the uniform prior distribution of $\boldsymbol{\theta}^0$. (b) Identification of $p = 20$ parameters via the EnKF algorithm. Reference values $\theta_i^*$, $i = 1, \ldots, 20$, estimates $(\bar{\theta}_e^k)_i$ and confidence intervals are reported in dotted red, solid blue and dotted blue lines, respectively. (c) 5% quantile, conditional mean and 95% quantile of the posterior distribution of $\boldsymbol{\theta}^K$. Numerical results were obtained using the finite element library redbKIT v2.1 (github.com/redbKIT/redbKIT/releases).

The numerical results obtained by this procedure are shown in Figure 10.3. The data were generated by the monodomain model with the relative conductivity field $\sigma^* = \sigma^*(\boldsymbol{x}; \boldsymbol{\theta}^*)$ shown in Figure 10.3(a); a uniform prior distribution $\boldsymbol{\theta}^0 \sim \mathcal{U}([0,1]^{20})$ is assumed. After executing the EnKF algorithm, we obtain the posterior distribution whose mean and 5%, 95% quantiles are shown in Figure 10.3(c). The uncertainty in the input parameters is greatly reduced, while the conditional mean of the posterior distribution correctly approximates the realization of the random field reported on the left, by which data exploited for the sake of parameter estimation have been generated.

# 11

# Reduced-order modelling

As seen in Chapters 8–10, several numerical strategies used for tackling PDE-constrained optimization, parameter estimation and uncertainty quantification problems arising in cardiovascular modelling involve the approximation of PDE systems for several input parameter values. On the other hand, the repeated evaluation of input/output maps to characterize different scenarios requires many queries to numerical models too. Furthermore, if quantitative outputs are meant to support clinicians and medical doctors in their decisions, each new numerical simulation should be carried out very rapidly (order of minutes, say) on deployed platforms rather than on huge parallel hardware architectures, possibly requiring limited data storage and memory capacity. Meeting all these requirements is a challenging task, with the result that traditional *high-fidelity*, or *full-order*, techniques (*e.g.* the finite element method) are ill-suited, despite the constant growth of computer resources available.

*Reduced-order models* (ROMs) are emerging methodologies aimed at reducing the computational complexity and costs entailed by the repeated solution of PDE problems (Antoulas 2005, Benner, Gugercin and Willcox 2015, Quarteroni and Rozza 2014). In the case of parametrized PDEs (*i.e.* PDEs depending on a vector of parameters $\boldsymbol{\mu} \in \mathcal{P} \subset \mathbb{R}^p$), the *reduced basis* (RB) method is a ROM that enables dramatic reduction of the dimension of the discrete problems arising from numerical approximation – from millions to hundreds, or thousands at most, of variables.

Describing the mathematical principles and numerical algorithms underlying the RB method would take us a long way; interested readers can find a detailed presentation in Quarteroni, Manzoni and Negri (2016), for example. Here we limit ourselves to sketch the main features of the RB method, using for the sake of generality an algebraic standpoint. We denote by $\mathbf{y}(t;\boldsymbol{\mu})$ the solution of a time-dependent non-linear problem ($\boldsymbol{\mu} \in \mathcal{P} \subset \mathbb{R}^p$ denotes a set of input parameters) of the form

$$M(\boldsymbol{\mu})\frac{\mathrm{d}\mathbf{y}(t;\boldsymbol{\mu})}{\mathrm{d}t} + A(\boldsymbol{\mu})\mathbf{y}(t;\boldsymbol{\mu}) + F(\mathbf{y}(t;\boldsymbol{\mu})) = \mathbf{f}(t;\boldsymbol{\mu}), \quad t \in (0,T], \\ \mathbf{y}(0;\boldsymbol{\mu}) = \mathbf{y}_0(\boldsymbol{\mu}), \tag{11.1}$$

stemming from the (*e.g.* finite element) discretization of a parametrized PDE, where $A(\boldsymbol{\mu}) \in \mathbb{R}^{N_h \times N_h}$, $M(\boldsymbol{\mu}) \in \mathbb{R}^{N_h \times N_h}$ and $F(\boldsymbol{\mu}) : \mathbb{R}^{N_h} \to \mathbb{R}^{N_h}$ are three operators corresponding to the linear, mass and non-linear terms of the PDE.

The dimensional reduction is made possible by exploiting the parametric dependence of the solution manifold, that is, the set $\mathcal{M}_h = \{\mathbf{y}(t;\boldsymbol{\mu}) : t \in (0,T], \boldsymbol{\mu} \in \mathcal{P}\}$, thanks to the evaluation of a database of solutions, or *snapshots*, for selected parameter values, and to a (Petrov–) Galerkin projection onto the RB space spanned by a set of RB functions. In the case of a stationary problem, these latter are the snapshots themselves if a *greedy* algorithm is used, or the first singular vectors of the snapshot matrix if *proper orthogonal decomposition* (POD) is used: see *e.g.* Quarteroni *et al.* (2016), Hesthaven, Rozza and Stamm (2016) and Cohen and DeVore (2015). For time-dependent problems, the parameter space can still be sampled by relying on one of the two techniques mentioned, whereas POD is usually exploited to reduce trajectories of the system over the time interval.

In a very broad sense, POD is a technique for reducing the dimensionality of a given dataset (and, generally speaking, of a system) by representing it onto an orthonormal basis which is optimal in a least-squares sense. The original variables are transformed into a new set of uncorrelated variables (called POD modes, or principal components), the first few of them ideally retaining most of the energy present in all of the original variables. A lower-dimensional representation of the data is thus obtained by retaining only the first few modes. In the theory of stochastic processes this procedure is known as Karhunen–Loève (KL) decomposition, whereas in multivariate statistics it goes under the name of Principal Component Analysis. From an algebraic standpoint, the POD method relies on the use of the singular value decomposition (SVD); for the sake of simplicity, we first consider the case of a steady problem, following the so-called *method of snapshots*. In this case, by considering a set of $n_s \ll N_h$ snapshot vectors $\{\mathbf{y}(\boldsymbol{\mu}_1), \dots, \mathbf{y}(\boldsymbol{\mu}_{n_s})\}$ belonging to $\mathbb{R}^{N_h}$, which form the snapshot matrix $U \in \mathbb{R}^{N_h \times n_s}$ sorting them as column vectors, we compute the SVD decomposition of $\mathbb{U}$,

$$V^{\mathrm{T}} U Z = \begin{pmatrix} \Sigma & 0 \\ 0 & 0 \end{pmatrix},$$

where $V = [\boldsymbol{\zeta}_1\ \boldsymbol{\zeta}_2\ \dots\ \boldsymbol{\zeta}_{N^h}] \in \mathbb{R}^{N_h \times N_h}$ and $Z = [\boldsymbol{\psi}_1\ \boldsymbol{\psi}_2\ \dots\ \boldsymbol{\psi}_{n_s}] \in \mathbb{R}^{n_s \times n_s}$ are orthogonal matrices and $\Sigma = \mathrm{diag}(\sigma_1, \dots, \sigma_r)$ with $\sigma_1 \geq \sigma_2 \geq \dots \geq \sigma_r$; here $r \leq n_s$ is the rank of $\mathbb{U}$, which is strictly smaller than $n_s$ if the snapshot vectors are not all linearly independent. For any $N \leq n_s$, the POD basis of dimension $N$ is defined as the set of the first $N$ left singular vectors $\boldsymbol{\zeta}_1, \dots, \boldsymbol{\zeta}_N$ of $U$ and denoted by $V_N$.

By construction, the POD basis is orthonormal. Moreover, it minimizes, over all possible $N$-dimensional orthonormal bases $W = [\mathbf{w}_1, \dots, \mathbf{w}_N] \in \mathbb{R}^{N_h \times N}$, the sum of the squares of the errors between each snapshot vector $\mathbf{y}_i$ and its projection onto the subspace spanned by $W$, that is,

$$\sum_{i=1}^{n_s} \|\mathbf{y}(\boldsymbol{\mu}_i) - V_N V_N^{\mathrm{T}} \mathbf{y}(\boldsymbol{\mu}_i)\|_2^2 = \min_{W \in \mathcal{V}_N} \sum_{i=1}^{n_s} \|\mathbf{y}(\boldsymbol{\mu}_i) - W W^{\mathrm{T}} \mathbf{y}(\boldsymbol{\mu}_i)\|_2^2 = \sum_{i=N+1}^{r} \sigma_i^2$$

where $\mathcal{V}_N = \{W \in \mathbb{R}^{N_h \times N} \ :\ W^{\mathrm{T}} W = I\}$ is the set of all $N$-dimensional orthonormal bases. The minimal POD dimension $N \leq r$ is selected so that the projection error is smaller than a desired tolerance $\varepsilon_{\mathrm{POD}}$; indeed, it is sufficient to choose $N$ as the smallest integer such that

$$\frac{\sum_{i=1}^{N} \sigma_i^2}{\sum_{i=1}^{r} \sigma_i^2} \geq 1 - \varepsilon_{\mathrm{POD}}^2,$$

that is the energy retained by the last $r - N$ modes is equal or smaller than $\varepsilon_{\mathrm{POD}}^2$.

In the case of time-dependent problems, the procedure above is applied to a snapshot matrix $U$ collecting snapshots $\mathbf{y}^n(\boldsymbol{\mu}_i)$ at different time instances $t^n$, $n = 1, \dots, N_t$ and different parameter values $\boldsymbol{\mu}_1, \dots, \boldsymbol{\mu}_{n_s}$. However, this can be computationally unbearable due to the large amount of data to be collected and stored; for this reason, POD is preferably performed in time, on each set of snapshots $\{\mathbf{y}^1(\boldsymbol{\mu}_i), \mathbf{y}^2(\boldsymbol{\mu}_i), \dots\}$, and then a further POD is performed to obtain the basis for the RB space.

In general, a RB method seeks an approximation $V_N \mathbf{y}_N(t; \boldsymbol{\mu}) \approx \mathbf{y}(t; \boldsymbol{\mu})$ to the solution of (11.1), where $\mathbf{y}_N(t; \boldsymbol{\mu})$ is the reduced state vector and $V_N = [\mathbf{v}_1, \dots, \mathbf{v}_N] \in \mathbb{R}^{N_h \times N}$ is a matrix stacking the RB functions by columns. One possible RB approximation of (11.1) might be

$$\begin{aligned} M_N(\boldsymbol{\mu}) \frac{\mathrm{d}\mathbf{y}_N(t; \boldsymbol{\mu})}{\mathrm{d}t} &+ A_N(\boldsymbol{\mu}) \mathbf{y}_N(t; \boldsymbol{\mu}) \\ &+ V_N^{\mathrm{T}} \mathbf{F}(V_N \mathbf{y}_N(t; \boldsymbol{\mu})) = \mathbf{f}_N(t; \boldsymbol{\mu}), \quad t \in (0, T] \\ &\qquad \mathbf{y}_N(0; \boldsymbol{\mu}) = \mathbf{y}_{N,0}(\boldsymbol{\mu}), \end{aligned} \tag{11.2}$$

where

$$A_N(\boldsymbol{\mu}) = V_N^{\mathrm{T}} A(\boldsymbol{\mu}) V_N, \quad M_N(\boldsymbol{\mu}) = V_N^{\mathrm{T}} M(\boldsymbol{\mu}) V_N, \quad \mathbf{f}_N(t;\boldsymbol{\mu}) = V_N^{\mathrm{T}} \mathbf{f}(t;\boldsymbol{\mu}).$$

The arrays appearing in (11.2) can be efficiently assembled in a rapid online phase by combining parameter-independent quantities stored during a more expensive offline phase, provided that the dependence of the high-fidelity arrays such as $A(\boldsymbol{\mu})$ and $\mathbf{f}(t;\boldsymbol{\mu})$ is affine. This is, *e.g.*, the case when $A(\boldsymbol{\mu})$ is expressed as a linear combination as follows:

$$A(\boldsymbol{\mu}) = \sum_{q=1}^{Q_a} \Theta_a^q(\boldsymbol{\mu}) A_q,$$

where $\Theta_a^q : \mathcal{P} \to \mathbb{R}$, $q = 1, \dots, Q_a$ are $\boldsymbol{\mu}$-dependent functions, and $A_q \in \mathbb{R}^{N_h \times N_h}$, $q = 1, \dots, Q_a$, are $\boldsymbol{\mu}$-independent matrices. In this way,

$$A_N(\boldsymbol{\mu}) = \sum_{q=1}^{Q_a} \Theta_a^q(\boldsymbol{\mu}) A_{N,q}, \qquad \text{with} \quad A_{N,q} = V_N^{\mathrm{T}} A_q V_N;$$

the arrays $A_{N,q}$, $q = 1, \dots, Q_a$, can be assembled offline and stored.

Suitable *hyper-reduction* techniques are instead required to manage non-affine and, above all, non-linear terms, in order to make their assembly independent of the dimension $N_h$ of the high-fidelity problem; see *e.g.* (Carlberg, Farhat, Cortial and Amsallem 2013). Indeed, the small dimension $N \ll N_h$ of system (11.2) does not warrant substantial computational savings as the assembly of the non-linear terms still involves computations whose complexity depends on $N_h$. If $\mathbf{F} : \mathbb{R}^{N_h} \to \mathbb{R}^{N_h}$ features a low-order polynomial non-linearity and the parametric dependence is affine, the assembly of the non-linear terms can be efficiently achieved via an offline-online decomposition. On the other hand, if $\mathbf{F}$ features a higher (or non-polynomial) non-linearity (and possibly a non-affine parametric dependence), a further level of reduction must be introduced by suitably employing techniques such as the *empirical interpolation method* (Barrault, Maday, Nguyen and Patera (2004) and Maday, Nguyen, Patera and Pau (2009)) or the *discrete empirical interpolation method* (Chaturantabut and Sorensen (2010) and Negri, Manzoni and Amsallem (2015)) with the aim of approximating the nonlinear/nonaffine terms and recovering an (approximate) affine structure.

We emphasize that a RB method requires the solution of some full-order – and therefore very expensive – discrete equations. The key idea is that these demanding calculations can be done offline, before the optimization with respect to the control parameters, or the parameter estimation, is attempted. In fact, the cost of each optimization step performed online is much smaller than that involving the full-order state approximation; similarly, computing the evolution of a particle set in the ensemble Kalman filter algorithm by querying the ROM can be performed in a way that is substantially less expensive. Numerical results shown in Chapters 8 and 10 have been obtained by exploiting suitable reduced order techniques to speed up the approximation of the partial differential equations modelling the problems.

Besides those contexts, the efficient solution of parameter-dependent PDE systems in cardiac modelling is of key importance in several circumstances. Examples include: the need of computing outputs of clinical interest in several different scenarios; the exploration of intra-patients variability affecting relevant physical and/or geometrical parameters. Here we report some numerical results, taken from Manzoni, Bonomi and Quarteroni (2018), obtained by means of the ROM framework described above in the case or parameter-dependent cardiac electrophysiology and mechanics problems solved in a patient-specific geometry.

Electrophysiology is modelled by the monodomain equation coupled with the minimal model of Bueno-Orovio (Bueno-Orovio *et al.* 2008). The electrical conductivities in the fibre direction ($\sigma_f$) and in the plane orthogonal to the former ($\sigma_s = \sigma_n$) are treated as parameters:

- $\sigma_f \in [30\, k\Omega^{-1} cm^{-1}, 80\, k\Omega^{-1} cm^{-1}]$;
- $\sigma_s = \sigma_n \in [10\, k\Omega^{-1} cm^{-1}, 30\, k\Omega^{-1} cm^{-1}]$.

The proposed ROM yields a speed-up of more than one order of magnitude: on a mesh with 248216 elements and $N_h = 45817$ degrees of freedom, the high-fidelity finite element approximation takes 0.12 s, while the ROM 12 times less. Provided we consider a sufficient number of basis functions for the state variables and of terms in the affine approximation of the $\boldsymbol{\mu}$-dependent quantities, the front propagation captured by the ROM is similar to the one obtained with the FOM. A comparison between the high-fidelity and the reduced solutions is reported in Figure 11.1; for the case at hand, the average (over a sample of parameter values) relative error between the ROM and the high-fidelity model is about 5%. The computed ROM makes the evaluation of several scenarios efficiently available. For instance, we report in Figure 11.2 the activation maps obtained for different parameter values; as expected, the duration of the depolarization phase is longer if electrical conductivities are smaller.

Regarding cardiac mechanics, we consider a quasi-incompressible, active-strain formulation of the mechanical problem, treating the myocardium as an hyperelastic material obeying the orthotropic model proposed in Holzapfel

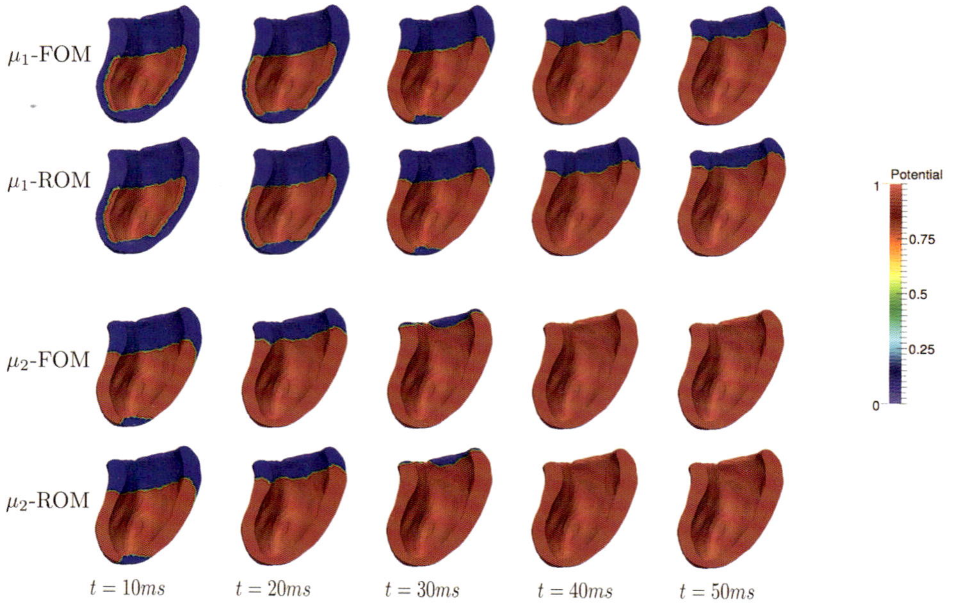


Figure 11.1 High-fidelity and reduced-order approximations of the electric potential (rescaled between 0 and 1) computed at different time instants for $\boldsymbol{\mu}_1 = [30, 10]$ and $\boldsymbol{\mu}_2 = [80, 30]$.

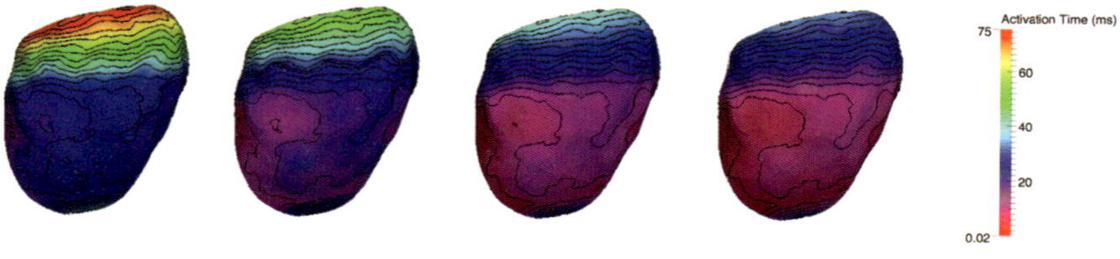


Figure 11.2 Activation maps for $\boldsymbol{\mu}_1 = [30, 10]$, $\boldsymbol{\mu}_2 = [45, 10]$, $\boldsymbol{\mu}_3 = [65, 30]$ and $\boldsymbol{\mu}_4 = [80, 30]$.

and Ogden (2009); see Section 6.2. In the present situation, the electromechanical coupling is not included in the ROM – that is, for each parameter value we use the high-fidelity approximation of the electrophysiology model and, in particular, of the fibres' shortening variable. We use the same patient-specific geometry as in the previous example, however we now consider a coarser mesh with 31027 elements and $N_h = 18567$ degrees of freedom. Here, the parameters are the electrical conductivities (similarly to the electrophysiology problem above) and the orientation of the fibres:

- $\sigma_f \in [30\, k\Omega^{-1}cm^{-1}, 80\, k\Omega^{-1}cm^{-1}]$;

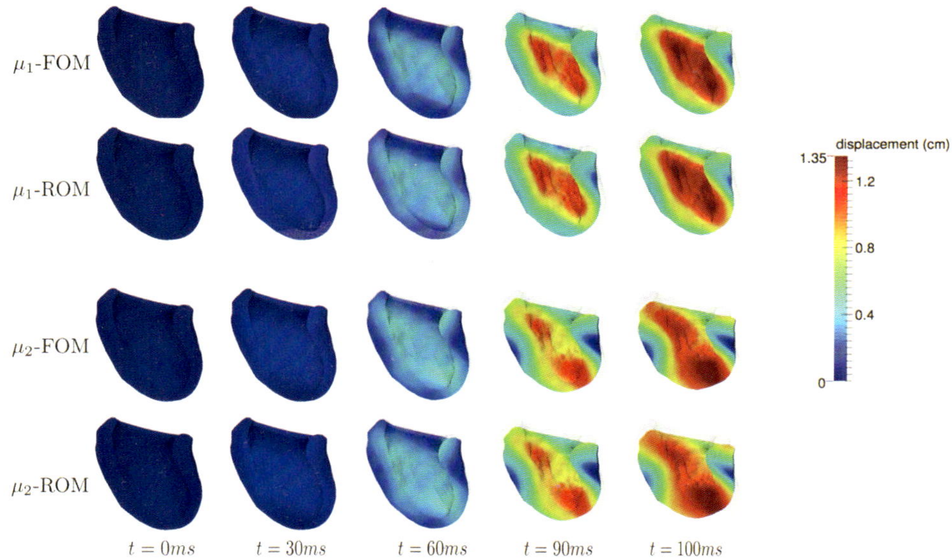


Figure 11.3 Section of the ventricle at different time instants, $\boldsymbol{\mu}_1 = [60, 10, 78^\circ]$ (first two rows), $\boldsymbol{\mu}_2 = [80, 30, 34^\circ]$ (last two rows), obtained with the high-fidelity and the reduced-order models.

- $\sigma_s = \sigma_n \in [10\, k\Omega^{-1}cm^{-1}, 30\, k\Omega^{-1}cm^{-1}]$;
- $\theta_{\max} \in [30^\circ, 80^\circ]$;
- $t \in [0, 100ms]$.

Time can be seen as an additional parameter since the problem here is quasi-static and needs to be solved at different time steps. Figure 11.3 highlights the displacement of the myocardium obtained with the high-fidelity and the reduced-order model on a longitudinal section of the ventricle, for two different parameters. In this case, the ROM yields a speed-up of about 20 times with respect to the 7 minutes of the high-fidelity model for each solution of the mechanical problem at a single time instant, on a single-core processor.

The proposed ROM correctly captures the high-fidelity solution as the relative error between the two is in this case about 2%. The associated ejection fraction (EF) is reported in Figure 11.4 by varying $\theta_{\max}$ and $\sigma_f - \sigma_s$; $\sigma_n$ only has a moderate effect on the solution. The quantity of blood ejected by the ventricle is larger when $\theta_{\max}$ and $\sigma_f$ assume large values. A similar parametric study, relating an output of clinical interest with relevant physical parameters, and showing the sensitivity of the former to the latter, would have been almost impossible to obtain without exploiting ROM modelling techniques such as the RB method, because of the overwhelming computa-

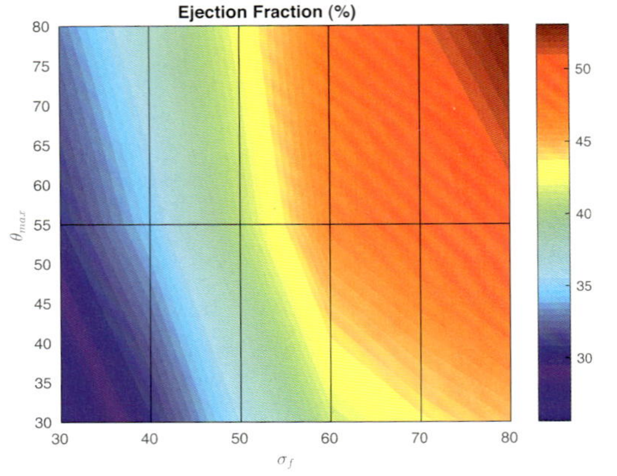


Figure 11.4 Ejection fraction as function of $\sigma_f$ and $\theta_{\max}$.

tional cost entailed by several queries to a high-fidelity computational model for cardiac mechanics.

We close this chapter by citing some notable applications of the RB method to problems of interest in cardiovascular modelling (this list is of course incomplete). Parametrized blood flows in idealized cardiovascular geometries have been considered by Lassila, Quarteroni and Rozza (2012),Manzoni, Quarteroni and Rozza (2012*a*), Ballarin *et al.* (2016), Ballarin *et al.* (2017), Colciago *et al.* (2014) and Negri (2016), taking into account more complex (and computationally challenging) patient-specific configurations; in all these cases, solutions of Navier–Stokes equations are computed with respect to inflow and/or geometric parameters. Applications to PDE-constrained optimization problems arising in the context of optimal design of prosthetic devices can be found, for example, in Manzoni *et al.* (2012*b*) and Lassila *et al.* (2013*a*). A reduced-order model based on POD is proposed for the bidomain equations of cardiac electrophysiology in Boulakia, Schenone and Gerbeau (2012), yielding the efficient approximation of a restitution curve and the estimation of ionic parameters and infarction locations from synthetic electrocardiograms with an evolutionary algorithm; Gerbeau, Lombardi and Schenone (2015) have proposed alternative options in this respect. More efficient strategies based on *local* reduced spaces to approximate the solution of problems whose dependence on parameters is rather involved have been used in Pagani *et al.* (2017). This is the case of the nonlinear electrophysiology problem, for which the presence of moving fronts in the solution and the high sensitivity of this latter to parameter variations make the application of standard RB techniques quite problematic. Regarding cardiac mechanics, a first attempt to solve (one-way coupled) electromechanics problems was instead considered in Bonomi, Manzoni and Quarteroni (2017), where a hyper-reduction framework for cardiac mechanics problems has been set and numerically tested. An overview of reduction and hyper-reduction techniques for both cardiac electrophysiology and mechanics can be found, for instance, in Manzoni *et al.* (2018).

Applications of POD to parameter estimation problems with sequential filtering techniques are given in Chapelle, Gariah, Moireau and Sainte-Marie (2013*b*), and an application of the RB method to the computational speed-up of Bayesian inverse problems related to blood flows modelling has been reported by Lassila *et al.* (2013*b*) and Manzoni *et al.* (2014). Variational parameter estimation problems arising in cardiac electrophysiology have been solved by means of POD in Yang and Veneziani (2017), whereas a convenient framework for dealing with uncertainty quantification – for sensitivity analysis, forward and backward UQ – can be found in (Pagani 2016).

We emphasize that while physical coefficients, boundary and/or initial conditions, as well as source terms, can usually be described in terms of input parameters in a straightforward way, the task of dealing with geometries of varying shape is much more involved. In this latter case, additional techniques providing flexible descriptions of complex shapes are required, possibly involving few parameters. Notable examples are given by *volume-based* representations, which operate on a control volume and define parametric maps by introducing a set of control points over the control volume; control point displacements, actually inducing a shape deformation, can thus be treated as input parameters. Within this class, free-form deformation techniques and interpolants constructed over a family of radial basis functions have been successfully employed; for further details see Manzoni *et al.* (2012*a*, 2012*b*) and Ballarin *et al.* (2016). A more general and automatic way of dealing with the efficient solution of parametrized PDEs defined on domains with variable shape has been used in Manzoni and Negri (2017), where a mesh motion technique relying on the solution of a solid extension problem is combined with the RB method, allowing to directly define global domain deformations starting from boundary parametrizations.

We also point out that the need to derive flexible and low-dimensional parametrizations is not confined to the realm of RB methods for parametrized PDEs. Indeed, it also arises when dealing with random inputs or fields; in this latter case, input uncertainties are usually parametrized with respect to a finite number of random variables, corresponding to the retained terms after truncating Karhunen–Loève or polynomial chaos expansions.

The analysis, development and application of reduced-order modelling techniques is a very active field in the numerical approximation of PDEs. Without any doubt, cardiovascular applications are one of the most relevant testing environments.

# References


S. Abboud, O. Berenfeld and D. Sadeh (1991), 'Simulation of high-resolution QRS complex using a ventricular model with a fractal conduction system: Effects of ischemia on high-frequency QRS potentials', *Circ. Res.* **68**, 1751–1760.

S. Ahmed and D. Giddens (1984), 'Pulsatile poststenotic flow studies with laser Doppler anemometry', *J. Biomech.* **17**, 695–705.

I. Akkerman, Y. Bazilevs, V. Calo, T. Hughes and S. Hulshoff (2008), 'The role of continuity in residual-based variational multiscale modeling of turbulence', *Comput. Mech.* **41**, 371–378.

F. Alauzet, B. Fabrèges, M. Fernández and M. Landajuela (2016), 'Nitsche-XFEM for the coupling of an incompressible fluid with immersed thin-walled structures', *Comput. Methods Appl. Mech. Engrg* **301**, 300–335.

R. Aliev and A. Panfilov (1996), 'A simple two-variable model of cardiac excitation', *Chaos Solitons Fract.* **7**, 293–301.

A. Álvarez, F. Alonso-Atienza, J. Rojo-Álvarez, A. Garcia-Alberola and M. Moscoso (2012), 'Shape reconstruction of cardiac ischemia from non-contact intracardiac recordings: A model study', *Math. Comput. Model.* **55**, 1770–1781.

D. Ambrosi and S. Pezzuto (2012), 'Active stress vs. active strain in mechanobiology: Constitutive issues', *J. Elasticity* **2**, 199–212.

D. Ambrosi, G. Arioli, F. Nobile and A. Quarteroni (2011), 'Electromechanical coupling in cardiac dynamics: The active strain approach', *SIAM J. Appl. Math.* **2**, 605–621.

B. Andreianov, M. Bendahmane, A. Quarteroni and R. Ruiz-Baier (2015), 'Solvability analysis and numerical approximation of linearized cardiac electromechanics', *Math. Models Methods Appl. Sci.* **25**, 959–993.

L. Antiga, J. Peiró and D. Steinman (2009), From image data to computational domains. Chapter 4 in *Cardiovascular Mathematics* (L. Formaggia, A. Quarteroni and A. Veneziani, eds), Springer, pp. 123–175.

L. Antiga, M. Piccinelli, L. Botti, B. Ene-Iordache, A. Remuzzi and D. Steinman (2008), 'An image-based modeling framework for patient-specific computational hemodynamics', *Med. Biol. Engrg Comput.* **46**, 1097–1112.

P.F. Antonietti, M. Verani, C. Vergara and S. Zonca (2018), 'Numerical solution of fluid–structure interaction problems by means of a high order Discontinuous Galerkin method on polygonal grids', MOX-Report 27-2018, Department of Mathematics, Politecnico di Milano.

A. Antoulas (2005), *Approximation of Large-Scale Dynamical Systems*, SIAM.

M. Asch, M. Bocquet and M. Nodet (2017), *Data Assimilation: Methods, Algorithms, and Applications*, SIAM.

M. Astorino and C. Grandmont (2009), 'Convergence analysis of a projection semi-implicit coupling scheme for fluid–structure interaction problems', *Numer. Math.* **45–46**, 3603–3612.

M. Astorino, F. Chouly and M. Fernández (2009), 'Robin based semi-implicit coupling in fluid–structure interaction: Stability analysis and numerics', *SIAM J. Sci. Comput.* **31**, 4041–4065.

M. Astorino, J.-F. Gerbeau, O. Pantz and K. Traoré (2010), 'Fluid–structure interaction and multi-body contact: Application to the aortic valves', *Comput. Methods Appl. Mech. Engrg* **116**, 721–767.

M. Astorino, J. Hamers, C. Shadden and J.-F. Gerbeau (2012), 'A robust and efficient valve model based on resistive immersed surfaces', *Int. J. Numer. Methods Biomed. Engrg* **28**, 937–959.

C. Augustin, G. Holzapfel and O. Steinbach (2014), 'Classical and all-floating FETI methods for the simulation of arterial tissues', *Int. J. Numer. Methods Engrg* **99**, 290–312.

F. Auricchio, A. Ferrara and S. Morganti (2012), 'Comparison and critical analysis of invariant-based models with respect to their ability in fitting human aortic valve data', *Ann. Solid Struct. Mech.* **4**, 1–14.

F. Auricchio, F. Lefieux, A. Reali and A. Veneziani (2016), 'A locally anisotropic fluid–structure interaction remeshing strategy for thin structures with application to a hinged rigid leaflet', *Int. J. Numer. Methods Engrg* **107**, 155–180.

A. Avolio (1980), 'Multi-branched model of the human arterial system', *Med. Biol. Engrg Comput.* **18**, 709–718.

L. Azzolin (2018), Electromechanical modeling of the human heart in bi-ventricle geometries. MSc thesis, Mathematical Engineering, Politecnico di Milano.

I. Babuška, F. Nobile and R. Tempone (2007), 'A stochastic collocation method for elliptic partial differential equations with random input data', *SIAM J. Numer. Anal.* **45**, 1005–1034.

I. Babuška, R. Tempone and G. Zouraris (2004), 'Galerkin finite element approximations of stochastic elliptic partial differential equations', *SIAM J. Numer. Anal.* **42**, 800–825.

S. Badia, F. Nobile and C. Vergara (2008*a*), 'Fluid–structure partitioned procedures based on Robin transmission conditions', *J. Comput. Phys.* **227**, 7027–7051.

S. Badia, F. Nobile and C. Vergara (2009), 'Robin–Robin preconditioned Krylov methods for fluid–structure interaction problems', *Comput. Methods Appl. Mech. Engrg* **198**, 2768–2784.

S. Badia, A. Quaini and A. Quarteroni (2008*b*), 'Modular vs. non-modular preconditioners for fluid–structure systems with large added-mass effect', *Comput. Methods Appl. Mech. Engrg* **197**, 4216–4232.

S. Badia, A. Quaini and A. Quarteroni (2008*c*), 'Splitting methods based on algebraic factorization for fluid–structure interaction', *SIAM J. Sci. Comput.* **30**, 1778–1805.

E. Bagci, Y. Vodovotz, T. Billiar, B. Ermentrout and I. Bahar (2008), 'Computational insights on the competing effects of nitric oxide in regulating apoptosis', *PLOS One* **3**, e2249.

J. Ball (1976), 'Convexity conditions and existence theorems in nonlinear elasticity', *Arch. Rat. Mech. Anal.* **63**, 337–403.

J. Ball (1977), Constitutive inequalities and existence theorems in nonlinear elastostatics. In *Nonlinear Analysis and Mechanics*, Vol. I (R. Knops, ed.), Pitman, pp. 187–241.

F. Ballarin, E. Faggiano, S. Ippolito, A. Manzoni, A. Quarteroni, G. Rozza and R. Scrofani (2016), 'Fast simulations of patient-specific haemodynamics of coronary artery bypass grafts based on a POD–Galerkin method and a vascular shape parametrization', *J. Comput. Phys.* **315**, 609–628.

F. Ballarin, E. Faggiano, A. Manzoni, A. Quarteroni, G. Rozza, S. Ippolito, C. Antona and R. Scrofani (2017), 'Numerical modeling of hemodynamics scenarios of patient-specific coronary artery bypass grafts', *Biomech. Model. Mechanobiol.* **16**, 1373–1399.

D. Balzani, D. Brands, A. Klawonn, O. Rheinbach and J. Schroder (2010), 'On the mechanical modeling of anisotropic biological soft tissue and iterative parallel solution strategies', *Arch. Appl. Mech.* **80**, 479–488.

D. Balzani, P. Neff, J. Schroder and G. Holzapfel (2006), 'A polyconvex framework for soft biological tissues: Adjustment to experimental data', *Int. J. Solids Struct.* **43**, 6052–6070.

H. Banks and K. Kunisch (1989), *Estimation Techniques for Distributed Parameter Systems*, Systems & Control: Foundations & Applications, Birkhäuser.

J. Banks, W. Henshaw and D. Schwendeman (2014), 'An analysis of a new stable partitioned algorithm for FSI problems, I: Incompressible flow and elastic solids', *J. Comput. Phys.* **269**, 108–137.

L. Barbarotta (2014), *A mathematical and numerical study of the left ventricular contraction based on the reconstruction of a patient specific geometry.* MSc thesis, Mathematical Engineering, Politecnico di Milano.

L. Barbarotta, S. Rossi, L. Dede' and A. Quarteroni (2018). 'Numerical validation of a transmurally heterogeneous orthotropic activation model for ventricular contraction', *Internat. J. Numer. Meth. Biomed. Engrg.* **34**, e3137.

A. Barker and X. Cai (2010*a*), 'Scalable parallel methods for monolithic coupling in fluid–structure interaction with application to blood flow modeling', *J. Comput. Phys.* **229**, 642–659.

A. Barker and X. Cai (2010*b*), 'Two-level Newton and hybrid Schwarz preconditioners for fluid–structure interaction', *SIAM J. Sci. Comput.* **32**, 2395–2417.

A. Barnard, W. Hunt, W. Timlake and E. Varley (1966), 'A theory of fluid flow in compliant tubes', *Biophys. J.* **6**, 717–724.

M. Barrault, Y. Maday, N. Nguyen and A. Patera (2004), 'An empirical interpolation method: application to efficient reduced-basis discretization of partial differential equations', *C. R. Math.* **339**(9), 667–672.

J. Bayer, R. Blake, G. Plank and N. Trayanova (2012), 'A novel rule-based algorithm for assigning myocardial fiber orientation to computational heart models', *Ann. Biomed. Engrg* **40**, 2243–2254.

Y. Bazilevs, V. Calo, J. Cottrell, T. Hughes, A. Reali and G. Scovazzi (2007), 'Variational multiscale residual-based turbulence modeling for large eddy simulation of incompressible flows', *Comput. Methods Appl. Mech. Engrg* **197**, 173–201.

Y. Bazilevs, V. Calo, Y. Zhang and T. Hughes (2006), 'Isogeometric fluid–structure interaction analysis with applications to arterial blood flow', *Comput. Mech.* **38**, 310–322.

Y. Bazilevs, J. Gohean, T. Hughes, R. Moser and Y. Zhang (2009), 'Patient-specific isogeometric fluid–structure interaction analysis of thoracic aortic blood flow due to implantation of the Jarvik 2000 left ventricular assist device', *Comput. Methods Appl. Mech. Engrg* **198**, 3534–3550.

Y. Bazilevs, K. Takizawa and T. Tezduyar (2012), *Computational Fluid–Structure Interaction: Methods and Applications*, Wiley.

G. Beeler and H. Reuter (1977), 'Reconstruction of the action potential of ventricular myocardial fibres', *J. Physiol.* **268**, 177–210.

H. Beirão da Veiga (2004), 'On the existence of strong solutions to a coupled fluid–structure evolution problem', *J. Math. Fluid Mech.* **6**, 21–52.

P. Benner, S. Gugercin and K. Willcox (2015), 'A survey of model reduction methods for parametric dynamical systems', *SIAM Review* **57**, 483–531.

J. Bentley and J. Friedman (1979), 'Data structures for range searching', *ACM Comput. Surv.* **11**, 397–409.

M. Benzi, G. Golub and J. Liesen (2005), Numerical solution of saddle point problems. In *Acta Numerica*, Vol. 14, Cambridge University Press, pp. 1–137.

L. Bertagna and A. Veneziani (2014), 'A model reduction approach for the variational estimation of vascular compliance by solving an inverse fluid–structure interaction problem', *Inverse Problems* **30**, 055006.

L. Bertagna, M. D'Elia, M. Perego and A. Veneziani (2014), Data assimilation in cardiovascular fluid–structure interaction problems: An introduction. In *Fluid–Structure Interaction and Biomedical Applications* (T. Bodnár, P. Galdi and Š. Nečasová, eds), Springer, pp. 395–481.

C. Bertoglio, P. Moireau and J.-F. Gerbeau (2012), 'Sequential parameter estimation for fluid–structure problems: Application to hemodynamics', *Int. J. Numer. Methods Biomed. Engrg* **28**, 434–455.

F. Bertrand, P. Tanguy and F. Thibault (1997), 'A three-dimensional fictitious domain method for incompressible fluid flow problems', *Int. J. Numer. Methods Fluids* **25**, 719–736.

R. Bevan, P. Nithiarasu, R. van Loon, I. Sazonov, H. Luckraz and A. Garnham (2010), 'Application of a locally conservative Galerkin (LCG) method for modelling blood flow through a patient-specific carotid bifurcation', *Int. J. Numer. Methods Fluids* **64**, 1274–1295.

J. Biehler, M. Gee and W. Wall (2015), 'Towards efficient uncertainty quantification in complex and large-scale biomechanical problems based on a Bayesian multi-fidelity scheme', *Biomech. Model. Mechanobiol.* **14**, 489–513.

P. Blanco and R. Feijóo (2013), 'A dimensionally-heterogeneous closed-loop model for the cardiovascular system and its applications', *Med. Engrg Phys.* **35**, 652–667.

P. Blanco, S. Deparis and A. Malossi (2013), 'On the continuity of mean total normal stress in geometrical multiscale cardiovascular problems', *J. Comput. Phys.* **51**, 136–155.

P. Blanco, R. Feijóo and S. Urquiza (2007), 'A unified variational approach for coupling 3D–1D models and its blood flow applications', *Comput. Methods Appl. Mech. Engrg* **196**, 4391–4410.

P. Blanco, M. Pivello, S. Urquiza and R. Feijóo (2009), 'On the potentialities of 3D–1D coupled models in hemodynamics simulations', *J. Biomech.* **42**, 919–930.

P. Blanco, S. Watanabe and R. Feijóo (2012), 'Identification of vascular territory resistances in one-dimensional hemodynamics simulations', *J. Biomech.* **45**, 2066–2073.

P. Blanco, S. Watanabe, M. Passos, P. Lemos, R. Feijóo *et al.* (2015), 'An anatomically detailed arterial network model for one-dimensional computational hemodynamics', *IEEE Trans. Biomed. Engrg* **62**, 736–753.

J. Blum, F.-X. Le Dimet and I. Navon (2009), Data assimilation for geophysical fluids. In *Handbook of Numerical Analysis*, Vol. 14: *Computational Methods for the Atmosphere and the Oceans* (R. Temam and J. Tribbia, eds), Elsevier, pp. 385–441.

T. Bodnár, G. Galdi and Š. Nečasová (2014), *Fluid–Structure Interaction and Biomedical Applications*, Springer.

J. Boese, M. Bock, S. Schoenberg and L. Schad (2000), 'Estimation of aortic compliance using magnetic resonance pulse wave velocity measurement', *Phys. Med. Biol.* **45**, 1703–1713.

D. Boffi and L. Gastaldi (2003), 'A finite element approach for the immersed boundary method', *Comput. Struct.* **81**, 491–501.

D. Boffi, F. Brezzi and M. Fortin (2013), *Mixed Finite Element Methods and Applications*, Springer.

D. Boffi, L. Gastaldi and L. Heltai (2007), 'Numerical stability of the finite element immersed boundary method', *Math. Models Methods Appl. Sci.* **17**, 1479–1505.

D. Boffi, L. Gastaldi, L. Heltai and C. Peskin (2008), 'On the hyper-elastic formulation of the immersed boundary method', *Comput. Methods Appl. Mech. Engrg* **197**, 2210–2231.

E. Boileau, P. Nithiarasu, P. Blanco, L. Muller, F. Fossan, L. Hellevik, W. Donders, W. Huberts, M. Willemet and J. Alastruey (2015), 'A benchmark study of numerical schemes for one-dimensional arterial blood flow modelling', *Int. J. Numer. Methods Biomed. Engrg* **31**, e02732.

C. Boldak, Y. Rolland and C. Toumoulin (2003), 'An improved model-based vessel tracking algorithm with application to computed tomography angiography', *Biocybern. Biomed.* **23**, 41–63.

D. Bonomi, A. Manzoni and A. Quarteroni (2017), 'A matrix DEIM technique for model reduction of nonlinear parametrized problems in cardiac mechanics' *Comput. Methods Appl. Mech. Engrg* **324**, 300–326.

D. Bonomi, C. Vergara, E. Faggiano, M. Stevanella, C. Conti, A. Redaelli, G. Puppini, G. Faggian, L. Formaggia and G. Luciani (2015), 'Influence of the aortic valve leaflets on the fluid-dynamics in aorta in presence of a normally functioning bicuspid valve', *Biomech. Model. Mechanobiol.* **6**, 1349–1361.

I. Borazjani, L. Ge and F. Sotiropoulos (2008), 'Curvilinear immersed boundary method for simulating fluid structure interaction with complex 3D rigid bodies', *J. Comput. Phys.* **227**, 7587–7620.

R. Bordas, K. Gillow, D. Gavaghan, B. Rodríguez and D. Kay (2012), 'A bidomain model of the ventricular specialized conduction system of the heart', *SIAM J. Appl. Math.* **72**, 1618–1643.

A. Borzì and V. Schulz (2011), *Computational Optimization of Systems Governed by Partial Differential Equations*, SIAM.

M. Boulakia, M. Fernández, J.-F. Gerbeau and N. Zemzemi (2008), 'Direct and inverse problems in electrocardiography', *AIP Conference Proceedings* **1048**, 113–117.

M. Boulakia, E. Schenone and J.-F. Gerbeau (2012), 'Reduced-order modeling for cardiac electrophysiology. application to parameter identification', *Int. J. Numer. Meth. Biomed. Engrg* **28**, 727–744.

Y. Bourgault, Y. Coudière and C. Pierre (2006), 'Existence and uniqueness of the solution for the bidomain model used in cardiac electrophysiology', *Nonlinear Analysis: Real World Applications* **10**, 458–482.

Y. Bourgault, M. Ethier and V. LeBlanc (2003), 'Simulation of electrophysiological waves with an unstructured finite element method', *ESAIM Math. Model. Numer. Anal.* **37**, 649–661.

M. Boyett, J. Frampton and M. Kirby (1991), 'The length, width and volume of isolated rat and ferret ventricular myocytes during twitch contractions and changes in osmotic strength', *Experimental Phys.* **76**, 259-270.

A. Brault, L. Dumas and D. Lucor (2016), 'Uncertainty quantification of inflow boundary condition and proximal arterial stiffness-coupled effect on pulse wave propagation in a vascular network', *Int. J. Numer. Methods Biomed. Engrg.* https://doi.org/10.1002/cnm.2859

S. Brenner and R. Scott (2008), *The Mathematical Theory of Finite Element Methods*, Springer.

A. Brooks and T. Hughes (1982), 'Streamline upwind/Petrov-Galerkin formulations for convective dominated flows with particular emphasis on the incompressible Navier-Stokes equations', *Comput. Methods Appl. Mech. Engrg.* **32**, 199–259.

A. Bueno-Orovio, E. Cherry and F. Fenton (2008), 'Minimal model for human ventricular action potentials in tissue', *J. Theoret. Biol.* **3**, 544–560.

E. Burman and M. Fernández (2009), 'Stabilization of explicit coupling in fluid–structure interaction involving fluid incompressibility', *Comput. Methods Appl. Mech. Engrg* **198**, 766–784.

E. Burman and M. Fernández (2014), 'An unfitted Nitsche method for incompressible fluid–structure interaction using overlapping meshes', *Comput. Methods Appl. Mech. Engrg* **279**, 497–514.

E. Burman, S. Claus, P. Hansbo, M. Larson and A. Massing (2015), 'CutFEM: Discretizing geometry and partial differential equations', *Int. J. Numer. Methods Engrg* **104**, 472–501.

I. Campbell, J. Ries, S. Dhawan, A. Quyyumi, W. Taylor and J. Oshinski (2012), 'Effect of inlet velocity profiles on patient-specific computational fluid dynamics simulations of the carotid bifurcation', *J. Biomech. Engrg* **134**, 051001.

T. Carew, R. Vaishnav and D. Patel (1968), 'Compressibility of the arterial wall', *Circ. Res.* **23**, 61–68.

K. Carlberg, C. Farhat, J. Cortial and D. Amsallem (2013), 'The GNAT method for nonlinear model reduction: effective implementation and application to computational fluid dynamics and turbulent flows', *J. Comput. Phys.*, **242**, 623–647.

J. Carr, W. Fright and R. Beatson (1997), 'Surface interpolation with radial basis functions for medical imaging', *IEEE Trans. Med. Imaging* **16**, 96–107.

P. Causin, J.-F. Gerbeau and F. Nobile (2005), 'Added-mass effect in the design of partitioned algorithms for fluid–structure problems', *Comput. Methods Appl. Mech. Engrg* **194**, 4506–4527.

I. Celik, U. Ghia, P. Roache, C. Freitas, H. Coleman and P. Raad (2008), 'Procedure for estimation and reporting of uncertainty due to discretization in CFD applications', *J. Fluids Engrg: Trans. ASME* **130**, 078001.

R. Chabiniok, P. Moireau, P.-F. Lesault, A. Rahmouni, J.-F. Deux and D. Chapelle (2012), 'Estimation of tissue contractility from cardiac cine-MRI using a biomechanical heart model', *Biomech. Model. Mechanobiol.* **11**, 609–630.

R. Chabiniok, V. Wang, M. Hadjicharalambous, L. Asner, J. Lee, M. Sermesant, E. Kuhl, A. Young, P. Moireau, M. Nash, D. Chapelle and D. Nordsletten (2016), 'Multiphysics and multiscale modelling, data–model fusion and integration of organ physiology in the clinic: Ventricular cardiac mechanics', *Interface Focus* **6**, 20150083.

D. Chapelle, M. Fragu, V. Mallet and P. Moireau (2013*a*), 'Fundamental principles of data assimilation underlying the Verdandi library: Applications to biophysical model personalization within euHeart', *Med. Biol. Engrg Comput.* **51**, 1221–1233.

D. Chapelle, A. Gariah, P. Moireau and J. Sainte-Marie (2013*b*), 'A Galerkin strategy with proper orthogonal decomposition for parameter-dependent problems: Analysis, assessments and applications to parameter estimation', *ESAIM Math. Model. Numer. Anal.* **47**, 1821–1843.

J. Charonko, R. Kumar, K. Stewart, W. Little and P. Vlachos (2013), 'Vortices formed on the mitral valve tips aid normal left ventricular filling', *Ann. Biomed. Engrg* **41**, 1049–1061.

S. Chaturantabut and S. Sorensen (2010), 'Nonlinear model reduction via Discrete Empirical Interpolation', *SIAM J. Sci. Comput.* **32**, 2737–2764.

G. Chavent (2010), *Nonlinear Least Squares for Inverse Problems: Theoretical Foundations and Step-by-Step Guide for Applications*, Scientific Computation, Springer.

J. Chen, X.-Y. Lu and W. Wang (2006), 'Non-Newtonian effects of blood flow on hemodynamics in distal vascular graft anastomoses', *J. Biomech.* **39**, 1983–1995.

P. Chen and C. Schwab (2015), 'Sparse-grid, reduced-basis Bayesian inversion', *Comput. Methods Appl. Mech. Engrg* **297**, 84–115.

P. Chen, A. Quarteroni and G. Rozza (2013), 'Simulation-based uncertainty quantification of human arterial network hemodynamics', *Int. J. Numer. Methods Biomed. Engrg* **29**, 698–721.

L. Cheng, J. Bodley and A. Pullan (2003), 'Comparison of potential- and activation-based formulations for the inverse problem of electrocardiology', *IEEE Trans. Biomed. Engrg* **50**, 11–22.

A. Cheng, F. Langer, F. Rodriguez, J.C. Criscione, G.T. Daughters, D.C. Miller and N.B. Ingels (2005), 'Transmural cardiac strains in the lateral wall of the ovine left ventricle', *Americ. J. Phys.-Heart Circ. Phys.* **288**, H1546-H1556.

Y. Cheng, H. Oertel and T. Schenkel (2005), 'Fluid–structure coupled CFD simulation of the left ventricular flow during filling phase', *Ann. Biomed. Engrg* **5**, 567–576.

C. Cherubini, S. Filippi, P. Nardinocchi and L. Teresi (2008), 'An electromechanical model of cardiac tissue: Constitutive issues and electrophysiological effects', *Prog. Biophys. Molec. Biol.* **2–3**, 562–573.

S. Cheung, K. K. L. Wong, G. H. Yeoh, W. Yang, J. Tu, R. Beare and T. Phan (2010), 'Experimental and numerical study on the hemodynamics of stenosed carotid bifurcation', *Australas. Phys. Engrg Sci. Med.* **33**, 319–328.

P. Chinchapatnam, K. Rhode, M. Ginks, C. Rinaldi, P. Lambiase, R. Razavi, S. Arridge and M. Sermesant (2008), 'Model-based imaging of cardiac apparent conductivity and local conduction velocity for diagnosis and planning of therapy', *IEEE Trans. Med. Imaging* **27**, 1631–1642.

J. Ching, J. Beck and K. Porter (2006), 'Bayesian state and parameter estimation of uncertain dynamical systems', *Probab. Engrg Mech.* **21**, 81–96.

C. Chnafa, S. Mendez and F. Nicoud (2014), 'Image-based large-eddy simulation in a realistic left heart', *Comput. Fluids* **94**, 173–187.

Y. Choi, J. Constantino, V. Vedula, N. Trayanova and R. Mittal (2015), 'A new MRI-based model of heart function with coupled hemodynamics and application to normal and diseased canine left ventricles', *Front. Bioeng. Biotechnol.* **3**, 140.

A. Chorin (1968), 'Numerical solution of the Navier–Stokes equations', *Math. Comp.* **22**, 745–762.

J. Chung and G. Hulbert (1993), 'A time integration algorithm for structural dynamics with improved numerical dissipation: The generalized-$\alpha$ method', *Trans. ASME J. Appl. Mech.* **60**, 371–375.

P. Ciarlet (1988), *Mathematical Elasticity*, Vol. 1: *Three Dimensional Elasticity*, Elsevier Science.

P. Ciarlet (2000), *Mathematical Elasticity*, Vol. 3: *Theory of Shells*, Elsevier Science.

P. Ciarlet (1978), *The Finite Element Method for Elliptic Problems*, NorthHolland, Amsterdam.

P. Ciarlet and J. Necas (1985), 'Unilateral problems in nonlinear, three-dimensional elasticity', *Arch. Rat. Mech. Anal.* **87**, 319–338.

S. Cimino, G. Pedrizzetti, G. Tonti, E. Canali, V. Petronilli, L. De Luca, C. Iacoboni and L. Agati (2012), 'In vivo analysis of intraventricular fluid dynamics in healthy hearts', *Europ. J. Mech. B/Fluids* **35**, 40–46.

R. Clayton and A. Panfilov (2008), 'A guide to modelling cardiac electrical activity in anatomically detailed ventricles', *Prog. Biophys. Molec. Biol.* **96**, 19–43.

R. Clayton, O. Bernus, E. Cherry, H. Dierckx, F. Fenton, L. Mirabella, A. Panfilov, F. Sachse, G. Seemann and H. Zhang (2011), 'Models of cardiac tissue electrophysiology: Progress, challenges and open questions', *Prog. Biophys. Molec. Biol.* **104**, 22–48.

C. Cocosco, T. Netsch, J. Sénégas, D. Bystrov, W. Niessen and M. Viergever (2004), Automatic cardiac region-of-interest computation in cine 3D structural MRI. In *Computer Assisted Radiology and Surgery: Proceedings of the 18th International Congress and Exhibition*, Vol. 1268 of International Congress Series, Elsevier, pp. 1126–1131.

R. Codina and S. Badia (2006), 'On some pressure segregation methods of fractional-step type for the finite element approximation of incompressible flow problems', *Comput. Methods Appl. Mech. Engrg* **195**, 2900–2918.

A. Cohen and R. DeVore (2015), Approximation of high-dimensional parametric PDEs. In *Acta Numerica*, Vol. 24, Cambridge University Press, pp. 1–159.

C. Colciago, S. Deparis and A. Quarteroni (2014), 'Comparisons between reduced order models and full 3D models for fluid–structure interaction problems in haemodynamics', *J. Comput. Appl. Math.* **2754**, 120–138.

P. Colli Franzone and L. Guerri (1993), 'Spreading excitation in 3-D models of the anisotropic cardiac tissue I: Validation of the Eikonal model', *Math. Biosci.* **113**, 145–209.

P. Colli Franzone and L. Pavarino (2004), 'A parallel solver for reaction-diffusion systems in computational electrocardiology', *Math. Models Methods Appl. Sci.* **14**, 883–911.

P. Colli Franzone and G. Savaré (2002), Degenerate evolution systems modeling the cardiac electric field at micro- and macroscopic level. In *Evolution Equa-*

*tions, Semigroups and Functional Analysis: In Memory of Brunello Terreni* (A. Lorenzi and B. Ruf, eds), Birkhäuser, pp. 49–78.

P. Colli Franzone, L. Guerri and S. Rovida (1990), 'Wavefront propagation in an activation model of the anisotropic cardiac tissue: Asymptotic analysis and numerical simulations', *J. Math. Biol.* **28**, 121–176.

P. Colli Franzone, L. Guerri, C. Viganotti and B. Taccardi (1985), 'Finite element approximation of regularized solution of the inverse potential problem of electrocardiography and applications to experimental data', *Calcolo* **12**, 91–186.

P. Colli Franzone, L. Pavarino and S. Scacchi (2014), *Mathematical Cardiac Electrophysiology*, Springer.

P. Colli Franzone, L. Pavarino and S. Scacchi (2016), 'Bioelectrical effects of mechanical feedbacks in a strongly coupled cardiac electro-mechanical model', *Math. Models Methods Appl. Sci.* **26**, 27–57.

P. Colli Franzone, L. Pavarino and B. Taccardi (2005), 'Simulating patterns of excitation, repolarization and action potential duration with cardiac bidomain and monodomain models', *Math. Biosci.* **197**, 35–66.

P. Colli Franzone, B. Taccardi and C. Viganotti (1978), 'An approach to inverse calculation of epicardial potentials from body surface maps', *Adv. Cardiol.* **21**, 50–54.

A. Collin, J.-F. Gerbeau, M. Hocini, M. Haïssaguerre and D. Chapelle (2013), 'Surface-based electrophysiology modeling and assessment of physiological simulations in atria'. In *International Conference on Functional Imaging and Modeling of the Heart*, pages 352-359, Springer, Berlin and Heidelberg.

C. Corrado, J.-F. Gerbeau and P. Moireau (2015), 'Identification of weakly coupled multiphysics problems: Application to the inverse problem of electrocardiography', *J. Comput. Phys.* **283**, 271–298.

K. Costa, J. Holmes and A. McCulloch (2001), 'Modelling cardiac mechanical properties in three dimensions', *Phil. Trans. Royal Soc.* A **359**, 1233–1250.

J.A. Cottrell, T.J.R. Hughes and Y. Bazilevs (2009), *Isogeometric Analysis: Toward Integration of CAD and FEA*, John Wiley & Sons.

M. Courtemanche, R.J. Ramirez and S. Nattel (1998), 'Ionic mechanisms underlying human atrial action potential properties: insights from a mathematical model', *American J. Phys.-Heart Circ. Phys.* **275**, H301–H321.

R. Crochiere and L.R. Rabiner (1983), *Multirate Digital Signal Processing*, Prentice–Hall.

P. Crosetto, S. Deparis, G. Fourestey and A. Quarteroni (2011), 'Parallel algorithms for fluid–structure interaction problems in haemodynamics', *SIAM J. Sci. Comput.* **33**, 1598–1622.

T. Cui, Y. Marzouk and K. Willcox (2015), 'Data-driven model reduction for the Bayesian solution of inverse problems', *Int. J. Numer. Methods Engrg* **102**, 966–990.

B. Dacorogna (2000), *Direct Methods in the Calculus of Variations*, Vol. 78 of Applied Mathematical Sciences, Springer.

H. Dal, S. Göktepe, M. Kaliske and E. Kuhl (2013), 'A fully implicit finite element method for bidomain models of cardiac electromechanics', *Comput. Methods Appl. Mech. Engrg* **253**, 323–336.

L. Dalong, A. Robertson, G. Lin and M. Lovell (2012) 'Finite element modeling of cerebral angioplasty using a structural multi-mechanism anisotropic damage model', *Int. J. Numer. Methods in Engrg* **92**, 457–474.

C. D'Angelo (2007), *Multiscale Modelling of Metabolism and Transport Phenomena in Living Tissues.* PhD thesis, Ecole Polytechnique Fédérale de Lausanne.

J. Degroote (2011), 'On the similarity between Dirichlet–Neumann with interface artificial compressibility and Robin–Neumann schemes for the solution of fluid–structure interaction problems', *J. Comput. Phys.* **230**, 6399–6403.

J. Degroote and J. Vierendeels (2011), 'Multi-solver algorithms for the partitioned simulation of fluid–structure interaction', *Comput. Methods Appl. Mech. Engrg* **25–28**, 2195–2210.

J. Degroote, A. Swillens, P. Bruggeman, Haelterman, P. Segers and J. Vierendeels (2010), 'Simulation of fluid–structure interaction with the interface artificial compressibility method', *Int. J. Numer. Methods Biomed. Engrg* **26**, 276–289.

M. D'Elia and A. Veneziani (2013), 'Uncertainty quantification for data assimilation in a steady incompressible Navier–Stokes problem', *ESAIM Math. Model. Numer. Anal.* **47**, 1037–1057.

M. D'Elia, M. Perego and A. Veneziani (2012), 'A variational data assimilation procedure for the incompressible Navier–Stokes equations in hemodynamics', *J. Sci. Comput.* **52**, 340–359.

H. Delingette, F. Billet, K. Wong, M. Sermesant, K. Rhode, M. Ginks, C. Rinaldi, R. Razavi and N. Ayache (2012), 'Personalization of cardiac motion and contractility from images using variational data assimilation', *IEEE Trans. Biomed. Engrg* **59**, 20–24.

S. Deparis (2004), *Numerical Analysis of Axisymmetric Flows and Methods for Fluid–Structure Interaction arising in Blood Flow Simulation.* PhD thesis, Ecole Polytechnique Fédérale de Lausanne.

S. Deparis, M. Discacciati, G. Fourestey and A. Quarteroni (2006), 'Fluid–structure algorithms based on Steklov–Poincaré operators', *Comput. Methods Appl. Mech. Engrg* **195**, 5797–5812.

S. Deparis, D. Forti, G. Grandperrin and A. Quarteroni (2016), 'FaCSI: A block parallel preconditioner for fluid–structure interaction in hemodynamics', *J. Comput. Phys.*, 700–718.

S. Deparis, G. Grandperrin and A. Quarteroni (2014), 'Parallel preconditioners for the unsteady Navier–Stokes equations and applications to hemodynamics simulations', *Comput. Fluids* **92**, 253–273.

M.D. De Tullio, A. Cristallo, E. Balaras and R. Verzicco (2009) 'Direct numerical simulation of the pulsatile flow through an aortic bileaflet mechanical heart valve', *J. Fluid Mech.* **622**, 259–290.

J. Dick, F. Kuo and I. Sloan (2013), High-dimensional integration: The quasi-Monte Carlo way. In *Acta Numerica*, Vol. 22, Cambridge University Press, pp. 133–288.

D. DiFrancesco (1993), 'Pacemaker mechanisms in cardiac tissue', *Annu. Rev. Physiol.* **55**, 455–472.

D. DiFrancesco and D. Noble (1985), 'A model of cardiac electrical activity incorporating ionic pumps and concentration changes', *Phil. Trans. Royal Soc. B* **307**, 353–398.

M. Dihlmann and B. Haasdonk (2016), 'A reduced basis Kalman filter for parametrized partial differential equations', *ESAIM Control Optim. Calc. Var.* **22**, 625–669.

H. Do, A. A. Owida, W. Yang and Y. Morsi (2011), 'Numerical simulation of the haemodynamics in end-to-side anastomoses', *Int. J. Numer. Methods Fluids* **67**, 638–650.

C. Dohrmann and O. Widlund (2009), 'An overlapping Schwarz algorithm for almost incompressible elasticity', *SIAM J. Numer. Anal.* **4**, 8811–8823.

S. Dokos, B. Smaill, A. Young and I. LeGrice (2002), 'Shear properties of passive ventricular myocardium', *Amer. J. Physiol.* **283**, H2650–H2659.

F. Domenichini, G. Pedrizzetti and B. Baccani, (2005) 'Three-dimensional filling flow into a model left ventricle', *J. Fluid Mech.* **539**, 179–198.

W. Donders, W. Huberts, F. van de Vosse and T. Delhaas (2015), 'Personalization of models with many model parameters: An efficient sensitivity analysis approach', *Int. J. Numer. Methods Biomed. Engrg* **31**, e02727.

J. Donea (1982), 'An arbitrary Lagrangian–Eulerian finite element method for transient dynamic fluid–structure interaction', *Comput. Methods Appl. Mech. Engrg* **33**, 689–723.

O. Dössel, D. Farina, M. Mohr, M. Reumann, G. Seemann and L.D. Weiss (2007), Modelling and imaging electrophysiology and contraction of the heart. In *Advances in Medical Engineering* (T.M. Buzug, D. Holz, J. Bongartz, M. Kohl-Bareis, U. Hartmann and S. Weber, eds), Springer.

O. Dössel and A. Loewe (2017), 'Computerized modeling of the human heart', *Zeitschrift für Medizinische Physik*, **27**, 167–169.

O. Dur, S. Coskun, K. Coskun, D. Frakes, L. Kara and K. Pekkan (2011), 'Computer-aided patient-specific coronary artery graft design improvements using CFD coupled shape optimizer', *Cardiovasc. Engr. Tech.* pp. 1–13.

D. Durrer, R. van Dam, G. Freud, M. Janse, F. Meijler and R. Arzbaecher (1970), 'Total excitation of the isolated human heart', *Circulation* **41**, 899–912.

V. Eck, W. Donders, J. Sturdy, J. Feinberg, T. Delhaas, L. Hellevik and W. Huberts (2016), 'A guide to uncertainty quantification and sensitivity analysis for cardiovascular applications', *Int. J. Numer. Methods Biomed. Engrg* **32**, e02755.

D. Einstein, K. Kunzelman, P. Reinhall, M. Nicosia and R. Cochran (2005), 'The effects of cellular contraction on aortic valve leaflet flexural stiffness', *J. Heart Valve Disease* **14**, 376–385.

C. Eitel, G. Hindricks, N. Dagres, P. Sommer and C. Piorkowski (2010), 'EnSite Velocity$^{\mathrm{TM}}$ cardiac mapping system: A new platform for 3D mapping of cardiac arrhythmias', *Expert Rev. Med. Devices* **7**, 185–192.

H. Elman and D. Silvester (1996), 'Fast nonsymmetric iterations and preconditioning for Navier–Stokes equations', *SIAM J. Sci. Comput.* **17**, 33–46.

H. Elman, D. Silvester and A. Wathen (2005), *Finite Elements and Fast Iterative Solvers*, Oxford Science Publications.

G. Enden and A. Popel (1992), 'A numerical study of the shape of the surface separating flow into branches in microvascular bifurcations', *J. Biomech. Engrg* **114**, 398–405.

T. Eriksson, A. Prassl, G. Plank and G. Holzapfel (2013), 'Modeling the dispersion in electromechanically coupled myocardium', *Int. J. Numer. Methods Biomed. Engrg* **29**, 1267–1284.

A. Ern and J.L.. Guermond (2004), *Theory and Practice of Finite Elements*, Springer.

O. Ernst, B. Sprungk and H.-J. Starkloff (2014), Bayesian inverse problems and Kalman filters. In *Extraction of Quantifiable Information from Complex Systems*, Vol. 102 of Lecture Notes in Computational Science and Engineering, Springer, pp. 133–159.

V. Ervin and H. Lee (2007), 'Numerical approximation of a quasi-Newtonian Stokes flow problem with defective boundary conditions', *SIAM J. Numer. Anal.* **45**, 2120–2140.

C. Ethier, D. Steinman, X. Zhang, S. Karpik and M. Ojha (1998), 'Flow waveform effects on end-to-side anastomotic flow patterns', *J. Biomech.* **31**, 609–617.

M. Ethier and Y. Bourgault (2008), 'Semi-implicit time-discretization schemes for the bidomain model', *SIAM J. Numer. Anal.* **5**, 2443–2468.

L. Euler (1775), Principia pro motu sanguinis per arterias determinando. In *Opera posthuma mathematica et physica anno 1844 detecta, editerunt P. H. Fuss et N. Fuss, Petropoli, apud Eggers et socios*, Vol. 1, pp. 814–823.

G. Evensen (1994), 'Sequential data assimilation with a nonlinear quasi-geostrophic model using Monte Carlo methods to forecast error statistics', *J. Geophys. Res.* **9**, 10143–10162.

G. Evensen (2003), 'The ensemble Kalman filter: Theoretical formulation and practical implementation', *Ocean Dynamics* **53**, 343–367.

G. Evensen (2009), 'The ensemble Kalman filter for combined state and parameter estimation', *IEEE Control Syst. Mag.* **29**, 83–104.

A. Fabbri, M. Fantini, R. Wilders and S. Severi (2017), 'Computational analysis of the human sinus node action potential: model development and effects of mutations', *J. Phys.* **595**, 2365–2396.

E. Faggiano, A. Antiga, G. Puppini, A. Quarteroni, G. Luciani and C. Vergara (2013), 'Helical flows and asymmetry of blood jet in dilated ascending aorta with normally functioning bicuspid valve', *Biomech. Model. Mechanobiol.* **4**, 801–813.

E. Faggiano, T. Lorenzi and A. Quarteroni (2014), 'Metal artefact reduction in computed tomography images by a fourth-order total variation flow', *Comput. Methods Biomech. Biomed. Engrg: Imaging & Visualization* **3-4**, 202–213.

C. Farhat and F. Roux (1991), 'A method of finite element tearing and interconnecting and its parallel solution algorithm', *Int. J. Numer. Methods Engrg* **32**, 1205–1227.

A. Fasano, R. Santos and A. Sequeira (2012), Blood coagulation: A puzzle for biologists, a maze for mathematicians. Chapter 3 in *Modeling of Physiological Flows* (D. Ambrosi, A. Quarteroni and G. Rozza, eds), Springer, pp. 41–75.

A. Fasano and A. Sequeira (2017), *Hemomath. The Mathematics of Blood*, MS & A Series, Springer.

M. Fedele, E. Faggiano, L. Barbarotta, F. Cremonesi, L. Formaggia and S. Perotto (2015), Semi-automatic three-dimensional vessel segmentation using a connected component localization of the region-scalable fitting energy. In *2015 9th International Symposium on Image and Signal Processing and Analysis (ISPA)*, IEEE, pp. 72–77.

M. Fedele, E. Faggiano, L. Dede' and A. Quarteroni (2017), 'A patient-specific aortic valve model based on moving resistive immersed implicit surfaces', *Biomech. Model. Mechanobiol.* **16**, 1779–1803.

F. Fenton and A. Karma (1998), 'Vortex dynamics in three-dimensional continuous myocardium with fiber rotation: Filament instability and fibrillation', *Chaos* **8**, 20–47.

M. Fernández (2013), 'Incremental displacement-correction schemes for incompressible fluid–structure interaction: Stability and convergence analysis', *Numer. Math.* **123**, 21–65.

M. Fernández and M. Moubachir (2005), 'A Newton method using exact Jacobians for solving fluid–structure coupling', *Comput. Struct.* **83**, 127–142.

M. Fernández and N. Zemzemi (2010), 'Decoupled time-marching schemes in computational cardiac electrophysiology and ECG numerical simulation', *Math. Biosci.* **226**, 58–75.

M. Fernández, J.-F. Gerbeau and C. Grandmont (2007), 'A projection semi-implicit scheme for the coupling of an elastic structure with an incompressible fluid', *Int. J. Numer. Methods Engrg* **69**, 794–821.

M. Fernández, V. Milisic and A. Quarteroni (2005), 'Analysis of a geometrical multiscale blood flow model based on the coupling of ODEs and hyperbolic PDEs', *Multiscale Model. Simul.* **4**, 215–236.

C. Figueroa, I. Vignon-Clementel, K. Jansen, T. Hughes and C. Taylor (2006), 'A coupled momentum method for modeling blood flow in three-dimensional deformable arteries', *Comput. Methods Appl. Mech. Engrg* **195**, 5685–5706.

L. Fin and R. Grebe (2003), 'Three dimensional modeling of the cerebrospinal fluid dynamics and brain interactions in the aqueduct of sylvius', *Comput. Methods Biomech. Biomed. Engrg* **3**, 163–170.

P. Fischer, F. Loth, S. Lee, S. Lee, D. Smith and H. Bassiouny (2007), 'Simulation of high-Reynolds number vascular flows', *Comput. Methods Appl. Mech. Engrg* **196**, 3049–3060.

G. Fishman (1996), *Monte Carlo: Concepts, Algorithms, and Applications*, Springer Series in Operations Research and Financial Engineering, Springer.

R. FitzHugh (1961), 'Impulses and physiological states in theoretical models of nerve membrane', *Biophys. J.* **1**, 445–466.

L. Formaggia and C. Vergara (2012), 'Prescription of general defective boundary conditions in fluid-dynamics', *Milan J. Math.* **80**, 333–350.

L. Formaggia, J.-F. Gerbeau, F. Nobile and A. Quarteroni (2001), 'On the coupling of 3D and 1D Navier–Stokes equations for flow problems in compliant vessels', *Comput. Methods Appl. Mech. Engrg* **191**, 561–582.

L. Formaggia, J.-F. Gerbeau, F. Nobile and A. Quarteroni (2002), 'Numerical treatment of defective boundary conditions for the Navier–Stokes equation', *SIAM J. Numer. Anal.* **40**, 376–401.

L. Formaggia, D. Lamponi and A. Quarteroni (2003), 'One-dimensional models for blood flow in arteries', *J. Engrg Math.* **47**, 251–276.

L. Formaggia, A. Moura and F. Nobile (2007), 'On the stability of the coupling of 3D and 1D fluid–structure interaction models for blood flow simulations', *M2AN Math. Model. Numer. Anal.* **41**, 743–769.

L. Formaggia, F. Nobile, A. Quarteroni and A. Veneziani (1999), 'Multiscale modelling of the circulatory system: A preliminary analysis', *Comput. Vis. Sci.* **2**, 75–83.

L. Formaggia, A. Quarteroni and A. Veneziani, eds (2009*a*), *Cardiovascular Mathematics: Modeling and Simulation of the Circulatory System*, Springer.

L. Formaggia, A. Quarteroni and C. Vergara (2013), 'On the physical consistency between three-dimensional and one-dimensional models in haemodynamics', *J. Comput. Phys.* **244**, 97–112.

L. Formaggia, A. Veneziani and C. Vergara (2008), 'A new approach to numerical solution of defective boundary value problems in incompressible fluid dynamics', *SIAM J. Numer. Anal.* **46**, 2769–2794.

L. Formaggia, A. Veneziani and C. Vergara (2009*b*), 'Flow rate boundary problems for an incompressible fluid in deformable domains: Formulations and solution methods', *Comput. Methods Appl. Mech. Engrg* **199**, 677–688.

M. Fornefett, K. Rohr and H. Stiehl (2001), 'Radial basis functions with compact support for elastic registration of medical images', *Image Vision Comput.* **19**, 87–96.

C. Forster, W. Wall and E. Ramm (2007), 'Artificial added mass instabilities in sequential staggered coupling of nonlinear structures and incompressible viscous flow', *Comput. Methods Appl. Mech. Engrg* **196**, 1278–1293.

D. Forti and L. Dede' (2015), 'Semi-implicit BDF time discretization of the Navier–Stokes equations with VMS-LES modeling in a high performance computing framework', *Comput. Fluids* **117**, 168–182.

A. Frangi, W. Niessen, R. Hoogeveen, T. van Walsum and M. Viergever (1999), 'Model-based quantitation of 3-D magnetic resonance angiographic images', *IEEE Trans. Med. Imaging* **18**, 946–956.

D. Frazier, W. Krassowska, P. Chen, P. Wolf, N. Danieley, W. Smith and R. Ideker (1988), 'Transmural activations and stimulus potentials in three-dimensional anisotropic canine myocardium', *Circ. Res.* **63**, 135–146.

T. Fritz, C. Wieners, G. Seemann, H. Steen and O. Dössel (2014), 'Simulation of the contraction of the ventricles in a human heart model including atria and pericardium', *Biomech. Model. Mechanobiol.* **13**, 627–641.

Y. Fung (1993), *Biomechanics: Mechanical Properties of Living Tissues*, Springer.

Y. C. Fung, K. Fronek and P. Patitucci (1979), 'Pseudoelasticity of arteries and the choice of its mathematical expression', *Amer. J. Physiol.* **237**, H620–H631.

K. Galvin and H. Lee (2013), 'Analysis and approximation of the cross model for quasi-Newtonian flows with defective boundary conditions', *Appl. Math. Comput.* **222**, 244–254.

K. Galvin, H. Lee and L. Rebholz (2012), 'Approximation of viscoelastic flows with defective boundary conditions', *J. Non-Newton. Fluid Mech.* **169/170**, 104–113.

M. Gee, U. Kuttler and W. Wall (2011), 'Truly monolithic algebraic multigrid for fluid–structure interaction', *Int. J. Numer. Methods Engrg* **85**, 987–1016.

R. van der Geest, E. Jansen, V. Buller and J. Reiber (1994), Automated detection of left ventricular epi- and endocardial contours in short-axis MR images. In *Computers in Cardiology 1994*, IEEE, pp. 33–36.

B. Geiger (1993), Three-dimensional modeling of human organs and its application to diagnosis and surgical planning. Technical Report RR-2105, INRIA.

S. Geneser, R. Kirby and R. MacLeod (2008), 'Application of stochastic finite element methods to study the sensitivity of ECG forward modeling to organ conductivity', *IEEE Trans. Biomed. Engrg* **55**, 31–40.

L. Gerardo-Giorda, L. Mirabella, F. Nobile, M. Perego and A. Veneziani (2009), 'A model-based block-triangular preconditioner for the bidomain system in electrocardiology', *J. Comput. Phys.* **228**, 3625–3639.

L. Gerardo-Giorda, F. Nobile and C. Vergara (2010), 'Analysis and optimization of Robin–Robin partitioned procedures in fluid–structure interaction problems', *SIAM J. Numer. Anal.* **48**, 2091–2116.

J.-F. Gerbeau, D. Lombardi and E. Schenone (2015), 'Reduced order model in cardiac electrophysiology with approximated lax pairs', *Adv. Comput. Math.* **41**, 1103–1130.

A. Gerbi (2018), *Numerical Approximation of Cardiac Electro-fluid-mechanical Models: Coupling Strategies for Large-scale Simulation*. PhD thesis, École Polytechnique Fédérale de Lausanne.

A. Gerbi, L. Dede' and A. Quarteroni (2018), 'A monolithic algorithm for the simulation of cardiac electromechanics in the human left ventricle', *Math. in Engrg.* **1**, 1–46.

A. Gerbi, L. Dede' and A. Quarteroni (2018), 'Segregated algorithms for the numerical simulation of cardiac electromechanics in the left human ventricle', MOX-Report 28-2018, Department of Mathematics, Politecnico di Milano.

P. Gervasio, F. Saleri and A. Veneziani (2006), 'Algebraic fractional-step schemes with spectral methods for the incompressible Navier–Stokes equations', *J. Comput. Phys.* **214**, 347–365.

R. Ghanem and P. Spanos (2003), *Stochastic Finite Elements: A Spectral Approach*, revised edition, Dover. Reprint of the Springer 1991 edition.

G. Gigante and C. Vergara (2015), 'Analysis and optimization of the generalized Schwarz method for elliptic problems with application to fluid–structure interaction', *Numer. Math.* **131**, 369–404.

M. Giles (2015), Multilevel Monte Carlo methods. In *Acta Numerica*, Vol. 24, Cambridge University Press, pp. 259–328.

S. Giordana, S. Sherwin, J. Peiró, D. Doorly, J. Crane, K. Lee, N. Cheshire and C. Caro (2005), 'Local and global geometric influence on steady flow in distal anastomoses of peripheral bypass grafts', *J. Biomech. Engrg* **127**, 1087–1098.

V. Girault and P. Raviart (1986), *Finite Element Methods for Navier–Stokes Equations*, Springer.

S. Glagov, C. Zarins, D. Giddens and D. Ku (1988), 'Hemodynamics and atherosclerosis: Insights and perspectives gained from studies of human arteries', *Arch. Pathol. Lab. Med.* **112**, 1018–1031.

R. Glowinski, T. Pan and J. Periaux (1997), 'A Lagrange multiplier/fictitious domain method for the numerical simulation of incompressible viscous flow around moving rigid bodies (I): Case where the rigid body motions are known *a priori*', *CR Acad. Sci.* I Math. **324**, 361–369.

R. Gnyaneshwar, R. Kumar and K. Balakrishnan (2002), 'Dynamic analysis of the aortic valve using a finite element model', *Ann. Thorac. Surg.* **73**, 1122–1129.

S. Goktepe and E. Kuhl (2010), 'Electromechanics of the heart: A unified approach to the strongly coupled excitation-contraction problem', *Comput. Mech.* **45**, 227–243.

A. Goshtasby and D. Turner (1995), 'Segmentation of cardiac cine MR images for extraction of right and left ventricular chambers', *IEEE Trans. Med. Imaging* **14**, 56–64.

C. Grandmont (1998), *Analyse Mathématique et Numérique de Quelques Problèmes d'Interaction Fluide–Structure*. PhD thesis, Laboratoire d'Analyse Numérique de Paris VI.

B. Griffith, R. Hornung, D. McQueen and C. Peskin (2007), 'An adaptive, formally second order accurate version of the immersed boundary method', *J. Comput. Phys.* **223**, 10–419.

B. Griffith, X. Luo, D. McQueen and C. Peskin (2009), 'Simulating the fluid dynamics of natural and prosthetic heart valves using the immersed boundary method', *Int. J. Appl. Mech.* **1**, 137–176.

L. Grinberg, E. Cheever, T. Anor, J. Madsen and G. Karniadakis (2010), 'Modeling blood flow circulation in intracranial arterial networks: A comparative 3D/1D simulation study', *Ann. Biomed. Engrg* **39**, 297–309.

L. Grinberg, A. Yakhot and G. Karniadakis (2009), 'Analyzing transient turbulence in a stenosed carotid artery by proper orthogonal decomposition', *Ann. Biomed. Engrg* **37**, 2200–2217.

J. Guccione, A. McCulloch and L. Waldman (1991), 'Passive material properties of intact ventricular myocardium determined from a cylindrical model', *J. Biomech. Engrg* **113**, 42–55.

B. Guerciotti, C. Vergara, L. Azzimonti, L. Forzenigo, A. Buora, P. Biondetti and M. Domanin (2015), 'Computational study of the fluid-dynamics in carotids before and after endarterectomy', *J. Biomech.* **195**, 2088–2099.

B. Guerciotti, C. Vergara, S. Ippolito, A. Quarteroni, C. Antona and R. Scrofani (2017), 'Computational study of the risk of restenosis in coronary bypasses', *Biomech. Model. Mechanobiol.* **16**, 313–332.

J. Guermond and L. Quartapelle (1998), 'On the approximation of the unsteady Navier–Stokes equations by finite element projection methods', *Numer. Math.* **80**, 207–238.

J. Guermond and J. Shen (2003), 'Velocity-correction projection methods for incompressible flows', *SIAM J. Numer. Anal.* **41**, 112–134.

J. Guermond and J. Shen (2006), 'An overview of projection methods for incompressible flows', *Comput. Methods Appl. Mech. Engrg* **195**, 6011–6045.

J. Guermond, P. Minev and J. Shen (2005), 'Error analysis of pressure-correction schemes for the time-dependent Stokes equations with open boundary conditions', *SIAM J. Numer. Anal.* **43**, 239–258.

J. Guermond, P. Minev and J. Shen (2006), 'An overview of projection methods for incompressible flows', *Comput. Methods Appl. Mech. Engrg* **195**, 6011–6045.

G. Guidoboni, R. Glowinski, N. Cavallini and S. Canic (2009), 'Stable loosely-coupled-type algorithm for fluid–structure interaction in blood flow', *J. Comput. Phys.* **228**, 6916–6937.

O. Gultekin, G. Sommer and G. Holzapfel (2016), 'An orthotropic viscoelastic model for the passive myocardium: Continuum basis and numerical treatment', *Comput. Methods Biomech. Biomed. Engrg* **19**, 1647–1664.

M. Gunzburger (2003), *Perspectives in Flow Control and Optimization*, Advances in Design and Control, SIAM.

M. Gunzburger, C. Webster and G. Zhang (2014), Stochastic finite element methods for partial differential equations with random input data. In *Acta Numerica*, Vol. 23, Cambridge University Press, pp. 521–650.

A. Gupta, L. von Kurowski, A. Singh, D. Geiger, C. Liang, M. Chiu, L. Adler, M. Haacke and D. Wilson (1993), Cardiac MR image segmentation using deformable models. In *Computers in Cardiology 1993*, IEEE, pp. 747–750.

V. Gurev, P. Pathmanathan, J. Fattebert, H. Wen, J. Magerlein, R. Gray, D. Richards and J. Rice (2015), 'A high-resolution computational model of the deforming human heart', *Biomech. Model. Mechanobiol.* **14**, 132–140.

C. Haggerty, L. Mirabella, M. Restrepo, D. de Zélicourt, J. Rossignac, F. Sotiropoulos, T. Spray, K. Kanter, M. Fogel and A. Yoganathan (2013), Patient-specific surgery planning for the fontan procedure. In *Computer Models in Biomechanics: From Nano to Macro* (G. Holzapfel and E. Kuhl, eds), Springer, pp. 217–228.

A. Hansbo and P. Hansbo (2002), 'An unfitted finite element method, based on Nitsche's method, for elliptic interface problems', *Comput. Methods Appl. Mech. Engrg* **191**, 5537–5552.

A. Hansbo, P. Hansbo and M. Larson (2003), 'A finite element method on composite grids based on Nitsche's method', *ESAIM: Math. Model. Numer. Anal.* **37**, 495–514.

I. Hariton, G. de Botton, T. Gasser and G. Holzapfel (2006), 'Stress-driven collagen fiber remodeling in arterial walls', *Biomech. Model. Mechanobiol.* **3**, 163–175.

J. de Hart, F. Baaijens, G. Peters and P. Schreurs (2003), 'A computational fluid–structure interaction analysis of a fiber-reinforced stentless aortic valve', *J. Biomech.* **36**, 699–712.

J. de Hart, G. Peters, P. Schreurs and F. Baaijens (2000), 'A two-dimensional fluid–structure interaction model of the aortic value', *J. Biomech.* **33**, 1079–1088.

H. Haruguchi and S. Teraoka (2003), 'Intimal hyperplasia and hemodynamic factors in arterial bypass and arteriovenous grafts: A review', *J. Artif. Organs* **6**, 227–235.

X. He, D. Ku and J. Moore Jr (1993), 'Simple calculation of the velocity profiles for pulsatile flow in a blood vessel using Mathematica', *Ann. Biomed. Engrg* **21**, 45–49.

M. Heil (2004), 'An efficient solver for the fully coupled solution of large-displacement fluid–structure interaction problems', *Comput. Methods Appl. Mech. Engrg* **193**, 1–23.

J. Hesthaven, G. Rozza and B. Stamm (2016), *Certified Reduced Basis Methods for Parametrized Partial Differential Equations*, Springer Briefs in Mathematics, Springer.

J. Heywood, R. Rannacher and S. Turek (1996), 'Artificial boundaries and flux and pressure conditions for the incompressible Navier–Stokes equations', *Int. J. Numer. Methods Fluids* **22**, 325–352.

D. Hilgemann and D. Noble (1987), 'Excitation–contraction coupling and extracellular calcium transients in rabbit atrium: Reconstruction of basic cellular mechanisms', *Proc. Royal Soc. London B* **230**, 163–205.

B. Hillen, H. Hoogstraten and L. Post (1986), 'A wave propagation model of blood flow in large vessels using an approximate velocity profile function', *J. Biomech.* **19**, 187–194.

M. Hintermüller, K. Kunisch, Y. Spasov and S. Volkwein (2004), 'Dynamical systems-based optimal control of incompressible fluids', *Int. J. Numer. Methods Fluids* **46**, 345–359.

M. Hinze, R. Pinnau, M. Ulbrich and S. Ulbrich (2009), *Optimization with PDE Constraints*, Vol. 23 of Mathematical Modelling: Theory and Applications, Springer.

M. Hirschvogel, M. Bassilious, L. Jagschies, S.M. Wildhirt and M.W. Gee (2017), 'A monolithic 3D-0D coupled closed-loop model of the heart and the vascular system: experiment-based parameter estimation for patient-specific cardiac mechanics', *Internat. J. Numer. Methods Biomed. Engng.* **33**, e2842.

C. Hirt, A. Amsden and J. Cook (1974), 'An arbitrary Lagrangian Eulerian computing method for all flow speeds', *J. Comput. Phys.* **69**, 277–324.

A. Hodgkin and A. Huxley (1952), 'A quantitative description of membrane current and its application to conduction and excitation in nerve', *J. Physiol.* **117**, 500–544.

G. Holzapfel (2000), *Nonlinear Solid Mechanics: A Continuum Approach for Engineering*, Wiley.

G. Holzapfel and T. Gasser (2000), 'A new constitutive framework for arterial wall mechanics and a comparative study of material models', *J. Elasticity* **61**, 1–48.

G. Holzapfel and T. Gasser (2001), 'A viscoelastic model for fiber-reinforced composites at finite strains: Continuum basis, computational aspects, and applications', *Comput. Methods Appl. Mech. Engrg* **190**, 4379–4403.

G. Holzapfel and R. Ogden (2009), 'Constitutive modelling of passive myocardium: A structurally based framework for material characterization', *Philos. Trans. Royal Soc. A* **367**, 3445–3475.

G. Holzapfel and R. Ogden (2010), 'Constitutive modelling of arteries', *Proc. Royal Soc. Lond. A: Math. Phys. Engrg Sci.* **466**, 1551–1596.

G. Holzapfel, T. Gasser and R. Ogden (2000), 'A new constitutive framework for arterial wall mechanics and a comparative study of material models', *J. Elast.* **61**, 1–48.

E. Hopf (1951), 'Über die Anfangswertaufgabe für die hydrodynamischen Grundgliechungen', *Math. Nachrichten* **4**, 213–231.

I. Hoteit, D. Pham and J. Blum (2002), 'A simplified reduced order Kalman filtering and application to altimetric data assimilation in Tropical Pacific', *J. Marine Systems* **36**, 101–127.

P. Houtemaker and F. Zhang (2016), 'Review of the ensemble Kalman filter for atmospheric data assimilation', *Monthly Weather Rev.* **122**, 4489–4532.

M. Hsu, D. Kamensky, Y. Bazilevs, M. Sacks and T. Hughes (2014), 'Fluid–structure interaction analysis of bioprosthetic heart valves: Significance of arterial wall deformation', *Comput. Mech.* **54**, 1055–1071.

W. Huberts, C. de Jonge, W. van der Linden, M. Inda, K. Passera, J. Tordoir, F. van de Vosse and E. Bosboom (2013*a*), 'A sensitivity analysis of a personalized pulse wave propagation model for arteriovenous fistula surgery, B: Identification of possible generic model parameters', *Med. Engrg Phys.* **35**, 827–837.

W. Huberts, C. de Jonge, W. van der Linden, M. Inda, J. Tordoir, F. van de Vosse and E. Bosboom (2013*b*), 'A sensitivity analysis of a personalized pulse wave propagation model for arteriovenous fistula surgery, A: Identification of most influential model parameters', *Med. Engrg Phys.* **35**, 810–826.

T. Hughes (1974), *A Study of the One-dimensional Theory of Arterial Pulse Propagation.* PhD thesis, University of California, Berkeley.

T. Hughes (1995), 'Multiscale phenomena: Green's function, the Dirichlet-to-Neumann formulation, subgrid scale models, bubbles and the origins of stabilized formulations', *Comput. Methods Appl. Mech. Engrg* **127**, 387–401.

T. Hughes (2000), *The Finite Element Method: Linear Static and Dynamic Finite Element Analysis*, Dover Publications, Mineola, NY.

T. Hughes and J. Lubliner (1973), 'On the one-dimensional theory of blood flow in the larger vessels', *Math. Biosci.* **18**, 161–170.

T. Hughes, L. Mazzei and K. Jansen (2000), 'Large eddy simulation and the variational multiscale method', *Comput. Vis. Sci.* **3**, 47–59.

G. Huiskamp (1998), 'Simulation of depolarization in a membrane- equations-based model of the anisotropic ventricle', *IEEE Trans. Biomed. Engrg* **45**, 847–855.

J.D. Humphrey and K.R. Rajagopal (2002), 'A constrained mixture model for growth and remodeling of soft tissues', *Math. Model. Meth. Appl. Sci.* **12**, 407–430.

J.D. Humphrey and F. Yin (1987), 'On constitutive relations and finite deformations of passive cardiac tissue, I: A pseudostrain-energy function', *J. Biomech. Engrg* **109**, 298–304.

J. Humphreys, P. Redd and J. West (2012), 'A fresh look at the Kalman filter', *SIAM Review* **54**, 801–823.

P. Hunter, M. Nash and G. Sands (1997), Computational electromechanics of the heart. In *Computational Biology of the Heart* (A. Panfilov and A. Holden, eds), Wiley-Blackwell, pp. 345–407.

M.-C. Hsu, D. Kamensky, F. Xu, J. Kiendl, C. Wang, M.C.H. Wu, J. Mineroff, A. Reali, Y. Bazilevs and M.S. Sacks (2015), 'Dynamic and fluid-structure interaction simulations of bioprosthetic heart valves using parametric design with T-splines and Fung-type material models', *Comput. Methods Appl. Mech. Engrg* **55**, 1211–1225.

H. Huxley and M. Kress (1985), 'Crossbridge behaviour during muscle contraction', *J. Muscle Res. & Cell Motility* **6**:153–161.

P. Iaizzo (2009), *Handbook of Cardiac Anatomy, Physiology, and Devices*, Springer.

K. Ide, P. Courtier, M. Ghil and A. Lorenc (1997), 'Unified notation for data assimilation: Operational, sequential and variational', *J. Met. Soc. Japan* **75**, 181–189.

M. Iglesias, K. Law and A. Stuart (2013), 'Ensemble Kalman methods for inverse problems', *Inverse Problems* **29**, 045001.

T. Ijiri, T. Ashihara, T. Yamaguchi, K. Takayama, T. Igarashi, T. Shimada, T. Namba, R. Haraguchi and K. Nakazawa (2008), 'A procedural method for modeling the Purkinje fibers of the heart', *J. Physiol. Sci.* **58**, 90–100.

J. Isaksen, Y. Bazilevs, T. Kvamsdal, Y. Zhang, J. Kaspersen, K. Waterloo, B. Romner and T. Ingebrigtsen (2008), 'Determination of wall tension in cerebral artery aneurysms by numerical simulation', *Stroke* **39**, 3172–3178.

R. Johnstone, E. Chang, R. Bardenet, T. de Boer, D. Gavaghan, P. Pathmanathan, R. Clayton and G. Mirams (2016), 'Uncertainty and variability in models of the cardiac action potential: Can we build trustworthy models?', *J. Molec. Cell. Cardiol.* **96**, 49–62.

S. Julier and J. Uhlmann (2004), 'Unscented filtering and nonlinear estimation', *Proc. IEEE* **92**, 401–422.

S. Julier, J. Uhlmann and H. Durrant-Whyte (1995), A new approach for filtering nonlinear systems. In *Proceedings of the 1995 American Control Conference*, Vol. 3, pp. 1628–1632.

S. Julier, J. Uhlmann and H. Durrant-Whyte (2000), 'A new method for the nonlinear transformation of means and covariance in filters and estimators', *IEEE Trans. Automat. Control* **45**, 477–482.

M. Juntunen and R. Stenberg (2009), 'Nitsche's method for general boundary conditions', *Math. Comp.* **78**, 1353–1374.

J. Kaipio and E. Somersalo (2005), *Statistical and Computational Inverse Problems*, Vol. 160 of Applied Mathematical Sciences, Springer.

R. Kalman (1960), 'A new approach to linear filtering and prediction problems', *ASME. J. Basic Engrg* **82**, 35–45.

D. Kamensky, M.-C. Hsu, D. Schillinger, J.A. Evans, A. Aggarwal, Y. Bazilevs, M.S. Sacks and T.J.R. Hughes (2015), 'An immersogeometric variational framework for fluid–structure interaction: Application to bioprosthetic heart valves', *Comput. Methods Appl. Mech. Engrg* **284**, 1005–1053.

G. Karniadakis, M. Israeli and S. Orszag (1991), 'High order splitting methods for the incompressible Navier–Stokes equations', *J. Comput. Phys.* **59**, 414–443.

J. Keener (1991), 'An eikonal-curvature equation for action potential propagation in myocardium', *J. Math. Biol.* **29**, 629–651.

J. Keener and K. Bogar (1998), 'A numerical method for the solution of the bidomain equations in cardiac tissue', *Chaos* **8**, 234–241.

S. Kefayati, D. Holdsworth and T. Poepping (2014), 'Turbulence intensity measurements using particle image velocimetry in diseased carotid artery models: Effect of stenosis severity, plaque eccentricity, and ulceration', *J. Biomech.* **47**, 253–263.

R. Keldermann, M. Nash and A. Panfilov (2009), 'Modeling cardiac mechano-electrical feedback using reaction-diffusion-mechanics systems', *Physica D: Nonlinear Phenomena* **238**, 1000–1007.

C. Kelley (1999), *Iterative Methods for Optimization*, SIAM.

D. Kelly, K. Law and A. Stuart (2014), 'Well-posedness and accuracy of the ensemble Kalman filter in discrete and continuous time', *Nonlinearity* **27**, 2579.

M. Kennedy and A. O'Hagan (2000), 'Predicting the output from a complex computer code when fast approximations are available', *Biometrika* **87**, 1–13.

B. Kerckoffs, O. Faris, P. Boveenderd, F. Prinzen, K. Smits and T. Arts (2003), 'Timing of depolarization and contraction in the paced canine left ventricle', *J. Cardiovasc. Electrophysiol.* **14**, S188–S195.

R. Keynton, M. Evancho, R. Sims, N. Rodway, A. Gobin and S. Rittgers (2001), 'Intimal hyperplasia and wall shear in arterial bypass graft distal anastomoses: An *in vivo* model study', *J. Biomech. Engrg* **123**, 464–473.

S. Khalafvand, L. Zhong and E. Ng (2014), 'Three-dimensional CFD/MRI modeling reveals that ventricular surgical restoration improves ventricular function by modifying intraventricular blood flow', *Int. J. Numer. Methods Biomed. Engrg* **30**, 1044–1056.

H. Kim, J. Lu, M. Sacks and K. Chandran (2008), 'Dynamic simulation of bioprosthetic heart valves using a stress resultant shell model', *J. Biomech.* **36**, 262–275.

H. Kim, I. Vignon-Clementel, C. Figueroa, J. Ladisa, K. Jansen, J. Feinstein and C. Taylor (2009), 'On coupling a lumped parameter heart model and a three-dimensional finite element aorta model', *Ann. Biomed. Engrg* **37**, 2153–2169.

R.E. Klabunde (2012), *Cardiovascular Physiology Concepts*, Philadelphia, PA, Lippincott Williams & Wilkins/Wolters Kluwer.

C. Kleinstreuer (2006), *Biofluid Dynamics: Principles and Selected Applications*, CRC Press.

P. Kohl and F. Sachs (2001), 'Mechanoelectric feedback in cardiac cells', *Philos. Trans. Royal Soc. A* **359**, 1173–1185.

P. Kohl, P. Hunter and D. Noble (1999), 'Stretch-induced changes in heart rate and rhythm: Clinical observations, experiments and mathematical models', *Prog. Biophys. Molec. Biol.* **71**, 91–138.

E. Konukoglu, J. Relan, U. Cilingir, B. Menze, P. Chinchapatnam, A. Jadidi, H. Cochet, M. Hocini, H. Delingette, P. Jaïs, M. Haïssaguerre, N. Ayache and M. Sermesant (2011), 'Efficient probabilistic model personalization integrating uncertainty on data and parameters: Application to eikonal-diffusion models in cardiac electrophysiology', *Prog. Biophys. Molec. Biol.* **107**, 134–146.

T. Korakianitis and Y. Shi (2006*a*), 'A concentrated parameter model for the human cardiovascular system including heart valve dynamics and atrioventricular interaction', *Med. Engrg Phys.* **28**, 613–628.

T. Korakianitis and Y. Shi (2006*b*), 'Numerical simulation of cardiovascular dynamics with healthy and diseased heart valves', *J. Biomech.* **39**, 1964–1982.

P. Koutsourelakis (2009), 'Accurate uncertainty quantification using inaccurate models', *SIAM J. Sci. Comput.* **31**, 3274–3300.

S. Krishnamoorthi, M. Sarkar and W.S. Klug (2013), 'Numerical quadrature and operator splitting in finite element methods for cardiac electrophysiology', *Internat. J. Numer. Methods Biomed. Engng.* **29**, 1243–1266.

A. Krishnamurthy, C. Villongco, J. Chuang, L. Frank, V. Nigam, E. Belezzuoli, P. Stark, D. Krummen, S. Narayan, J. Omens, A. McCulloch and R. Kerckhoffs (2013), 'Patient-specific models of cardiac biomechanics', *J. Comput. Phys.* **244**, 4–21.

R. Kufahl and M. Clark (1985), 'A circle of Willis simulation using distensible vessels and pulsatile flow', *J. Biomech. Engrg* **107**, 112–122.

E. Kuhl and G. Holzapfel (2006), 'A continuum model for remodeling in living structures', *J. Mater. Sci.* **21**, 8811–8823.

K. Kunisch and A. Rund (2015), 'Time optimal control of the monodomain model in cardiac electrophysiology', *IMA J. Appl. Math.* **80**, 1664–1683.

K. Kunisch and B. Vexler (2007), 'Optimal vortex reduction for instationary flows based on translation invariant cost functionals', *SIAM J. Control Optim.* **46**, 1368–1397.

K. Kunzelman and R. Cochran (1990), 'Mechanical properties of basal and marginal mitral valve chordae tendineae', *ASAIO Trans.* **36**, M405.

K. Kunzelman, R. Cochran, C. Chuong, W. Ring, Verrier and R. Eberhart (1993), 'Finite element analysis of the mitral valve', *J. Heart Valve Disease* **2**, 326–340.

U. Kuttler and W. Wall (2008), 'Fixed-point fluid–structure interaction solvers with dynamic relaxation', *Comput. Mech.* **43**, 61–72.

U. Kuttler, M. Gee, C. Forster, A. Comerford and W. Wall (2010), 'Coupling strategies for biomedical fluid–structure interaction problems', *Int. J. Numer. Methods Biomed. Engrg* **26**, 305–321.

A. Laadhari and A. Quarteroni (2016), 'Numerical modeling of heart valves using resistive Eulerian surfaces', *Int. J. Numer. Methods Biomed. Engrg* **32**, e02743.

R. Lal, B. Mohammadi and F. Nicoud (2017), 'Data assimilation for identification of cardiovascular network characteristics', *Int. J. Numer. Methods Biomed. Engrg* **33**, e2824.

R. Lancellotti, C. Vergara, L. Valdettaro, S. Bose and A. Quarteroni (2017), 'Large eddy simulations for blood fluid-dynamics in real stenotic carotids', *Int. J. Numer. Methods Biomed. Engrg* **33**, e2868.

S. Land, S. Niederer, J. Aronsen, E. Espe, L. Zhang, W. Louch, I. Sjaastad, O. Sejersted and N. Smith (2012), 'An analysis of deformation-dependent electromechanical coupling in the mouse heart', *J. Physiol.* **590**, 4553–4569.

M. Landajuela, C. Vergara, A. Gerbi, L. Dede', L. Formaggia and A. Quarteroni (2018) 'Numerical approximation of the electromechanical coupling in the left ventricle with inclusion of the Purkinje network', *Internat. J. Numer. Methods Biomed. Engng.*, https://doi.org/10.1002/cnm.2984

T. Lassila, A. Manzoni, A. Quarteroni and G. Rozza (2013*a*), 'Boundary control and shape optimization for the robust design of bypass anastomoses under uncertainty', *ESAIM Math. Model. Numer. Anal.* **47**, 1107–1131.

T. Lassila, A. Manzoni, A. Quarteroni and G. Rozza (2013*b*), 'A reduced computational and geometrical framework for inverse problems in haemodynamics', *Int. J. Numer. Methods Biomed. Engrg* **29**, 741–776.

T. Lassila, A. Quarteroni and G. Rozza (2012), 'A reduced basis model with parametric coupling for fluid–structure interaction problems', *SIAM J. Sci. Comput.* **34**, A1187–A1213.

K. Law, A. Stuart and K. Zygalakis (2015), *Data Assimilation: A Mathematical Introduction*, Vol. 62 of Texts in Applied Mathematics, Springer.

T. Le and F. Sotiropoulos (2013), 'Fluid–structure interaction of an aortic heart valve prosthesis driven by an animated anatomic left ventricle', *J. Comput. Phys.* **224**, 41–62.

F.-X. Le Dimet and O. Talagrand (1986), 'Variational algorithms for analysis and assimilation of meteorological observations: Theoretical aspects', *Tellus A* **38**, 97–110.

O. Le Maître and O. Knio (2010), *Spectral Methods for Uncertainty Quantification: With Applications to Computational Fluid Dynamics*, Springer.

H. Lee (2011), 'Optimal control for quasi-Newtonian flows with defective boundary conditions', *Comput. Methods Appl. Mech. Engrg* **200**, 2498–2506.

J. Lee, A. Cookson, I. Roy, E. Kerfoot, L. Asner, G. Vigueras, T. Sochi, S. Deparis, C. Michler, N. Smith and D. Nordsletten (2016), 'Multiphysics computational modeling in CHeart', *SIAM J. Sci. Comput.* **38**, C150–C178.

S. Lee, S. Lee, P. Fischer, H. Bassiouny and F. Loth (2008), 'Direct numerical simulation of transitional flow in a stenosed carotid bifurcation', *J. Biomech.* **41**, 2551–2561.

M. Legato (1973), 'Ultrastructure of the atrial, ventricular, and Purkinje cell, with special reference to the genesis of arrhythmias', *Circulation* **47**, 178–189.

C. Leguy, A. Bosboom, A. Belloum, A. Hoeks and F. van de Vosse (2011), 'Global sensitivity analysis of a wave propagation model for arm arteries', *Med. Engrg Phys.* **33**, 1008–1016.

M. Lei, J. Archie and C. Kleinstreuer (1997), 'Computational design of a bypass graft that minimizes wall shear stress gradients in the region of the distal anastomosis', *J. Vasc. Surg.* **25**, 637–646.

J. Leiva, P. Blanco and G. Buscaglia (2011), 'Partitioned analysis for dimensionally-heterogeneous hydraulic networks', *Multiscale Model. Simul.* **9**, 872–903.

J. Leray (1934), 'Sur le mouvement d'un liquide visqueux emplissant l'espace', *Acta Math.* **63**, 193–248.

D. Lesage, E. Angelini, I. Bloch and G. Funka-Lea (2009), 'A review of 3D vessel lumen segmentation techniques: Models, features and extraction schemes', *Med. Image Anal.* **13**, 819–845.

A. Leuprecht, K. Perktold, M. Prosi, T. Berk, W. Trubel and H. Schima (2002), 'Numerical study of hemodynamics and wall mechanics in distal end-to-side anastomoses of bypass grafts', *J. Biomech.* **2**, 225–236.

R. LeVeque (1992), *Numerical Methods for Conservation Laws*, Vol. 132 of Lectures in Mathematics, Birkhäuser.

C. Li and C. Vuik (2004), 'Eigenvalue analysis of the simple preconditioning for incompressible flow', *Numer. Linear Algebra Appl.* **11**, 511–523.

D. Li and A. Robertson (2013), 'A structural multi-mechanism damage model for cerebral arterial tissue', *J. Biomech. Engrg* **131**, 101013.

F. Liang and H. Liu (2006), 'Simulation of hemodynamic responses to the valsalva maneuver: An integrative computational model of the cardiovascular system and the autonomic nervous system', *J. Physiol. Sci.* **1**, 45–65.

J. Lions and G. Prodi (1959), 'Un théorème d'existence et d'unicité dans les équations de Navier–Stokes en dimension 2', *CR Acad. Sci. Paris* **248**, 3519–3521.

Y. Liu, C. Charles, M. Gracia, H. Gregersen and G. S. Kassab (2007), 'Surrounding tissues affect the passive mechanics of the vessel wall: Theory and experiment', *Amer. J. Physiol.: Heart Circ. Physiol.* **293**, H3290–H3300.

D. Lombardi (2014), 'Inverse problems in 1D hemodynamics on systemic networks: A sequential approach', *Int. J. Numer. Methods Biomed. Engrg* **30**, 160–179.

M. Lorenzo-Valdés, G. Sanchez-Ortiz, A. Elkington, R. Mohiaddin and D. Rueckert (2004), 'Segmentation of 4D cardiac MR images using a probabilistic atlas and the EM algorithm', *Med. Image Anal.* **8**, 255–265.

F. Loth, P. Fischer and H. Bassiouny (2008), 'Blood flow in end-to-side anastomoses', *Annu. Rev. Fluid. Mech.* **40**, 367–393.

C. Luo and Y. Rudy (1991), 'A model of the ventricular cardiac action potential: Depolarization, repolarization, and their interaction', *Circ. Res.* **68**, 1501–1526.

C. Luo and Y. Rudy (1994*a*), 'A dynamic model of the cardiac ventricular action potential, I: Simulations of ionic currents and concentration changes', *Circ. Res.* **74**, 1071–1096.

C. Luo and Y. Rudy (1994*b*), 'A dynamic model of the cardiac ventricular action potential, II: Afterdepolarizations, triggered activity, and potentiation', *Circ. Res.* **74**, 1097–1113.

M. Lykaser and B. Nielsen (2006), 'Towards a level-set framework for infarction modeling: An inverse problem', *Int. J. Numer. Anal. Model.* **3**, 377–394.

M. MacLachlan, B. Nielsen, M. Lysaker and A. Tveito (2006), 'Computing the size and location of myocardial ischemia using measurements of ST-segment shift', *IEEE Trans. Biomed. Engrg* **53**, 1024–1031.

Y. Maday (2009), Analysis of coupled models for fluid–structure interaction of internal flows. Chapter 8 in *Cardiovascular Mathematics* (A. Quarteroni, L. Formaggia and A. Veneziani), Springer, pp. 279–306.

Y. Maday, N. Nguyen, A. Patera and G. Pau (2009), 'A general multipurpose interpolation procedure: the magic points', *Commun. Pure Appl. Anal.* **8**(1), 383–404.

A. Mahmoud, A. El-Barkouky, H. Farag, J. Graham and A. Farag (2013), A non-invasive method for measuring blood flow rate in superficial veins from a single thermal image. In *2013 IEEE Conference on Computer Vision and Pattern Recognition Workshops (CVPRW)*, IEEE, pp. 354–359.

A. Malossi (2012), *Partitioned Solution of Geometrical Multiscale Problems for the Cardiovascular System: Models, Algorithms, and Applications.* PhD thesis, Ecole Polytechnique Fédérale de Lausanne. Thesis 5453.

A. Malossi, P. Blanco and S. Deparis (2012), 'A two-level time step technique for the partitioned solution of one-dimensional arterial networks', *Comput. Methods Appl. Mech. Engrg* **237–240**, 212–226.

A. Malossi, P. Blanco, P. Crosetto, S. Deparis and A. Quarteroni (2013), 'Implicit coupling of one-dimensional and three-dimensional blood flow models with compliant vessels', *Multiscale Model. Simul.* **11**, 474–506.

T. Mansi, I. Voigt, B. Georgescu, X. Zheng, E. Mengue, M. Hackl, R. Ionasec, T. Noack, J. Seeburger and D. Comaniciu (2012), 'An integrated framework for finite-element modeling of mitral valve biomechanics from medical images: Application to MitralClip intervention planning', *Med. Image Anal.* **16**, 1330–1346.

A. Manzoni (2012), *Reduced Models for Optimal Control, Shape Optimization and Inverse Problems in Haemodynamics*. PhD thesis, Ecole Polytechnique Fédérale de Lausanne.

A. Manzoni, D. Bonomi and A. Quarteroni (2018), 'Reduced order modeling for cardiac electrophysiology and mechanics: new methodologies, challenges & perspectives', MOX-Report 29-2018, Department of Mathematics, Politecnico di Milano.

A. Manzoni, T. Lassila, A. Quarteroni and G. Rozza (2014), A reduced-order strategy for solving inverse Bayesian shape identification problems in physiological flows. In *Modeling, Simulation and Optimization of Complex Processes, HPSC 2012: Proceedings of the Fifth International Conference on High Performance Scientific Computing* (G. Bock, P. Hoang, R. Rannacher and P. Schlöder, eds), Springer, pp. 145–155.

A. Manzoni and F. Negri (2017), Efficient reduction of PDEs defined on domains with variable shape. In *Model Reduction of Parametrized Systems* (P. Benner, M. Ohlberger, A. Patera, G. Rozza and K. Urban, eds), Springer, pp. 183–199.

A. Manzoni, S. Pagani and T. Lassila (2016), 'Accurate solution of Bayesian inverse uncertainty quantification problems combining reduced basis methods and reduction error models', *SIAM/ASA J. Uncert. Quant.* **4**, 380–412.

A. Manzoni, A. Quarteroni and G. Rozza (2012*a*), 'Model reduction techniques for fast blood flow simulation in parametrized geometries', *Int. J. Numer. Methods Biomed. Engrg* **28**, 604–625.

A. Manzoni, A. Quarteroni and G. Rozza (2012*b*), 'Shape optimization of cardiovascular geometries by reduced basis methods and free-form deformation techniques', *Int. J. Numer. Methods Fluids* **70**, 646–670.

S. Marchesseau, H. Delingette, M. Sermesant and N. Ayache (2012), 'Fast parameter calibration of a cardiac electromechanical model from medical images based on the unscented transform', *Biomech. Model. Mechanobiol.* **12**, 815–831.

S. Marchesseau, H. Delingette, M. Sermesant, R. Cabrera-Lozoya, C. Tobon-Gomez, P. Moireau, R. Figueras i Ventura, K. Lekadir, A. Hernandez, M. Garreau, E. Donal, C. Leclercq, S. Duckett, K. Rhode, C. Rinaldi, A. Frangi, R. Razavi, D. Chapelle and N. Ayache (2013), 'Personalization of a cardia electromechanical model using reduced order unscented Kalman filtering from regional volumes', *Med. Image Anal.* **17**, 816–829.

K. Mardal, B. Nielsen, X. Cai and A. Tveito (2007), 'Semi-implicit time-discretization schemes for the bidomain modelan order optimal solver for the discretized bidomain equations', *Numer. Linear Algebra Appl.* **14**, 83–98.

K. Margaris and R. Black (2012), 'Modelling the lymphatic system: Challenges and opportunities', *J. Royal Soc. Interface* **69**, 601–612.

G. Marom (2015), 'Numerical methods for fluid–structure interaction models of aortic valves', *Arch. Comput. Methods Engrg* **22**, 595–620.

A. Marsden (2014), 'Optimization in cardiovascular modeling', *Annu. Rev. Fluid Mech.* **46**, 519–546.

A. Marsden, J. Feinstein and C. Taylor (2008), 'A computational framework for derivative-free optimization of cardiovascular geometries', *Comput. Methods Appl. Mech. Engrg* **197**, 1890–1905.

V. Martin, F. Clément, A. Decoene and J.-F. Gerbeau (2005), 'Parameter identification for a one-dimensional blood flow model', *ESAIM Proc.* **14**, 174–200.

A. Masci, M. Alessandrini, D. Forti, F. Menghini, L. Dede', C. Tommasi, A. Quarteroni and C. Corsi (2017), A patient–specific computational fluid dynamics model of the left atrium in atrial fibrillation: development and initial evaluation. In *Functional Imaging and Modelling of the Heart. FIMH 2017* (M. Pop and G. Wright eds), Lecture Notes in Computer Science, **10263**, Springer, Cham, pp. 392-400.

K. Matthys, J. Alastruey, J. Peiró, A. Khir, P. Segers, P. Verdonck, K. Parker and S. Sherwin (2007), 'Pulse wave propagation in a model human arterial network: Assessment of 1-D numerical simulations against *in vitro* measurements', *J. Biomech.* **40**, 3476–3486.

B. Maury (2013), *The Respiratory System in Equations*, Springer.

K. May-Newman and F. Yin (1998), 'A constitutive law for mitral valve tissue', *J. Biomech. Engrg* **120**, 38–47.

K. May-Newman, C. Lam and F. Yin (2009), 'A hyperelastic constitutive law for aortic valve tissue', *J. Biomech. Engrg* **131**, 081009.

F. Menghini, L. Dede', D. Forti and A. Quarteroni (2017), 'Hemodynamics in a left atrium based on a Variational Multiscale-LES numerical model', MOX-Report 47-2017, Department of Mathematics, Politecnico di Milano.

F. Menghini, L. Dede' and A. Quarteroni (2018), 'Variational Multiscale LES modeling of blood flow in an idealized left human heart', MOX-Report 19-2018, Department of Mathematics, Politecnico di Milano.

W. Merryman, H. Huang, F. Schoen and M. Sacks (2006), 'The effects of cellular contraction on aortic valve leaflet flexural stiffness', *J. Biomech.* **39**, 88–96.

V. Meschini, M. De Tullio, G. Querzoli and R. Verzicco (2018), 'Flow structure in healthy and pathological left ventricles with natural and prosthetic mitral valves', *J. Fluid Mech.* **834**, 271–307.

F. Migliavacca and G. Dubini (2005), 'Computational modeling of vascular anastomoses', *Biomech. Model. Mechanobiol.* **3**, 235–250.

F. Migliavacca, R. Balossino, G. Pennati, G. Dubini, T. Hsia, M. de Leval and E. Bove (2006), 'Multiscale modelling in biofluidynamics: Application to reconstructive paediatric cardiac surgery', *J. Biomech.* **39**, 1010–1020.

J. Mitchell and J. Wang (2014), 'Expanding application of the Wiggers diagram to teach cardiovascular physiology', *Adv. Physiology Education* **38**, 170–175.

R. Mittal and G. Iaccarino (2005), 'Immersed boundary methods', *Annu. Rev. Fluid Mech.* **37**, 239–261.

R. Mittal, J. Seo, V. Vedula, Y. Choi, H. Liu, H. Huang, S. Jain, L. Younes, T. Abraham and R. George (2016), 'Computational modeling of cardiac hemodynamics: Current status and future outlook', *J. Comput. Phys.* **305**, 1065–1082.

P. Moireau and D. Chapelle (2011), 'Reduced-order unscented Kalman filtering with application to parameter identification in large-dimensional systems', *ESAIM Control Optim. Calc. Var.* **17**, 380–405.

P. Moireau, C. Bertoglio, N. Xiao, C. Figueroa, C. Taylor, D. Chapelle and J.-F. Gerbeau (2013), 'Sequential identification of boundary support parameters in a fluid–structure vascular model using patient image data', *Biomech. Model. Mechanobiol.* **12**, 475–496.

P. Moireau, D. Chapelle and P. Le Tallec (2008), 'Joint state and parameter estimation for distributed mechanical systems', *Comput. Methods Appl. Mech. Engrg* **197**, 659–677.

P. Moireau, D. Chapelle and P. Le Tallec (2009), 'Filtering for distributed mechanical systems using position measurements: perspectives in medical imaging', *Inverse Problems* **25**, 035010.

P. Moireau, N. Xiao, M. Astorino, C. Figueroa, D. Chapelle, C. Taylor and J.-F. Gerbeau (2012), 'External tissue support and fluid–structure simulation in blood flows', *Biomech. Model. Mechanobiol.* **11**, 1–18.

J. Moore, D. Steinman and C. Ethier (1997), 'Computational blood flow modelling: Errors associated with reconstructing finite element models from magnetic resonance images', *J. Biomech.* **31**, 179–184.

H. Moradkhani, S. Sorooshian, H. Gupta and P. Houser (2005), 'Dual state-parameter estimation of hydrological models using ensemble Kalman filter', *Adv. Water Resour.* **28**, 135–147.

U. Morbiducci, R. Ponzini, G. Rizzo, M. Cadioli, A. Esposito, F. De Cobelli, A. Del Maschio, F. Montevecchi and A. Redaelli (2009), '*In vivo* quantification of helical blood flow in human aorta by time-resolved three-dimensional cine phase contrast magnetic resonance imaging', *Ann. Biomed. Engrg* **37**, 516–531.

S. Morganti, F. Auricchio, D.J. Benson, F.I. Gambarin, S. Hartmann, T.J.R. Hughes and A. Reali (2015), 'Patient-specific isogeometric structural analysis of aortic valve closure', *Comput. Methods Appl. Mech. Engrg* **284**, 508–520.

D. Mozaffarian, E. Benjamin, A. Go, D. Arnett, M. Blaha, M. Cushman, S. Das, S. de Ferranti, J.-P. Després, H. Fullerton, V. Howard, M. Huffman, C. Isasi, M. Jiménez, S. Judd, B. Kissela, J. Lichtman, L. Lisabeth, S. Liu, R. Mackey, D. Magid, D. McGuire, E. Mohler, C. Moy, P. Muntner, M. Mussolino, K. Nasir, R. Neumar, G. Nichol, L. Palaniappan, D. Pandey, M. Reeves, C. Rodriguez, W. Rosamond, P. Sorlie, J. Stein, A. Towfighi, T. Turan, S. Virani, D. Woo, R. Yeh and M. Turner (2015), 'Heart disease and stroke statistics: 2016 update', *Circulation* **133**, 447–454.

J. Muller, O. Sahni, X. Lia, K. Jansen, M. Shephard and C. Taylor (2005), 'Anisotropic adaptive finite element method for modelling blood flow', *Comput. Methods Biomech. Biomed. Engrg* **8**, 295–305.

L. Muller and E. Toro (2013), 'Well-balanced high-order solver for blood flow in networks of vessels with variable properties', *Int. J. Numer Methods Biomed. Engrg* **29**, 1388–1411.

L. Muller and E. Toro (2014), 'A global multiscale mathematical model for the human circulation with emphasis on the venous system', *Int. J. Numer. Methods Biomed. Engrg* **30**, 681–725.

M. Munteanu, L. Pavarino and S. Scacchi (2009), 'A scalable Newton–Krylov–Schwarz method for the bidomain reaction-diffusion system', *SIAM J. Sci. Comput.* **31**, 3861–3883.

M. Murillo and X. Cai (2004), 'A fully implicit parallel algorithm for simulating the non-linear electrical activity of the heart', *Numer. Linear Algebra Appl.* **2/3**, 261–277.

A. Muszkiewicz, O. Britton, P. Gemmell, E. Passini, C. Sánchez, X. Zhou, A. Carusi, T. Quinn, K. Burrage, A. Bueno-Orovio and B. Rodriguez (2016), 'Variability in cardiac electrophysiology: Using experimentally-calibrated populations of models to move beyond the single virtual physiological human paradigm', *Prog. Biophys. Molec. Biol.* **120**, 115–127.

C. Nagaiah, K. Kunisch and G. Plank (2011), 'Numerical solution for optimal control of the reaction-diffusion equations in cardiac electrophysiology', *Comput. Optim. Appl.* **49**, 149–178.

C. Nagaiah, K. Kunisch and G. Plank (2013*a*), 'On boundary stimulation and optimal boundary control of the bidomain equations', *Math. Biosci.* **245**, 206–215.

C. Nagaiah, K. Kunisch and G. Plank (2013*b*), 'Optimal control approach to termination of re-entry waves in cardiac electrophysiology', *J. Math. Biol.* **67**, 1–30.

C. Nagaiah, K. Kunisch and G. Plank (2016), 'PDE constrained optimization of electrical defibrillation in a 3D ventricular slice geometry', *Int. J. Numer. Methods Biomed. Engrg* **32**, e02742.

A. Nagler, C. Bertoglio, M. Gee and W. Wall (2013), Personalization of cardiac fiber orientations from image data using the unscented Kalman filter. In *Functional Imaging and Modeling of the Heart* (S. Ourselin, D. Rueckert and N. Smith, eds), Vol. 7945 of Lecture Notes in Computer Science, Springer, pp. 132–140.

A. Nagler, C. Bertoglio, C. Stoeck, S. Kozerke and W. Wall (2015), Cardiac fibers estimation from arbitrarily spaced diffusion weighted MRI. In *Functional Imaging and Modeling of the Heart: FIMH 2015* (H. van Assen *et al.*, eds), Vol. 9126 of Lecture Notes in Computer Science, Springer.

M. Nash and A. Panfilov (2004), 'Electromechanical model of excitable tissue to study reentrant cardiac arrhythmias', *Prog. Biophys. Molec. Biol.* **2/3**, 501–522.

F. Negri (2016), *Efficient Reduction Techniques for the Simulation and Optimization of Parametrized Systems: Analysis and Applications.* PhD thesis, Ecole Polytechnique Fédérale de Lausanne.

F. Negri, A. Manzoni and D. Amsallem (2015), 'Efficient model reduction of parametrized systems by matrix discrete empirical interpolation', *J. Comp. Phys.* **303**, 431–454.

M. Nestola, E. Faggiano, C. Vergara, R. Lancellotti, S. Ippolito, C. Antona, A. Quarteroni and R. Scrofani (2017), 'Computational comparison of aortic root stresses in presence of stentless and stented aortic valve bio-prostheses', *Comput. Methods Biomech. Biomed. Engrg* **20**, 171–181.

N. Newmark (1959), 'A method of computation for structural dynamics', *J. Engrg Mech.* **85**, 67–94.

N. Nichols (2010), Mathematical concepts of data assimilation. In *Data Assimilation: Making Sense of Observations* (W. Lahoz, B. Khattatov and R. Menard, eds), Springer, pp. 13–39.

W. Nichols and M. O'Rourke, eds (2005), *McDonald's Blood Flow in Arteries*, Hodder Arnold.

S. Niederer and N. Smith (2007), 'A mathematical model of the slow force response to stretch in rat ventricular myocytes', *Biophys. J.* **92**, 4030–4044.

S. Niederer and N. Smith (2008), 'An improved numerical method for strong coupling of excitation and contraction models in the heart', *Prog. Biophys. Molec. Biol.* **96**, 90–111.

S. Niederer, P. Hunter and N. Smith (2006), 'A quantitative analysis of cardiac myocyte relaxation: A simulation study', *Biophysical Journal* **90**, 1697–1722.

S. Niederer, E. Kerfoot, A. Benson, M. Bernabeu, O. Bernus, C. Bradley, E. Cherry, R. Clayton, F. Fenton, A. Garny *et al.* (2011), 'Verification of cardiac tissue electrophysiology simulators using an $N$-version benchmark', *Phil. Trans. R. Soc. A* **369**, 4331–4351.

B. Nielsen, X. Cai and M. Lykaser (2007*a*), 'On the possibility for computing the transmembrane potential in the heart with a one shot method: An inverse problem', *Math. Biosciences* **210**, 523–553.

B. Nielsen, M. Lykaser and A. Tveito (2007*b*), 'On the use of the resting potential and level-set methods for identifying ischemic heart disease: An inverse problem', *J. Comput. Phys.* **220**, 772–790.

J. Nitsche (1970/71), 'Über ein Variationsprinzip zur lösung von Dirichlet-Problemen bei verwendung von Teilräumen, die keinen Randbedingungen unterworfen sind', *Abhandlungen aus dem Mathematischen Seminar der Universität Hamburg* **36**, 9–15.

F. Nobile (2001), *Numerical Approximation of Fluid–structure Interaction Problems with Application to Haemodynamics.* PhD thesis, Ecole Polytechnique Fédérale de Lausanne. Thesis 2458.

F. Nobile and C. Vergara (2008), 'An effective fluid–structure interaction formulation for vascular dynamics by generalized Robin conditions', *SIAM J. Sci. Comput.* **30**, 731–763.

F. Nobile and C. Vergara (2012), 'Partitioned algorithms for fluid–structure interaction problems in haemodynamics', *Milan J. Math.* **80**, 443–467.

F. Nobile, M. Pozzoli and C. Vergara (2013), 'Time accurate partitioned algorithms for the solution of fluid–structure interaction problems in haemodynamics', *Comput. Fluids* **86**, 470–482.

F. Nobile, M. Pozzoli and C. Vergara (2014), 'Inexact accurate partitioned algorithms for fluid–structure interaction problems with finite elasticity in haemodynamics', *J. Comput. Phys.* **273**, 598–617.

F. Nobile, R. Tempone and C. Webster (2008), 'A sparse grid stochastic collocation method for partial differential equations with random input data', *SIAM J. Numer. Anal.* **46**, 2309–2345.

J. Nocedal (1992), Theory of algorithms for unconstrained optimization. In *Acta Numerica*, Vol. 1, Cambridge University Press, pp. 199–242.

D. Nordsletten, M. McCormick, P. Kilner, P. Hunter, D. Kayand and N. Smith (2011*a*), 'Fluid–solid coupling for the investigation of diastolic and systolic human left ventricular function', *Int. J. Numer. Methods Biomed. Engrg* **27**, 1017–1039.

D. Nordsletten, S. Niederer, M. Nash, P. Hunter and N. Smith (2011*b*), 'Coupling multi-physics models to cardiac mechanics', *Prog. Biophys. Molec. Biol.* **104**, 77–88.

A. Oberai, N. Gokhale and G. Feijóo (2003), 'Solution of inverse problems in elasticity imaging using the adjoint method', *Inverse Problems* **19**, 297–313.

T. O'Donnell, M. Jolly and A. Gupta (1998), 'A cooperative framework for segmentation using 2D active contours and 3D hybrid models as applied to branching cylindrical structures', *Proc. IEEE Int. Conf. Computer Vision* pp. 454–459.

M. Olufsen, C. Peskin, W. Kim, E. Pedersen, A. Nadim and J. Larsen (2000), 'Numerical simulation and experimental validation of blood flow in arteries with structured-tree outflow conditions', *Ann. Biomed. Engrg* **28**, 1281–1299.

S. Orszag, M. Israeli and M. Deville (1986), 'Boundary conditions for incompressible flows', *J. Sci. Comput.* **1**, 75–111.

H. Osnes and J. Sundnes (2012), 'Uncertainty analysis of ventricular mechanics using the probabilistic collocation method', *IEEE Trans. Biomed. Engrg* **59**, 2171–2179.

A. Owida, H. Do and Y. Morsi (2012), 'Numerical analysis of coronary artery bypass grafts: An over view', *Comput. Methods Programs Biomed.* **108**, 689–705.

M. Padala, M. Sacks, S. Liou, K. Balachandran, Z. He and A. Yoganathan (2010), 'Mechanics of the mitral valve strut chordae insertion region', *J. Biomech. Engrg* **132**, 081004.

S. Pagani (2016), *Reduced Order Models for Inverse Problems and Uncertainty Quantification in Cardiac Electrophysiology.* PhD thesis, Mathematical Models and Methods in Engineering, Department of Mathematics, Politecnico di Milano.

S. Pagani, A. Manzoni and A. Quarteroni (2017), 'A reduced basis ensemble Kalman filter for state/parameter identification in large-scale nonlinear dynamical systems', *SIAM/ASA J. Uncert. Quant.* **5**, 890–921.

S. Pagani, A. Manzoni and A. Quarteroni (2018), 'Numerical approximation of parametrized problems in cardiac electrophysiology by a local reduced basis method', *Comput. Methods Appl. Mech. Engrg.* **340**, 530–558.

S. Palamara, C. Vergara, D. Catanzariti, E. Faggiano, M. Centonze, C. Pangrazzi, M. Maines and A. Quarteroni (2014), 'Computational generation of the Purkinje network driven by clinical measurements: The case of pathological propagations.', *Int. J. Numer. Meth. Biomed. Engrg* **30**, 1558–1577.

S. Palamara, C. Vergara, E. Faggiano and F. Nobile (2015), 'An effective algorithm for the generation of patient-specific Purkinje networks in computational electrocardiology', *J. Comput. Phys.* **283**, 495–517.

A. Panfilov (1999), 'Three-dimensional organization of electrical turbulence in the heart', *Phys. Rev. E* **59**, R6251–R6254.

S. Pant, B. Fabrèges, J.-F. Gerbeau and I. Vignon-Clementel (2014), 'A methodological paradigm for patient-specific multi-scale CFD simulations: From clinical measurements to parameter estimates for individual analysis', *Int. J. Numer. Meth. Biomed. Engrg* **30**, 1614–1648.

G. Papadakis (2009), 'Coupling 3D and 1D fluid–structure-interaction models for wave propagation in flexible vessels using a finite volume pressure-correction scheme', *Comm. Numer. Methods Engrg* **25**, 533–551.

S. Patankar and D. Spalding (1972), 'A calculation procedure for heat, mass and momentum transfer in three-dimensional parabolic flows', *Int. J. Heat Mass Transfer* **15**, 1787–1806.

A.S. Patelli, L. Dede', T. Lassila, A. Bartezzaghi and A. Quarteroni (2017), 'Isogeometric approximation of cardiac electrophysiology models on surfaces: an accuracy study with application to the human left atrium', *Comput. Methods Appl. Mech. Engrg.* **317**, 248–273.

P. Pathmanathan, S. Chapman, D. Gavaghan and J. Whiteley (2010), 'Cardiac electromechanics: The effect of contraction model on the mathematical problem and accuracy of the numerical scheme', *Quart. J. Mech. Appl. Math.* **63**, 375–399.

P. Pathmanathan, G. Mirams, J. Southern and J. Whiteley (2011), 'The significant effect of the choice of ionic current integration method in cardiac electrophysiological simulations', *Int. J. Numer. Methods Biomed. Engrg* **27**, 1751–1770.

L. Pavarino and S. Scacchi (2008), 'Multilevel additive Schwarz preconditioners for the bidomain reaction-diffusion system', *SIAM J. Sci. Comput* **31**, 420–443.

L. Pavarino, S. Scacchi and S. Zampini (2015), 'Newton–Krylov–BDDC solvers for nonlinear cardiac mechanics', *Comput. Methods Appl. Mech. Engrg.* **295**, 562–580.

T. Pedley (1980), *The Fluid Mechanics of Large Blood Vessels*, Cambridge Monographs on Mechanics and Applied Mathematics, Cambridge University Press.

L. Pegolotti (2017), Isogeometric Analysis of cardiac electrophysiology: application to the human atria. MSc thesis, Computational Science and Engineering, École Polytechnique Fédérale de Lausanne.

L. Pegolotti, L. Dede' and A. Quarteroni (2019), 'Isogeometric analysis of the electrophysiology in the human heart: numerical simulation of the bidomain equations on the atria', *Comput. Methods Appl. Mech. Engrg.* **343**, 52–73.

J. Peiró and A. Veneziani (2009), Reduced models of the cardiovascular system. Chapter 10 in *Cardiovascular Mathematics* (A. Quarteroni, L. Formaggia and A. Veneziani, eds), Springer, pp. 347–394.

J. Peiró, L. Formaggia, M. Gazzola, A. Radaelli and V. Rigamonti (2007), 'Shape reconstruction from medical images and quality mesh generation via implicit surfaces', *Int. J. Numer. Methods Fluids* **53**, 1339–1360.

M. Pennacchio and V. Simoncini (2002), 'Efficient algebraic solution of reaction-diffusion systems for the cardiac excitation process', *J. Comput. Appl. Math.* **145**, 49–70.

P. Perdikaris and G. Karniadakis (2015), 'Model inversion via multi-fidelity Bayesian optimization: A new paradigm for parameter estimation in haemodynamics, and beyond', *J. Royal Soc. Interface* **13**, 20151107.

M. Perego, A. Veneziani and C. Vergara (2011), 'A variational approach for estimating the compliance of the cardiovascular tissue: An inverse fluid–structure interaction problem', *SIAM J. Sci. Comput.* **33**, 1181–1211.

K. Perktold and D. Hilbert (1986), 'Numerical simulation of pulsatile flow in a carotid bifurcation model', *J. Biomed. Engrg* **8**, 193–199.

K. Perktold, E. Thurner and T. Kenner (1994), 'Flow and stress characteristics in rigid walled and compliant carotid artery bifurcation models', *Med. Biol. Engrg Comput.* **32**, 19–26.

P. Perona and J. Malik (1990), 'Scale-space and edge detection using anisotropic diffusion', *IEEE Trans. Pattern Anal. Mach. Intel.* **12**, 629–639.

C. Peskin (1972), 'Flow patterns around heart valves: A numerical method', *J. Comput. Phys.* **10**, 252–271.

C. Peskin (1989), 'Fiber architecture of the left ventricular wall: An asymptotic analysis', *Comm. Pure Appl. Math.* **42**, 1126–1131.

C. Peskin (2002), The immersed boundary method. In *Acta Numerica*, Vol. 11, Cambridge University Press, pp. 479–517.

C. Petitjean and J.-N. Dacher (2011), 'A review of segmentation methods in short axis cardiac MR images', *Med. Image Anal.* **15**, 169–184.

S. Pezzuto (2013), *Mechanics of the Heart: Constitutive Issues and Numerical Experiments*. PhD thesis, Department of Mathematics, Politecnico di Milano.

D. Pham (2001), 'Stochastic methods for sequential data assimilation in strongly nonlinear systems', *Monthly Weather Rev.* **129**, 1194–1207.

D. Pham, C. Xu and J. Prince (2000), 'Current methods in medical image segmentation', *Annu. Rev. Biomed. Engrg* **2**, 315–337.

M. Piccinelli, C. Vergara, L. Antiga, L. Forzenigo, P. Biondetti and M. Domanin (2013), 'Impact of hemodynamics on lumen boundary displacements in abdominal aortic aneurysms by means of dynamic computed tomography and computational fluid dynamics', *Biomech. Model. Mechanobiol.* **12**, 1263–1276.

C. Pierre (2012), 'Preconditioning the bidomain model with almost linear complexity', *J. Comput. Phys.* **231**, 82–97.

S. Piperno and C. Farhat (2001), 'Partitioned prodecures for the transient solution of coupled aeroelastic problems, II: Energy transfer analysis and three-dimensional applications', *Comput. Methods Appl. Mech. Engrg* **190**, 3147–3170.

G. Plank, M. Liebmann, R. dos Santos, E. Vigmond and G. Haase (2007), 'Algebraic multigrid preconditioner for the cardiac bidomain model', *IEEE Trans. Biomed. Engrg* **54**, 585–596.

R. Ponzini, C. Vergara, A. Redaelli and A. Veneziani (2006), 'Reliable CFD-based estimation of flow rate in haemodynamics measures', *Ultrasound Med. Biol.* **32**, 1545–1555.

R. Ponzini, C. Vergara, G. Rizzo, A. Veneziani, A. Roghi, A. Vanzulli, O. Parodi and A. Redaelli (2010), 'Womersley number-based estimates of blood flow rate in Doppler analysis: *In vivo* validation by means of phase contrast magnetic resonance imaging', *IEEE Trans. Biomed. Engrg* **57**, 1807–1815.

A. Porpora, P. Zunino, C. Vergara and M. Piccinelli (2012), 'Numerical treatment of boundary conditions to replace lateral branches in haemodynamics', *Int. J. Numer. Methods Biomed. Engrg* **28**, 1165–1183.

M. Potse, B. Dubé, J. Richer, A. Vinet and R. Gulrajani (2006), 'A comparison of monodomain and bidomain reaction-diffusion models for action potential propagation in the human heart', *IEEE Trans. Biomed. Engrg* **53**, 2425–2435.

S. Pravdin, V. Berdyshev, A. Panfilov, L. Katsnelson, O. Solovyova and V. Markhasin (1989), 'Mathematical model of the anatomy and fibre orientation field of the left ventricle of the heart', *Biomed. Engrg OnLine* **12**, 54.

G. Prodi (1962), 'Teoremi di tipo locale per il sistema di Navier–Stokes e stabilitá delle soluzioni stazionarie', *Rendiconti del Seminario Matematico della Universitá di Padova* **32**, 374–397.

V. Prot, B. Skallerud and G. Holzapfel (2007), 'Transversely isotropic membrane shells with application to mitral valve mechanics. constitutive modelling and finite element implementation', *Int. J. Numer. Methods Engrg* **71**, 987–1008.

A. Pullan, L. Cheng, M. Nash, C. Bradley and D. Paterson (2001), 'Noninvasive electrical imaging of the heart: Theory and model development', *Ann. Biomed. Engrg* **29**, 817–836.

A. Pullan, L. Cheng, M. Nash, A. Ghodrati, R. MacLeod and D. Brooks (2010), The inverse problem of electrocardiography. In *Comprehensive Electrocardiology* (P. Macfarlane *et al.*, eds), Springer, pp. 299–344.

S. Puwal and B. Roth (2007), 'Forward Euler stability of the bidomain model of cardiac tissue', *IEEE Trans. Biomed. Engrg* **5**, 951–953.

Z. Qu and A. Garfinkel (1998), 'An advanced algorithm for solving partial differential equation in cardiac conduction', *IEEE Trans. Biomed. Engrg* **46**, 1166–1168.

A. Quarteroni, ed. (2015), *Modeling the Heart and the Circulatory System*, Springer.

A. Quarteroni and L. Formaggia (2004), Mathematical modelling and numerical simulation of the cardiovascular system. In Handbook of Numerical Analysis, Vol. 12: *Computational Models for the Human Body*, Elsevier, pp. 3–127.

A. Quarteroni and G. Rozza (2003), 'Optimal control and shape optimization of aorto-coronaric bypass anastomoses', *Math. Models Methods Appl. Sci.* **13**, 1801–1823.

A. Quarteroni and G. Rozza, eds (2014), *Reduced Order Methods for Modeling and Computational Reduction*, Vol. 9 of Modeling, Simulation and Applications, Springer.

A. Quarteroni and A. Valli (1999), *Domain Decomposition Methods for Partial Differential Equations*, Oxford Science Publications, Oxford.

A. Quarteroni and A. Valli (1994), *Numerical Approximation of Partial Differential Equations*, Springer.

A. Quarteroni and A. Veneziani (1997), Modeling and simulation of blood flow problems. In *Computational Science for the 21st Century* (M.-O. Bristeau *et al.*, eds), Wiley.

A. Quarteroni and A. Veneziani (2003), 'Analysis of a geometrical multiscale model based on the coupling of ODE and PDE for blood flow simulations', *Multiscale Model. Simul.* **1**, 173–195.

A. Quarteroni, T. Lassila, S. Rossi and R. Ruiz-Baier (2017), 'Integrated heart-coupling multiscale and multiphysics models for the simulation of the cardiac function', *Comput. Methods Appl. Mech. Engrg* **314**, 345–407.

A. Quarteroni, A. Manzoni and F. Negri (2016), *Reduced Basis Methods for Partial Differential Equations. An Introduction*, Vol. 92 of Unitext, Springer.

A. Quarteroni, S. Ragni and A. Veneziani (2001), 'Coupling between lumped and distributed models for blood flow problems', *Comput. Vis. Sci.* **4**, 111–124.

A. Quarteroni, R. Sacco and F. Saleri (2000*a*), *Numerical Mathematics*, Springer.

A. Quarteroni, F. Saleri and A. Veneziani (1999), 'Analysis of the Yosida method for the incompressible Navier–Stokes equations', *J. Math. Pures Appl.* **78**, 473–503.

A. Quarteroni, F. Saleri and A. Veneziani (2000*b*), 'Factorization methods for the numerical approximation of Navier–Stokes equations', *Comput. Methods Appl. Mech. Engrg* **188**, 505–526.

A. Quarteroni, M. Tuveri and A. Veneziani (2000*c*), 'Computational vascular fluid dynamics: Problems, models and methods', *Comput. Vis. Sci.* **2**, 163–197.

A. Quarteroni, A. Veneziani and C. Vergara (2016*c*), 'Geometric multiscale modeling of the cardiovascular system, between theory and practice', *Comput. Methods Appl. Mech. Engrg* **302**, 193–252.

G. Querzoli, S. Fortini and A. Cenedese (2010), 'Effect of the prosthetic mitral valve on vortex dynamics and turbulence of the left ventricular flow', *Phys. Fluids* **22**, 041901.

M. Raghavan and D. Vorp (2000), 'Towards a biomechanical tool to evaluate rupture potential of abdominal aortic aneurysm: Identification of a finite strain constitutive model and evaluation of its applicability', *J. Biomech.* **33**, 475–482.

R. Rannacher (1992), *On Chorin's Projection Method for Incompressible Navier–Stokes Equations*, Vol. 1530 of Lecture Notes in Mathematics, Springer, pp. 167–183.

S. Raya and J. Udupa (1990), 'Shape-based interpolation of multidimensional objects', *IEEE Trans. Med. Imaging* **9**, 32–42.

V. Rayz, S. Berger and D. Saloner (2007), 'Transitional flows in arterial fluid dynamics', *Comput. Methods Appl. Mech. Engrg* **196**, 3043–3048.

F. Regazzoni, L. Dede' and A. Quarteroni (2017), 'Active contraction of cardiac cells: a reduced model for sarcomere dynamics with cooperative interactions', MOX-Report 42-2017, Department of Mathematics, Politecnico di Milano.

T. Rees, H. Dollar and A. Wathen (2010), 'Optimal solvers for PDE-constrained optimization', *SIAM J. Sci. Comput.* **32**, 271–298.

J. Relan, P. Chinchapatnam, M. Sermesant, K. Rhode, M. Ginks, H. Delingette, C. Rinaldi, R. Razavi and N. Ayache (2011), 'Coupled personalization of cardiac electrophysiology models for prediction of ischaemic ventricular tachycardia', *Interface Focus* **1**, 396–407.

P. Reymond, F. Merenda, F. Perren, D. Rufenacht and N. Stergiopulos (2009), 'Validation of a one-dimensional model of the systemic arterial tree', *Amer. J. Physiol.: Heart Circ. Physiol.* **297**, H208–H222.

C. Robert and G. Casella (2004), *Monte Carlo Statistical Methods*, second edition, Springer.

A. Robertson, A. Sequeira and R. Owens (2009), Rheological models for blood. Chapter 6 in *Cardiovascular Mathematics* (L. Formaggia, A. Quarteroni and A. Veneziani, eds), Springer, pp. 211–241.

D. Robertson, J. Yuan, G. Wang and M. Vannier (1997), 'Total hip prosthesis metal-artifact suppression using iterative deblurring reconstruction', *J. Comput. Assist. Tomogr.* **21**, 293–298.

J. Rogers and A. McCulloch (1994), 'A collocation-Galerkin finite element model of cardiac action potential propagation', *IEEE Trans. Biomed. Engrg* **41**, 743–757.

S. Rossi (2014), *Anisotropic Modeling of Cardiac Mechanical Activation*. PhD thesis, Ecole Polytechnique Fédérale de Lausanne.

S. Rossi, T. Lassila, R. Ruiz-Baier, A. Sequeira and A. Quarteroni (2014), 'Thermodynamically consistent orthotropic activation model capturing ventricular systolic wall thickening in cardiac electromechanics', *Europ. J. Mech. A: Solids* **48**, 129–142.

S. Rossi, R. Ruiz-Baier, L. Pavarino, and A. Quarteroni (2012), 'Orthotropic active strain models for the numerical simulation of cardiac biomechanics', *Internat. J. Numer. Methods Biomed. Engng.* **28**,761–788.

B. Roth (1991), 'Action potential propagation in a thick strand of cardiac muscle', *Circ. Res.* **68**, 162–173.

B. Roth (1997), 'Electrical conductivity values used with the bidomain model of cardiac tissue', *IEEE Trans. Biomed. Engrg* **44**, 326–328.

O. Rousseau (2010), *Geometrical Modeling of the Heart*. PhD thesis, Université d'Ottawa.

Y. Rudy and B. Messinger-Rapport (1988), 'The inverse problem in electrocardiography: Solutions in terms of epicardial potentials', *Crit. Rev. Biomed. Engrg* **16**, 215–268.

Y. Rudy and J. Silva (2006), 'Computational biology in the study of cardiac ion channels and cell electrophysiology', *Quart. Rev. Biophys.* **39**, 57–116.

R. Ruiz-Baier, A. Gizzi, S. Rossi, C. Cherubini, A. Laadhari, S. Filippi and A. Quarteroni (2014), 'Mathematical modelling of active contraction in isolated cardiomyocytes', *Math. Med. Bio.* **31**, 259–283.

Y. Saad (1996), *Iterative Methods for Sparse Linear Systems*, PWS Publishing Company, Boston.

A. Saltelli, M. Ratto, T. Andres, F. Campolongo, J. Cariboni, D. Gatelli, M. Salsana and S. Tarantola (2008), *Global Sensitivity Analysis: The Primer*, Wiley.

S. Sankaran and A. Marsden (2010), 'The impact of uncertainty on shape optimization of idealized bypass graft models in unsteady flow', *Phys. Fluids* **22**, 121902.

S. Sankaran and A. Marsden (2011), 'A stochastic collocation method for uncertainty quantification and propagation in cardiovascular simulations', *J. Biomech. Engrg* **133**, 031001.

S. Sankaran, L. Grady and C. Taylor (2015), 'Impact of geometric uncertainty on hemodynamic simulations using machine learning', *Comput. Methods Appl. Mech. Engrg* **297**, 167–190.

S. Sankaran, H. Kim, G. Choi and C. Taylor (2016), 'Uncertainty quantification in coronary blood flow simulations: Impact of geometry, boundary conditions and blood viscosity', *J. Biomech.* **49**, 2540–2547.

R. dos Santos, G. Plank, S. Bauer and E. Vigmond (2005), Preconditioning techniques for the bidomain equations. In *Domain Decomposition Methods in Science and Engineering* (R. Kornhuber *et al.*, eds), Vol. 40 of Lecture Notes in Computational Science and Engineering, Springer, pp. 571–580.

S. Särkkä (2013), *Bayesian Filtering and Smoothing*, Cambridge University Press.

S. Savader, G. Lund and F. Osterman (1997), 'Volumetric evaluation of blood flow in normal renal arteries with a Doppler flow wire: A feasibility study', *J. Vasc. Intervent. Radiol.* **8**, 209–214.

I. Sazonov, S. Yeo, R. Bevan, X. Xie, R. van Loon and P. Nithiarasu (2011), 'Modelling pipeline for subject-specific arterial blood flow: A review', *Int. J. Numer. Methods Biomed. Engrg* **27**, 1868–1910.

D. Schiavazzi, G. Arbia, C. Baker, A. Hlavacek, T. Hsia, A. Marsden, I. Vignon-Clementel and the Modeling Of Congenital Hearts Alliance (MOCHA) investigators (2016), 'Uncertainty quantification in virtual surgery hemodynamics predictions for single ventricle palliation', *Int. J. Numer. Methods Biomed. Engrg* **32**, 02737.

R. Schilling, N. Peters and D. Davies (1998), 'Simultaneous endocardial mapping in the human left ventricle using a noncontact catheter comparison of contact and reconstructed electrograms during sinus rhythm', *Circulation* **98**, 887–898.

R. Sebastian, V. Zimmerman, D. Romero and A. Frangi (2011), 'Construction of a computational anatomical model of the perpheral cardiac conduction system', *IEEE Trans. Biomed. Engrg* **58**, 90–100.

J. Seo, V. Vedula, T. Abraham, A. Lardo, F. Dawoud, H. Luo and R. Mittal (2014), 'Effect of the mitral valve on diastolic flow patterns', *Phys. Fluids* **26**, 121901.

M. Sermesant, R. Chabiniok, P. Chinchapatnam, T. Mansi, F. Billet, P. Moireau, J. Peyrat, K. Wong, J. Relan, K. Rhode, M. Ginks, P. Lambiase, H. Delingette, M. Sorine, C. Rinaldi, D. Chapelle, R. Razavi and N. Ayache (2012), 'Patient-specific electromechanical models of the heart for the prediction of pacing acute effects in CRT: A preliminary clinical validation', *Med. Image Anal.* **16**, 201–215.

M. Sermesant, P. Moireau, O. Camara, J. Sainte-Marie, R. Andriantsimiavona, R. Cimrman, D. Hill, D. Chapelle and R. Razavi (2006), 'Cardiac function estimation from MRI using a heart model and data assimilation: Advances and difficulties', *Med. Image Anal.* **10**, 642–656.

J. Sethian (1999), *Level Set Methods and Fast Marching Methods*, Cambridge University Press.

S. Sherwin, L. Formaggia, J. Peiró and V. Franke (2003*a*), 'Computational modelling of 1D blood flow with variable mechanical properties and its application to the simulation of wave propagation in the human arterial system', *Int. J. Numer. Methods Fluids* **43**, 673–700.

S. Sherwin, V. Franke, J. Peiró and K. Parker (2003*b*), 'One-dimensional modelling of a vascular network in space-time variables', *J. Engrg Math.* **47**, 217–259.

J.C. Simo and R.L. Taylor (1991), 'Quasi-incompressible finite elasticity in principal stretches. Continuum basis and numerical algorithms', *Comput. Methods Appl. Mech. Engrg* **85**, 273–310.

D. Simon (2006), *Optimal State Estimation: Kalman, H-Infinity, and Nonlinear Approaches*, Wiley.

N. Smith, D. Nickerson, E. Crampin and P. Hunter (2004), Multiscale computational modelling of the heart. In *Acta Numerica*, Vol. 13, Cambridge University Press, pp. 371–431.

R. Spilker and C. Taylor (2010), 'Tuning multidomain hemodynamic simulations to match physiological measurements', *Ann. Biomed. Engrg* **38**, 2635–2648.

R.J. Spiteri and S. Torabi Ziaratgahi (2016), 'Operator splitting for the bidomain model revisited', *J. Comput. Appl. Math.* **296**, 550–563.

T. Stankovičová, V. Bito, F. Heinzel, K. Mubagwa and K. Sipido (2003), 'Isolation and morphology of single Purkinje cells from the porcine heart', *Gen. Physiol. Biophys.* **22**, 329–340.

B. Steele, J. Wan, J. Ku, T. Hughes and C. Taylor (2003), '*In vivo* validation of a one-dimensional finite-element method for predicting blood flow in cardiovascular bypass grafts', *IEEE Trans. Biomed. Engrg* **50**, 649–656.

D. Steinman, J. Thomas, H. Ladak, J. Milner, B. Rutt and J. Spence (2001), 'Reconstruction of carotid bifurcation hemodynamics and wall thickness using computational fluid dynamics and MRI', *Magnet. Reson. Med.* **47**, 149–159.

N. Stergiopulos, B. Westerhof and N. Westerhof (1999), 'Total arterial inertance as the fourth element of the windkessel model', *Amer. J. Physiol.: Heart Circ. Physiol.* **276**, H81–H88.

N. Stergiopulos, B. Westerhof, J. Meister and N. Westerhof (1996), The four-element windkessel model. In *Bridging Disciplines for Biomedicine: Proceedings of the 18th Annual International Conference of the IEEE*, Vol. 4, pp. 1715–1716.

J. Stijnen, J. de Hart, P. Bovendeerd and F. van de Vosse (2004), 'Evaluation of a fictitious domain method for predicting dynamic response of mechanical heart valves', *Int. J. Numer. Methods Fluids* **19**, 835–850.

J. Stroud, S. Berger and D. Saloner (2002), 'Numerical analysis of flow through a severely stenotic carotid artery bifurcation', *J. Biomech. Engrg* **124**, 9–20.

A. Stuart (2010), Inverse problems: A Bayesian perspective. In *Acta Numerica*, Vol. 19, Cambridge University Press, pp. 451–559.

S. Sugiura, T. Washio, A. Hatano, J. Okada, H. Watanabe and T. Hisada (2012), 'Multi-scale simulations of cardiac electrophysiology and mechanics using the University of Tokyo heart simulator', *Progr. Biophys. Molecular Biol.* **110**:380–389.

T. Sullivan (2015), *Introduction to Uncertainty Quantification*, Vol. 63 of Texts in Applied Mathematics, Springer.

W. Sun, B. Starly, J. Nam and A. Darling (2005), 'Bio-CAD modeling and its applications in computer-aided tissue engineering', *Comput. Aided Design* **11**, 1097–1114.

G. Sundaram, K. Balakrishnan and R. Kumar (2015), 'Aortic valve dynamics using a fluid structure interaction model: The physiology of opening and closing', *J. Biomech.* **48**, 1737–1744.

J. Sundnes, G.T. Lines, X. Cai, B.F. Nielsen, K.-A. Mardal and A. Tveito (2007), *Computing the Electrical Activity in the Heart*, Springer.

J. Sundnes, G. Lines and A. Tveito (2005), 'An operator splitting method for solving the bidomain equations coupled to a volume conductor model for the torso', *Math. Biosci.* **2**, 233–248.

J. Sundnes, S. Wall, H. Osnes, T. Thorvaldsen and A. McCulloch (2014), 'Improved discretisation and linearisation of active tension in strongly coupled cardiac electro-mechanics simulations', *Comput. Methods Biomech. Biomed. Engrg* **6**, 604–615.

E. Swim and P. Seshaiyer (2006), 'A nonconforming finite element method for fluid–structure interaction problems', *Comput. Methods Appl. Mech. Engrg* **195**, 2088–2099.

A. Tagliabue, L. Dede' and A. Quarteroni (2017*a*), 'Complex blood flow patterns in an idealized left ventricle: a numerical study', *Chaos* **27**, 093939.

A. Tagliabue, L. Dede' and A. Quarteroni (2017*b*), 'Fluid dynamics of an idealized left ventricle: The extended Nitsche's method for the treatment of heart valves as mixed time varying boundary conditions', *Int. J. Numer. Meth. Fluids* **85**, 135–164.

A. Tagliabue, L. Dede' and A. Quarteroni (2016), 'Nitsche's method for parabolic partial differential equations with mixed time varying boundary conditions', *ESAIM: M2AN* **50**, 541–563.

H. Talbot, S. Cotin, R. Razavi, C. Rinaldi and H. Delingette (2015), Personalization of cardiac electrophysiology model using the unscented Kalman filtering. In *Computer Assisted Radiology and Surgery: CARS 2015.*

A. Tarantola (2004), *Inverse Problem Theory and Methods for Model Parameter Estimation*, SIAM.

C. Taylor and C. Figueroa (2009), 'Patient-specific modeling of cardiovascular mechanics', *Annu. Rev. Biomed. Engrg* **11**, 109–134.

C. Taylor, T. Hughes and C. Zarins (1996), 'Finite element analysis of pulsatile flow in the abdominal aorta under resting and exercise conditions', *Amer. Soc. Mech. Engineers, Bioengineering Division* **33**, 81–82.

C. Taylor, T. Hughes and C. Zarins (1998), 'Finite element modeling of blood flow in arteries', *Comput. Methods Appl. Mech. Engrg* **158**, 155–196.

R. Temam (1984), *Navier-Stokes Equations. Theory and Numerical Analysis*, North-Holland.

R. Temam (1969), 'Sur l'approximation de la solution des équations de Navier–Stokes par la méthode des pas fractionaires (I)', *Arch. Rat. Mech. Anal.* **32**, 135–153.

T. Tezduyar, S. Sathe, T. Cragin, B. Nanna, B. Conklin, J. Pausewang and M. Schwaab (2007), 'Modelling of fluid–structure interactions with the space–time finite elements: Arterial fluid mechanics', *Int. J. Numer. Methods Fluids* **54**, 901–922.

J. Thompson, B. Soni and N. Weatherill, eds (1999), *Handbook of Grid Generation*, CRC Press.

L. Timmermans, P. Minev and F. van de Vosse (1996), 'An approximate projection scheme for incompressible flow using spectral elements', *Int. J. Numer. Methods Fluids* **22**, 673–688.

K. Tomlinson, P. Hunter and A. Pullan (2002), 'A finite element method for an eikonal equation model of myocardial excitation wavefront propagation', *SIAM J. Appl. Math.* **1**, 324–350.

E. Toro (2016), 'Brain venous haemodynamics, neurological diseases and mathematical modelling: A review', *Appl. Math. Comput.* **272**, 542–579.

A. Toselli and O. Widlund (2005), *Domain Decomposition Methods – Algorithms and Theory*, Springer-Verlag, Berlin Heidelberg.

N. Trayanova (2006), 'Defibrillation of the heart: Insights into mechanisms from modelling studies', *Exp. Physiol.* **91**, 323–337.

N. Trayanova, W. Li, J. Eason and P. Kohl (2004), 'Effect of stretch-activated channels on defibrillation efficacy', *Heart Rhythm* **1**, 67–77.

P. Trenhago, L. Fernandes, L. Müller, P. Blanco and R. Feijóo (2016), 'An integrated mathematical model of the cardiovascular and respiratory systems', *Int. J. Numer. Methods Biomed. Engrg* **32**, e02736.

P. Tricerri, L. Dede', S. Deparis, A. Quarteroni, A. Robertson and A. Sequeira (2015), 'Fluid–structure interaction simulations of cerebral arteries modeled by isotropic and anisotropic constitutive laws', *Comput. Mech.* **55**, 478–498.

P. Tricerri, L. Dede', A. Gambaruto, A. Quarteroni and A. Sequeira (2016), 'A numerical study of isotropic and anisotropic constitutive models with relevance to healthy and unhealthy cerebral arterial tissues', *Internat. J. Engng. Sci.* **101**, 126–155.

F. Tröltzsch (2010), *Optimal Control of Partial Differential Equations: Theory, Methods and Applications*, Vol. 112 of Graduate Studies in Mathematics, AMS.

C. Tu and C. Peskin (1992), 'Stability and instability in the computation of flows with moving immersed boundaries: A comparison of three methods', *SIAM J. Sci. Statist. Comput.* **6**, 1361–1376.

S. Turek (1999), *Efficient Solvers for Incompressible Flow Problems*, Vol. 6 of Lecture Notes in Computational Science and Engineering, Springer.

K. ten Tusscher and A. Panfilov (2006), 'Cell model for efficient simulation of wave propagation in human ventricular tissue under normal and pathological conditions', *Phys. Med. Biol.* **51**, 6141–6156.

M. Unser (1999), 'Splines: A perfect fit for signal and image processing', *IEEE Trans. Signal Process. Mag.* **16**, 22–38.

T. Usyk, I. LeGrice and A. McCulloch (2002), 'Computational model of three-dimensional cardiac electromechanics', *Comput. Vis. Sci.* **4**, 249–257.

A. Veneziani (1998*a*), 'Boundary conditions for blood flow problems'. In *Proceedings of ENUMATH* (R. Rannacher *et al.*, eds), World Scientific.

A. Veneziani (1998*b*), *Mathematical and Numerical Modeling of Blood Flow Problems*. PhD thesis, University of Milan.

A. Veneziani (2003), 'Block factorized preconditioners for high-order accurate in time approximation of the Navier–Stokes equations', *Numer. Methods Partial Differ. Equations* **19**, 487–510.

A. Veneziani and C. Vergara (2005), 'Flow rate defective boundary conditions in haemodynamics simulations', *Int. J. Numer. Methods Fluids* **47**, 803–816.

A. Veneziani and C. Vergara (2007), 'An approximate method for solving incompressible Navier–Stokes problems with flow rate conditions', *Comput. Methods Appl. Mech. Engrg* **196**, 1685–1700.

A. Veneziani and C. Vergara (2013), 'Inverse problems in cardiovascular mathematics: Toward patient-specific data assimilation and optimization', *Int. J. Numer. Methods Biomed. Engrg* **29**, 723–725.

A. Veneziani and U. Villa (2013), 'ALADINS: An ALgebraic splitting time ADaptive solver for the Incompressible Navier–Stokes equations', *J. Comput. Phys.* **238**, 359–375.

C. Vergara (2011), 'Nitsche's method for defective boundary value problems in incompressibile fluid-dynamics', *J. Sci. Comput.* **46**, 100–123.

C. Vergara, M. Lange, S. Palamara, T. Lassila, A. Frangi and A. Quarteroni (2016), 'A coupled 3D–1D numerical monodomain solver for cardiac electrical activation in the myocardium with detailed Purkinje network', *J. Comput. Phys.* **308**, 218–238.

C. Vergara, S. Palamara, D. Catanzariti, F. Nobile, E. Faggiano, C. Pangrazzi, M. Centonze, M. Maines, A. Quarteroni and G. Vergara (2014), 'Patient-specific generation of the Purkinje network driven by clinical measurements of a normal propagation', *Med. Biol. Engrg Comput.* **52**, 813–826.

C. Vergara, R. Ponzini, A. Veneziani, A. Redaelli, D. Neglia and O. Parodi (2010), 'Womersley number-based estimation of flow rate with Doppler ultrasound: Sensitivity analysis and first clinical application', *Comput. Methods Programs Biomed.* **98**, 151–160.

C. Vergara, F. Viscardi, L. Antiga and G. Luciani (2012), 'Influence of bicuspid valve geometry on ascending aortic fluid-dynamics: A parametric study', *Artificial Organs* **36**, 368–378.

J. A. Vierendeels, K. Riemslagh, E. Dick and P. Verdonck (2000), 'Computer simulation of intraventricular flow and pressure gradients during diastole', *J. Biomech. Engrg* **6**, 667–674.

E. Vigmond, F. Aguel and N. Trayanova (2002), 'Computational techniques for solving the bidomain equations in three dimensions', *IEEE Trans. Biomed. Engrg* **49**, 1260–1269.

E. Vigmond and C. Clements (2007), 'Construction of a computer model to investigate sawtooth effects in the Purkinje system', *IEEE Trans. Biomed. Engrg* **54**, 389–399.

E. Vigmond, R. dos Santos, A. Prassl, M. Deo and G. Plank (2008), 'Solvers for the cardiac bidomain equations', *Prog. Biophys. Molec. Biol.* **96**, 3–18.

I. Vignon-Clementel, C. Figueroa, K. Jansen and C. Taylor (2006), 'Outflow boundary conditions for three-dimensional finite element modeling of blood flow and pressure waves in arteries', *Comput. Methods Appl. Mech. Engrg* **195**, 3776–3996.

N. Virag, V. Jacquemet, C. Henriquez, S. Zozor, O. Blanc, J.-M. Vesin, E. Pruvot and L. Kappenberger (2002), 'Study of atrial arrhythmias in a computer model based on magnetic resonance images of human atria', *Chaos* **12**, 754–763.

F. Viscardi, C. Vergara, L. Antiga, S. Merelli, A. Veneziani, G. Puppini, G. Faggian, A. Mazzucco and G. Luciani (2010), 'Comparative finite element model analysis of ascending aortic flow in bicuspid and tricuspid aortic valve', *Artificial Organs* **34**, 1114–1120.

H. U. Voss, J. Timmer and J. Kurths (2004), 'Nonlinear dynamical system identification from uncertain and indirect measurements', *Int. J. Bifurc. Chaos* **14**, 1905–1933.

J. Voss (2013), *An Introduction to Statistical Computing: A Simulation-Based Approach*, Wiley.

J. Vossoughi, R. Vaishnav and D. Patel (1980), 'Compressibility of the myocardial tissue'. In *Advances in Bioengineering 1980: Papers Presented at the Winter Annual Meeting of the American Society of Mechanical Engineers* (V.C. Mow, ed.), ASME, pp. 45–48.

E. Votta, T. Le, M. Stevanella, L. Fusinic, E. Caiani, A. Redaelli and F. Sotiropoulos (2013), 'Toward patient-specific simulations of cardiac valves: State-of-the-art and future directions', *J. Biomech.* **46**, 217–228.

E. Votta, F. Maisano, S. Bolling, O. Alfieri, F. Montevecchi and A. Redaelli (2007), 'The geoform disease-specific annuloplasty system: A finite element study', *Ann. Thorac. Surg.* **84**, 92–101.

G. Waiter, F. McKiddie, T. Redpath, S. Semple and R. Trent (1999), 'Determination of normal regional left ventricular function from cine-MR images using a semi-automated edge detection method', *Magnet. Reson. Imaging* **17**, 99–107.

W. Wall, L. Wiechert, A. Comerford and S. Rausch (2010), 'Towards a comprehensive computational model for the respiratory system', *Int. J. Numer. Methods Biomed. Engrg* **26**, 807–827.

M. Wallman, N. Smith and B. Rodriguez (2014), 'Computational methods to reduce uncertainty in the estimation of cardiac conduction properties from electroanatomical recordings', *Med. Image Anal.* **18**, 228–240.

D. Wang, R. Kirby, R. MacLeod and C. Johnson (2013), 'Inverse electrocardiographic source localization of ischemia: An optimization framework and finite element solution', *J. Comput. Phys.* **250**, 403–424.

K. Wang, R. Dutton and C. Taylor (1999), 'Improving geometric model construction for blood flow modeling', *IEEE Engrg Med. Biol. Mag.* **18**, 33–39.

L. Wang, K. L. Wong, H. Zhang, H. Liu and P. Shi (2011), 'Noninvasive computational imaging of cardiac electrophysiology for 3-D infarct', *IEEE Trans. Biomed. Engrg* **58**, 1033–1043.

L. Wang, H. Zhang, K. Wong and P. Shi (2009), A reduced-rank square root filtering framework for noninvasive functional imaging of volumetric cardiac electrical activity. In *2009 IEEE International Conference on Acoustics, Speech and Signal Processing*, pp. 533–536.

H. Watanabe, T. Hisada, S. Sugiura, J. Okada and H. Fukunari (2002), 'Computer simulation of blood flow, left ventricular wall motion and their interrelationship by fluid–structure interaction finite element method', *JSME Int. J. C: Mechanical Systems, Machine Elements and Manufacturing* **45**, 1003–1012.

H. Watanabe, S. Sugiura and T. Hisada (2004), 'Multiphysics simulation of left ventricular filling dynamics using fluid–structure interaction finite element method', *Biophys. J.* **87**, 2074–2085.

D. Watson (1981), 'Computing the $n$-dimensional Delaunay tessellation with application to Voronoi polytopes', *Comput. J.* **24**, 167–172.

N. Weatherill and O. Hassan (1994), 'Efficient three-dimensional Delaunay triangulation with automatic point creation and imposed boundary constraints', *Int. J. Numer. Methods Engrg* **37**, 2005–2039.

E. Weinberg and M. Kaazempur-Mofrad (2006), 'A large-strain finite element formulation for biological tissues with application to mitral valve leaflet tissue mechanics', *J. Biomech.* **39**, 1557–1561.

J. Wenk, L. Ge, Z. Zhang, M. Soleimani, D. Potter, A. Wallace, E. Tseng, M. Ratcliffe and J. Guccione (2013), 'Mechanics of the mitral valve strut chordae insertion region', *Comput. Methods Biomech. Biomed. Engrg* **16**, 807–818.

N. Westerhof, J. Lankhaar and B. Westerhof (2009), 'The arterial windkessel', *Med. Biol. Engrg Comput.* **47**, 131–141.

C. Wiggers (1915), *Circulation in Health and Disease*, Lea & Febiger, Philadelphia PA.

J. Wong and E. Kuhl (2014), 'Generating fibre orientation maps in human heart models using Poisson interpolation', *Comput. Methods Biomech. Biomed. Engrg* **17**, 1217–1226.

J. Wong, S. Goktepe and E. Kuhl (2013), 'Computational modeling of chemo-electro-mechanical coupling: A novel implicit monolithic finite element approach', *Int. J. Numer. Methods Biomed. Engrg* **29**, 1104–1133.

J. Xi, P. Lamata, J. Lee, P. Moireau, D. Chapelle and N. Smith (2011), 'Myocardial transversely isotropic material parameter estimation from *in-silico* measurements based on a reduced-order unscented Kalman filter', *J. Mech. Behav. Biomed. Materials* **4**, 1090–1102.

F. Xie, Z. Qu, J. Yang, A. Baher, J. Weiss and A. Garfinkel (2004), 'A simulation study of the effects of cardiac anatomy in ventricular fibrillation', *J. Clin. Invest.* **113**, 686–693.

F. Xiong and C. Chong (2008), 'A parametric numerical investigation on haemodynamics in distal coronary anastomoses', *Med. Engrg Phys.* **30**, 311–320.

D. Xiu and J. Hesthaven (2005), 'High-order collocation methods for differential equations with random inputs', *SIAM J. Sci. Comput.* **27**, 1118–1139.

D. Xiu and G. Karniadakis (2002*a*), 'Modeling uncertainty in steady state diffusion problems via generalized polynomial chaos', *Comput. Methods Appl. Mech. Engrg* **191**, 4927–4948.

D. Xiu and G. Karniadakis (2002*b*), 'The Wiener–Askey polynomial chaos for stochastic differential equations', *SIAM J. Sci. Comput.* **24**, 619–644.

D. Xiu and S. Sherwin (2007), 'Parametric uncertainty analysis of pulse wave propagation in a model of a human arterial network', *J. Comput. Phys.* **226**, 1385–1407.

Y. Yamashita (1982), 'Theoretical studies on the inverse problem in electrocardiography and the uniqueness of the solution', *IEEE Trans. Biomed. Engrg* **BME-29**, 719–725.

K. Yanagihara, A. Noma and H. Irisawa (1980), 'Reconstruction of sino-atrial node pacemaker potential based on the voltage clamp experiments', *Japan. J. Physiol* **30**, 841–857.

H. Yang and A. Veneziani (2015), 'Estimation of cardiac conductivities in ventricular tissue by a variational approach', *Inverse Problems* **31**, 115001.

H. Yang and A. Veneziani (2017), Efficient estimation of cardiac conductivities via POD-DEIM model order reduction. *Appl. Numer. Math.* **115**, pp 180–199.

P. Yim, J. Cebral, R. Mullick, H. Marcos and P. Choyke (2001), 'Vessel surface reconstruction with a tubular deformable model', *IEEE Trans. Med. Imaging* **20**, 1411–1421.

F.C. Yin, C.C. Chan and R.M. Judd (1996), 'Compressibility of perfused passive myocardium', *Americ. J. Phys.-Heart Circ. Phys.* **271**, H1864–H1870.

M. Yin, X. Luo, T. Wang and P. Watton (2009), 'Effects of flow vortex on a chorded mitral valve in the left ventricle', *Int. J. Numer. Methods Biomed. Engrg* **26**, 381–404.

H. Younis, M. Kaazempur-Mofrad, R. Chan, A. Isasi, D. Hinton, A. Chau, L. Kim and R. Kamm (2004), 'Hemodynamics and wall mechanics in human carotid bifurcation and its consequences for atherogenesis: Investigation of inter-individual variation', *Biomech. Model. Mechanobiol.* **3**, 17–32.

Y. Yu, H. Baek and G. Karniadakis (2013), 'Generalized fictitious methods for fluid–structure interactions: Analysis and simulations', *J. Comput. Phys.* **245**, 317–346.

S. Zhao, X. Xu, A. Hughes, S. Thom, A. Stanton, B. Ariff and Q. Long (2000), 'Blood flow and vessel mechanics in a physiologically realistic model of a human carotid arterial bifurcation', *J. Biomech.* **33**, 975–984.

F. Zhu and J. Tian (2003), 'Modified fast marching and level-set method for medical image segmentation', *J. X-Ray Sci. Technol.* **11**, 193–204.

O. Zienkiewicz and R. Taylor (2005), *The Finite Element Method for Solid and Structural Mechanics*, sixth edition, Butterworth–Heinemann.

S. Zonca (2018), *Unfitted Numerical Methods for Fluid–Structure Interaction arising between an Incompressible Fluid and an Immersed Thick Structure.* PhD thesis, Politecnico di Milano.

S. Zonca, L. Formaggia and C. Vergara (2018), 'An unfitted formulation for the interaction of an incompressible fluid with a thick structure via an XFEM/DG approach', *SIAM J. Sci. Comput.* **40**, B59–B84.

P. Zunino (2009), 'Numerical approximation of incompressible flows with net flux defective boundary conditions by means of penalty techniques', *Comput. Methods Appl. Mech. Engrg* **198**, 3026–3038.

# Index